OXFORD MEDICAL PUBLICATIONS

Oxford Handbook of
Clinical Diagnosis

Oxford Handbook of
Clinical
Diagnosis

Huw Llewelyn

Hock Aun Ang

Keir Lewis

Anees Al-Abdulla

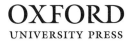

OXFORD
UNIVERSITY PRESS

OXFORD
UNIVERSITY PRESS

Great Clarendon Street, Oxford OX2 6DP

Oxford University Press is a department of the University of Oxford.
It furthers the University's objective of excellence in research, scholarship,
and education by publishing worldwide in

Oxford New York

Auckland Cape Town Dar es Salaam Hong Kong Karachi
Kuala Lumpur Madrid Melbourne Mexico City Nairobi
New Delhi Shanghai Taipei Toronto

With offices in

Argentina Austria Brazil Chile Czech Republic France Greece
Guatemala Hungary Italy Japan Poland Portugal Singapore
South Korea Switzerland Thailand Turkey Ukraine Vietnam

Oxford is a registered trade mark of Oxford University Press
in the UK and in certain other countries

Published in the United States
by Oxford University Press, Inc., New York

British Library Cataloguing in Publication Data
Data available

Library of Congress Cataloging in Publication Data
Data available

Typeset by Newgen Imaging Systems (P) Ltd., Chennai, India
Printed in Italy
on acid-free paper by
Legoprint

ISBN 0–19–263249–3   978–0–19–263249–4

10 9 8 7 6 5 4 3 2 1

Contents

The contents of each chapter is detailed on each chapter's first page.

For Angela

Preface

This book explains how to use a history, examination and preliminary tests to arrive at a diagnosis in a transparent way. The diagnosis is a title for what we imagine is happening to a patient physically and socially. It allows us to anticipate what may happen next, how this can be influenced by intervention and to share with the patient and colleagues in various disciplines what we are doing.

The book allows the diagnostician to focus on symptoms, physical signs and initial test results that are likely to lead to a diagnosis. This is based on the principle that 'diagnostic leads' with short differential diagnoses will be more informative than those features with long lists of causes.

Each diagnosis on a page resembles an entry from an evidence-based past medical history. The reader scans down the page to see which of the entries are compatible with the patient's findings so far. The compatible findings can then be used as evidence for the diagnosis to be shared with the patient or other members of the multidisciplinary team. Such information can also be shared by using computer systems.

Readers are encouraged to be critical about the contents of the book, to make changes in the Oxford Handbook spirit and to let us know of any significant differences in opinion, or errors.

HL

Some important questions and answers about this book

1. Why is this book different to other textbooks?

Most medical books describe a disease process and give physiological, biochemical and other explanations for the causes and complications and how these processes can be treated. They also describe what symptoms, signs and test results occur. When a patient presents with new symptoms and other findings, the reader must somehow work out which of all the conditions that they have read about, the patient has. This book is different. It lists the causes of findings that are the best clues (or 'leads') and then outlines some findings, which when used in combination with the lead, suggest the diagnosis with a reasonably high probability, or confirm it. The number of findings is usually small for two reasons. The first reason is that many findings occur often in many other diseases and are therefore 'non-specific'; it is only a few that form powerful predictors. The second reason is practical—it is only possible to build up experience of small combinations of findings because it is difficult to find many patients with the same large combination of findings.

The diagnostic findings given in this book are based mostly on an impression of what other doctors expect in the form of evidence for a diagnosis during clinical discussions (or in an evidence-based past medical history). Ideally these findings should have been shown to form the best combinations that identify patients who respond well to treatment compared to placebo in clinical trials. Failing this, they should be the combinations recognised by convention as being the best (known as diagnostic criteria). In the absence of both these situations one has to resort to impressions of what most doctors would think reasonable.

The usefulness of 'suggestive' findings would also require more studies on their frequency of occurrence in association with different diagnostic criteria in various clinical settings (see the answer to question 16 and p 676).

2. Does this book claim to reveal all the mysteries of diagnosis?

No; the way in which our minds work is a mystery and so also is much of the diagnostic process. Diagnosis is based on the Greek to 'know through'. In the context of medicine, it is to see through the patient's symptoms and other findings to imagine and understand what may be happening in terms of current theories applied to medicine. The decision of what to do is made by using the diagnosis to infer what will probably happen next and how the process can be changed by various available interventions. Doctors learn to do this by experience so that as they take a history and examine the patients, it 'dawns' on them what may be going on, what may happen next and what they should do. In essence, their diagnosis is a title or label for what they are imagining in terms of current processes and future events.

The process is uncertain. Philosophically, we can only show that other diagnoses or hypotheses are improbable and that the patient's findings are probably explained by only one known diagnosis. However, there may be some other processes not yet discovered by basic medical research, with which the patient's findings are also compatible. Therefore, the outcomes of actions based on a presumed diagnosis have to be monitored and the diagnosis and decision revised if necessary. The process is often cyclical so that the doctor is supplementing the patient's own reparative and homeostatic feedback processes.

The diagnostician has to be alert to new concerns, symptoms and other findings and has to be able to interpret them to arrive at new diagnoses and decisions. Surgeons may have to do this as they are operating on a patient; even what may appear to be a simple routine procedure may produce surprises and require a quick, innovative and skilled response. Diagnosis is thus bound up with 'clinical management'. Doctors depend on such rapid intuitive processes to get through their day with the speed and efficiency required of them.

In some cases a doctor will listen to the patient, conduct an examination and decide what to do (e.g. giving a pain-relieving drug, pressing on a bleeding wound or sending the patient quickly to hospital) without consciously thinking of a diagnosis. It is only on reflection that he or she will offer an explanation and describe what was imagined subconsciously at the time the decision was made. This is often described as 'empirical' medicine.

3. What approach to diagnosis does this book describe?

In addition to our private inner thoughts and diagnoses, we have to use transparent thought processes to explain to others what we are doing. This is how we explain to patients what we think is wrong, why and what should be done. It is also central to team work involving members of other disciplines who have to help to provide the medical care arising from the various diagnoses that apply to a patient. It is also essential when handing over care to other teams, which is an increasingly prominent feature of modern medicine.

So, however mysteriously the mind works, the decisions, diagnoses and the evidence also have to be communicated very clearly to doctors, nurses and others in the team, the patients and their supporters. The diagnosis may also have to be coded for clinical audit, activity analysis and payment. The evidence and reasoning has to be communicated in order that others can understand and if necessary continue the thought processes. This is the public, explicit form of diagnosis and decision making as opposed to the private, rapid, intuitive process that often leads to diagnoses and decisions in the first place.

The explicit diagnostic thought process can also be used to arrive at the diagnosis in the first place. This has to be done very often by those with little experience but not infrequently by those with wide experience when they inevitably meet new situations. The book describes how this is done.

4. Do doctors traditionally use the transparent methods in this book?

Yes, when they write out a traditional 'Past Medical History' (PMH). There is a current tendency to only provide a list of the past and current diagnoses and problems. If this list is wrong then mistakes can be perpetuated if other doctors copy it uncritically. However, a traditional PMH is based on 'particular' evidence from that 'particular patient'. This means that each diagnosis is a heading, which is followed by an outline of the particular patient's evidence and then the management (see p 657).

Other doctors can check its accuracy more easily than a bare list. The following is an example:

Non-ST elevated myocardial infarction in October 2005
Evidence: Chest pain for 4 hours on 1/10/05, Troponin 2.7 u/l 1/10/05, ECG: no St elevation but inverted T waves in leads V4 to V6 and AVL on 1/10/05.
Management: Analgesia, oxygen, low molecular weight heparin, cardiac monitoring and cardiac rehabilitation protocol. Secondary prevention regimen started 2/10/05.

The PMH can also be set out in table format[1], especially when it is being drafted:

Non-ST elevated myocardial infarction in October 2005	*Evidence:* Chest pain for 4 hours on 1/10/05, Troponin 2.7 u/l 1/10/05, *ECG:* no St elevation but inverted T waves in leads V4 to V6 and AVL on 1/10/05.	*Management:* Analgesia, oxygen, low molecular weight heparin, cardiac monitoring and cardiac rehabilitation protocol. Secondary prevention regimen started 2/10/05.

Each page in the book is represented by a 'lead' such as chest pain. The differential diagnoses on each page are the possible diagnoses and evidence that may be written later in the PMH when the diagnosis is finalised. The reader can scan down this page to see which of these diagnoses and their evidence are compatible with the findings so far.

5. Is there is a simple concept on which transparent diagnosis is based?

Yes—the idea of small predictive combinations of information. If a group of patients with a combination of features turn out to have some diagnosis with a known frequency, then if more features are added, the frequency of the outcome in the new combination will increase, decrease or remain the same. However, the original frequency will represent the average of the new frequencies in the groups formed by subdividing the original group. Thus, a small combination of features that predicts an outcome with a very high frequency can be very useful.

This book outlines findings that form useful combinations for diagnosis and thus predict the outcome of treatment. It does not specify the detailed logical structure of the combinations. Before this can be done, it would be necessary to conduct systematic studies during day-to-day care at the same time as data is collected for audit. Thus all the 'total evidence' of positive and negative findings is taken into account but 'central evidence' is identified within it, which is used to summarise the 'total evidence'[2]. If different combinations of 'central evidence' point to different diagnoses, then these may be simultaneous or differential diagnoses.

1 Llewelyn D.E.H., Ewins D.L., Horn J., Evans T.G.R., McGregor A.M. (1988). Computerised updating of clinical summaries: new opportunities for clinical practice and research? *British Medical Journal*, **297**; 1504–6.
2 Llewelyn, D.E.H., (1988). Assessing the validity of diagnostic tests and clinical decisions. MD thesis. University of London.

6. What are 'leads' and how are they used?

A 'lead' is a finding associated with a limited number of conditions and which is thus easier to investigate. The titles of the pages of the book represent such 'leads'. If a healthy student has experienced a symptom that resolved spontaneously, then it is unlikely to be a good lead. An unusual or disturbing symptom or physical sign may well be a good lead. In the same way extreme results of measurement are often good leads.

If the reader discovers a good 'lead' when taking the history or examining the patient, then by turning to the appropriate page, he or she will be able to scan down the page to see if the patient had other features that form a combination that point to one of the diagnoses.

If the patient's findings are compatible with a number of different pre-dictive combinations, then these will represent the differential diagnoses (provided that they are also capable of causing the presenting complaint). The approach of assembling a combination of findings by selecting items of information that occur commonly in one cause but rarely in others rarely is the probabilistic version of 'logic by elimination'[1, 2, 3]. 'Leads' have also been referred to as 'pivots'[4].

7. At what points in a medical career is this book useful?

This is a book and an approach that can be used throughout a medical career. It can be used by students beginning the medical course to learn the principles of interpreting clinical information. It can be referred to at any time during the medical course when 'clerking' patients or when tackling diagnostic exercises on paper.

This handbook is also designed to help doctors to deal with problems clearly by using a logical and flexible approach when they are on strange territory. More importantly, it also helps students and doctors to defend their diagnoses and decisions and if necessary, to help them to explain their reasoning to patients, nurses and other doctors verbally or in evidence-based past medial histories.

A traditional current past medical history that summarises diagnostic evidence for others (see p 657) would be very helpful when handing over a patient's care to another team, especially when transferring a patient between specialities with mutually unfamiliar conventions of diagnostic evidence. Such an approach would also reduce unnecessary duplication

1 Llewelyn D.E.H. (1975). A concept of diagnosis: A relationship between logic and limits of probability. Clinical Science and Molecular Medicine, 49; 7.

2 Llewelyn D.E.H. (1979). Mathematical analysis of the diagnostic relevance of clinical findings. Clinical Science, 57(5); 477–9.

3 Llewelyn D.E.H. (1981). Applying the principle of logical elimination to probabilistic diagnosis. Medical Informatics, 6(1); 25

4 Eddy D.M., Clanton C.H. (1982). The art of diagnosis: solving the clinicopathological conference. New England Journal of Medicine, 306; 1263–8.

and wasting of resources and might be used on computer systems for health care.

8. In what situations can this book be used?

The book can be used in a number of situations. It can be read after taking a history, examining a patient, arriving at diagnoses and a management plan. The latter will include a 'positive finding summary' or problem list, proposed investigations and initial treatments. The positive findings can then be looked up in this book, beginning with most striking or severe, to see if you have considered important causes and ways of confirming them.

It can be used for problem based learning. Thus, after trying to solve a problem without the aid of this book, use this book for a second attempt. Make your own notes on the blank pages if you find that a cause or important finding has not been mentioned. As with other Oxford Handbooks, we would welcome suggestions. Some diseases are only common in examinations (partly because they provide physical signs that are reliably stable over many years). They are often rare in clinical practice except in specialised departments.

9. How does the structure of the book work?

The main part of the book describes the findings that can emerge at each step of the history and examination and as a result of doing the preliminary tests. Each page will describe the list of the main differential diagnoses to be considered for a lead that is starting point for the diagnostic reasoning process. Alongside each diagnosis there is an outline of the typical evidence that suggests the diagnosis with sufficient probability to justify doing confirmatory tests. It may then outline the typical results of doing these tests to provide reasonable evidence to confirm the diagnosis. There will be some duplication in that these details will be repeated for the reader's convenience each time the diagnosis is listed as a cause of a symptom or sign.

10. How can the book help with revision?

When you read the book, imagine that you have come across a patient with the finding(s) forming the title for that page. Cover the differential diagnoses on the left hand side of the page with your hand or a bookmark to see if you can predict the diagnosis from reading the findings on the right hand side of the page. This is the direction in which your mind should be working when you are trying to help your patients by solving their medical problems. You can then read the whole page for an 'overview'. You should always try to recall what you know already about something before reading about it, in order to learn in an integrated way.

11. Can a transparent diagnostic approach improve the diagnostic accuracy of an experienced doctor?

It is a common experience that if we try to give a carefully reasoned justification for an intuitive opinion, especially by writing it down, we may find that we cannot justify it easily and will reconsider our opinion. Conversely, if our explicitly reasoned justification confirms our intuitive opinion, then we will feel more confident in its success. This is illustrated by what happened when the data assembled by the late Professor Tim de Dombal was analysed. The surgeon was 'correct' in his intuitive diagnosis 235/300 = 78.3% of the time and a transparent logical approach using small combinations of findings was correct 230/300 = 76.6% of the time. However, the surgeon and transparent logical approach agreed about the diagnosis in 221/300 of cases. When there was agreement in these 221 instances, the diagnosis was correct in 200/221= 90.5% of cases[1].

12. How can the reasoning used in this book reassure patients?

When patients see a new doctor, they are asked to give an account of their past medical history and have some responsibility for being able to do so. The doctor often has to struggle to work out what is going on by wading through voluminous notes, computer print-outs and electronic records. It would be so much more reassuring for the patient if the preceding doctor had given the patient a typed, up-to-the-minute traditional evidence based PMH to hand to the next doctor who would be able to look up the evidence used easily by referring to the date at which it was discovered. It is now recognised good practice to give copies of letters to patients. A typed current PMH would help patients to understand such letters by putting them in context. The typed PMH would also act as a focus for giving logical explanations to the patient, allowing the patient to make informed choices and thus to give a more enlightened informed consent.

There is often concern that patients are losing confidence in the medical profession. However, if a doctor is prepared to give a written evidence-based past medical history to patients, then the doctor is effectively inviting those patients to show this explanation to other doctors if they wish. This degree of transparency makes it difficult to hide errors and so it would be sensible to produce such current evidence based past medical

1 Llewelyn, D.E.H., (1988). Assessing the validity of diagnostic tests and clinical decisions. MD thesis. University of London.

histories by referring to example past medical histories or standard text based on locally validated guidelines. If what is proposed is at variance with the guidelines, then the original diagnosis, evidence and management can be reconsidered. This would allow the conclusions to be 'audited' before they are finalised and communicated to the patient.

13. Can this approach improve the use of 'clinical guidelines'?

Guidelines can be re-written as a series of anticipated 'Past Medical Histories' along the lines described in this book. After a diagnosis has been made and the treatments started, a current PMH can be written as soon as possible. This PMH can then be compared with a manual of guideline-based PMHs. As this is done, decisions are 'audited' against the guidelines immediately, when there is still time to reconsider a decision before much damage has been done by any errors.

The guideline-based PMH can also be stored as word-processed standard texts. A current past medical history can be written by copying the standard text into the patient's PMH and then edited. Again, as this is done, decisions are 'audited' by the decision maker against the guidelines immediately.

14. How does this approach relate to diagnostic algorithms?

The suggestive and confirmatory evidence under each diagnosis represents the findings that would have been chosen by following the path down a diagnostic algorithm in order to arrive at the diagnosis. However, instead of locking the reader into a fixed sequence, this book allows the reader to scan the different diagnoses and recognise which findings on the page best fit those of the patient. The confirmatory evidence should be compatible with only one diagnosis.

15. How comprehensive is the information about each diagnosis?

There is not enough space in a hand-book of this kind to describe all the combinations of evidence that might point to a diagnosis. Therefore, each page describes 'some' of the differential diagnoses and for each of these, an outline of 'typical' findings that are suggestive and confirmatory. This provides a start to which further information can be added by the reader in the Oxford Handbook spirit.

The diagnostic 'causes' of a lead are usually listed in the order of their frequency in those patients with the 'lead'. (Sometimes they are grouped together because of causal similarity e.g. into 'cardiac causes' and not in an order of frequency.) A major factor in determining this order is the prevalence of those with the diagnosis in the overall study population. Therefore, the order of the diagnoses on the page may vary between clinical settings. Readers should try to insert the order number of the diagnostic causes in terms of probability in their own clinical settings.

16. Why can the clinical setting affect diagnostic probabilities?

The probability of a diagnosis such as *NSTEMI* given the presence of some findings such as *chest pain with T wave changes* is by convention the same as the frequency of patients with the diagnostic criterion in a group of patients with the findings. In some settings there may be additional patients with another mimicking condition that also causes the same findings. This means that there will be more patients in the study population with the findings of *chest pain with T wave changes* and fewer of them will have a *NSTEMI*, illustrated by the following example.

If 90 patients in a study population have a *NSTEMI* and 30 in the population have a combination of the three features of *NSTEMI with chest pain and T wave changes* then the 'likelihood' of getting these three features in those patients with a *NSTEMI* is 30/90 = 33%. It is also the likelihood of seeing the two findings of *chest pain and T wave changes* because we know already of course before we make this likely prediction that they have a *NSTEMI*.

If 40 different patients in the population have the combination of *chest pain and T wave changes* and that 30 have a combination of the three features of *NSTEMI with chest pain and T wave changes*, then 30 out of the 40 = 30/40 = 75% of patients with this combination in the study population will have a *NSTEMI* (and obversely, 10 out of 40 = 10/40 = 25% do not). So the combination of *chest pain and T wave changes* predicts a *NSTEMI* with a probability of 30/40 = 75% or 0.75.

If in a different clinical setting, the total number of patients in the population with *chest pain and T wave changes* were 60 (instead of 40), then the combination of *chest pain and T wave changes* would predict a *NSTEMI* (and chest pain and T wave changes that we know before making the prediction) with a probability of 30/60 = 50% or 0.5.

We can repeat the above 'verbal reasoning' by using simple arithmetic. If the total study population in the above example was 1000, then the 'prevalence' of the 90 patients with *NSTEMI* in the population of 1000 would be 90/1000 = 9%. We know from the above 'verbal reasoning' that the likelihood of finding patients with the combination of *chest pain and T wave changes* in those with *NSTEMI* is 30/90 = 33%. If the prevalence of the 40 patients with the combination of *chest pain and T wave changes* in the population of 1000 is 40/1000 = 4%, then *chest pain and T wave changes* predict *NSTEMI* with a 'predictive' probability of:

$90/1000 \times \mathbf{30}/90 \div \mathbf{40}/1000 = 30/40 = 75\%$

(Note how the 90s and 1000s cancel each other out:)

$90/\mathbf{1000} \times \mathbf{30}/90 \div \mathbf{40}/\mathbf{1000} = 30/40 = 75\%$

However, if in the different clinical setting, the prevalence of patients with the combination of *chest pain with T wave changes* is 60 patients out of a population of 1000 is 60/1000 = 6%, then this combination of findings predicts *NSTEMI* with a 'predictive' probability of:

90/1000 × **30**/90 ÷ **60**/1000 = **30**/60 = 50%

This simple arithmetic relationship between the 'predictiveness' and the other proportions is known as 'Bayes theorem' (see p 676).

17. Is the information in this book evidence-based?

Each diagnosis in the book is followed by typical evidence of the kind usually mentioned in a traditional PMH. This is the 'particular evidence that applies to a 'particular' patient with that diagnosis. In this sense, the information in the book is all 'evidence-based'. However, there is also scientific evidence based on observations made on groups of patients. In clinical medicine, most of this is about the efficacy of treatment, rather than diagnostic tests.

Most general scientific evidence about symptoms, signs and tests is based on measuring the 'sensitivity' and 'specificity' of findings. These indices describe a finding's ability to predict the result of the confirmatory 'gold standard' test. However, there is little scientific evidence in the medical literature on the validity of the tests that are used as gold standards and which are the best for this purpose. For example we do not know whether the 24 hour albumin excretion rate is a better 'gold standard' than the albumin-creatinine ratio for diagnosing 'Incipient diabetic nephropathy' and thus predicting which diabetic patients with a controlled BP go on to develop nephropathy within 2 years (see p 673).

There are two levels of evidence given for each diagnosis: 'suggestive' and 'confirmatory'. Confirmatory evidence should be validated with clinical trials that allow the effect of different entry criteria for treatment efficacy to be assessed. We can then assess the ability of other findings to predict the presence of 'gold standard' selection criteria using indices such as 'sensitivity' and 'specificity'.

It is possible to cite particularised evidence for all diagnoses and decisions in medicine. This is also possible for alternative medicine such as herbal remedies and homeopathy. The patient can be asked what an alternative practitioner had said by way of explanation (the diagnosis) and the evidence. The evidence would include the original complaint, how the diagnosis was confirmed and how the original symptoms were progressing. It is also important to identify the alternative treatments, as they may interact with conventional treatments. Having identified such alternative diagnoses and treatments, the patient can also be offered other diagnoses and treatments of conventional medicine based on careful general scientific evidence and invited to choose.

18. What is meant by 'facts', 'opinions' and 'evidence' in the book?

Evidence is an account of real events that supports what we believe. It is made up of 'facts'. Thus, facts are also accounts of real events. Real events are transient and immediately become memories that are easily forgotten or distorted. Evidence is usually shared with others and because of this it has to be recorded carefully using conventions that other people will also accept. One of these conventions is that the record of a fact must bear a time and date so that it can be corroborated (e.g. by questioning other witnesses). If such details are omitted, then this may arouse suspicion even if there is no need to seek corroboration. In many cases a listener would judge that the probability of corroboration or replicating the finding would be high.

Most evidence takes the form of contemporaneous notes or printed numerical values from a measuring device. In other cases, a finding is preserved e.g. an X-ray, a photograph, or a video recording with sound. However, all these methods are subject to error or some other distortion and the method of detection and recording has to follow appropriate conventions if they are to be accepted by others. In this book, 'evidence' is described as being 'suggestive' or 'confirmatory' of a diagnosis and when it is applied to a real patient, will have to bear a date or time. Evidence about a single patient may be termed 'particular' evidence, whereas evidence about a group of patients may be termed 'general evidence'.

The principle of replication also applies to general evidence. For example, 1/77 (1.3%) of normative diabetic patients taking placebo with an albumin excretion rate (AER) starting between 20 and 40 µg/minute had nephropathy within 2 years[1]. This would be 'general scientific evidence'.

If we took the pile of 77 records from the study we could simulate repeat studies by selecting a set of notes at random from the pile, examining, returning it and doing this 77 times. If a large number of such 'simulated studies' were done, then from the binomial distribution there would be a 99.7% chance of finding nephropathy in 0/77 or 1/77 or 2/77 or 3/77 or 4/77 of patients with a controlled BP in different simulated studies (i.e. from 0% (0/77) to 5.2% (4/77)). There is thus a 99.7% chance of replicating the finding of 1/77 by a repeat result being between 0/77 and 4/77 inclusive. By comparison, the standard 95% confidence interval for 1/77 is 0.03% to 7.02% and the 99% confidence interval for 1/77 is 0.01% to 9.37%. However, the probability of replication between two limits are more similar to the percentage 'confidence' interval if the numbers in the study are high and the observed result is near to 50%.

A fact is an account of an observation but an opinion is a prediction about something that has not yet (or even cannot) be seen. If an opinion can be checked by observation, it can be founded on evidence (it is 'substantiable'). If it can never be observed it cannot be founded on evidence (it is 'unsubstantiable'). An opinion can thus be 'substantiated' if it can be based on past evidence. For example, if an individual patient's

1 Llewelyn D.E.H., Garcia-Puig J. (2004). How different urinary albumin excretion rates can predict progression to nephropathy and the effect of treatment in hypertensive diabetics. *JRAAS*, **5**; 141–5.

AER is between 20 and 40µg/minute, then an opinion that such a diabetic patient with a controlled BP is unlikely to develop nephropathy would be well founded or 'substantiated' by the 'fact' that of 77 such past patients only one went on to get nephropathy in a particular study.

19. How do these ideas relate to statistical and other models of diagnosis?

Statistical and other mathematical methods (many based on Bayes theorem) generate a value much like a diagnostic test. These may be calculated estimates of some biological value e.g. a 'calculated' glomerular filtration rate, a diagnostic score or an estimated probability. All these 'numerical outputs' of a calculation can be treated in the same way as direct measurements by calibrating them against the frequency of some outcome (e.g. the proportion who progress to requiring dialysis within 2 years—see figure on p 673). The numerical outputs could then be incorporated into the 'suggestive' or 'confirmatory' evidence for the diagnosis.

Decision Analysis [1,2] is essentially a process that estimates the result of a detailed therapeutic clinical trial on a hypothetical group of patients in a transparent way when a real detailed trial is not available or impracticable. The analysis is usually applied to an individual patient who thus is identical to all those in the hypothetical group. The approach uses available estimates of outcome frequencies in the medical literature from related studies and also estimates from the patient of the range of personal well-being that should be gained from each outcome. The analysis involves calculating the average degree of well being for each treatment outcome in a transparent way. Doctors may do this for an individual patient by estimating the outcome of such a hypothetical trial without making calculations. This approach is not covered in this book.

20. How might the approach fit in with electronic patient records?

An electronic patient record (EPR) can overload the user with information just as easily as voluminous paper records. A current or latest evidence-based PMH could act as an introduction to the contents of a patient's records, whether they are electronic or paper-based. By referring to the time and dates of a current PMH, then the user would know what information to focus upon to follow the reasoning process of the person who originally entered information into the record.

1 Dowie J., Elstein A. (1988). *Professional judgement. A reader in clinical decision making.* Cambridge University Press, Cambridge.
2 Llewelyn H., Hopkins A. (1993). *Analysing how we reach clinical decisions.* Royal College of Physicians of London. London.

The 'current PMH' might in future be built into an EPR. Details of test results in an electronic current PMH might be accessed using hypertext connections. It could also be typed out and given to a patient to show to the next doctor or copied into the patient's own electronic health record, such as 'Health-Space', e.g. on *www.healthspace.nhs.uk*.

Acknowledgements

This book is based on ideas and teaching methods developed originally at King's College Hospital, London. We also thank staff and students at Luton & Dunstable Hospital, Eastbourne District General Hospital, Newham University Hospital and the Whittington Hospital in London for their helpful advice and comments. We are grateful to Dr Charlotte Fowler, Mr Jiten Tolia and Mr John Pickles of Luton & Dunstable Hospital for their assistance with the sections on the chest X-ray, eyes and ENT respectively. We are grateful to Dr Lois Davies and Dr James Jones for reviewing early drafts and to Dr Rhys Llewelyn for his advice on later drafts and for suggesting the questions and answers linked to the preface. We are grateful to the staff at OUP for their support and patience, particularly Esther Browning, Martin Baum, Catherine Barnes, Georgia Pinteau and Kate Martin.

Abbreviations

OHCM	Oxford Handbook of Clinical Medicine, sixth edition
OHCS	Oxford Handbook of Clinical Specialties, seventh edition
±	with/without
+ve	positive
−ve	negative
↑	increased
↓	decreased
°	degrees
>	greater than
<	less than
1°	primary
2°	secondary
5-HIAA	5-hydroxyindole acetic acid
A&E	accident and emergency
AAU	accident unit
ABG/s	arterial blood gas/gases
AFB	acid-fast bacillus
ALT	alanine transaminase
ANA	anti-nuclear antibody
ANCA	anti-neutrophil cytoplasmic antibody
A-P	anterior to posterior
ARDS	acute respiratory distress syndrome
AS	aortic stenosis
ASOT	anti-streptolysin O titre
AST	asparate transaminase
AV	atrioventricular
β-hCG	β-human chorionic gonadotrophin
BM	bone marrow
BMI	body mass index
BP	blood pressure
bpm	beats per minute
cANCA	cytoplasmic anti-neutrophil cytoplasmic antibody
CAPD	continuous ambulatory peritoneal dialysis
CCF	congestive cardiac failure
CK-MB	creatine kinase MB isoenzyme
CNS	central nervous system
COPD	chronic obstructive pulmonary disease
CPK	creatine phosphokinase
CRP	C-reactive protein
CSF	cerebrospinal fluid

CT	computerised tomography
CTPA	computerised tomography pulmonary angiogram
CVA	cerebrovascular accident
CVS	cardiovascular system
CXR	chest X-ray
DC	direct current
DIC	disseminated intravascular coagulation
D-dimer	dextrorotatory dimer
DH	drug history
dL	decilitre
DOB	date of birth
DVT	deep vein thrombosis
ECG	electrocardiogram
ECT	electroconvulsive treatment
EEG	electroencephalogram
ELISA	enzyme-linked immunosorbent assay
ERCP	endoscopic retrograde cholangiopancreatography
ESR	erythrocyte sedimentation rate
FBC	full blood count
FDP/s	fibrogen degredation product/s
FEV_1	forced expiratory volume (1 second)
FH	family history
FL	Fluorescence
FSH	follicular stimulating hormone
FT3	free T3
FT4	free T4
FVC	forced vital capacity
G6PD	glucose-6-phosphate dehydrogenase
GALS	Gait, Arms, Legs, Spine
γGT	γ glutamyl transpeptidase
GCS	Glasgow Coma Scale
GI	gastrointestinal
GP	general practitioner
Gr/g	gram
Grm/dL	grams/decilitre
GTT	glucose tolerance test
GU	genitourinary
Hb	haemoglobin
HBsAG	hepatitis B surface antigen
hCG	human chorionic gonadotrophin
HCV	hepatitis C virus
Hg	mercury
HIV	human immunodeficiency virus
HLA-B27	human lymphocyte antigen B27
HOCM	hypertrophic cardiomyopathy
HPC	history of each presenting complaint
HR-CT	high resolution computerised tomography

IgM	immunoglobin M
IHD	ischaemic heart disease
IM	intramuscular
I-P	inter-phalangeal
IV	intravenous
IVU	intravenous urography
JVP	jugular venous pressure
K	potassium
L	litre
LFT	liver function test
LH	luteinizing hormone
LIF	left iliac fossa
LMN	lower motor neurone
LRT	lower respiratory tract
LV	left ventricle
MCP	metacarpophalangeal
MI	myocardial infarction
mmHg	millimetres of mercury
mmol	millimoles
MS	multiple sclerosis
MSU	midstream urine
Na	sodium
NAD	no abnormality detected
NSAIDS	non-steroidal anti-inflammatory drugs
NSAP	non-specific abdominal pain
od	*omni die* (once daily)
OGD	oesophagogastroduodenoscopy
OHCD	*Oxford Handbook of Clinical Diagnosis*
P2	pulmonary component of 2nd heart sound
P-A	posterior to anterior
PA	pernicious anaemia
PAS	periodic acid Schiff
PC	presenting complaints
PCR	polymerase chain reaction
PE	pulmonary embolism
PEFR	peak expiratory flow rate
PMH	past medical history
PND	paroxysmal nocturnal dyspnoea
po	*per os* (by mouth)
PR	*per rectum* (by the rectum)
PSA	Prostatic-specific antigen
PUO	pyrexia of unknown origin
PV	*per vaginam* (by the vagina)
qds	*quater die sumendus* (to be taken 4 times a day)
R factor	rheumatoid factor

RA	rheumatoid arthritis
RBB	right bundle branch
RBC	red blood cells
RLQ	right lower quadrant
RS	respiratory system
RUQ	right upper quadrant
RV	right ventricle
SH	social history
SLE	systemic lupus erythematosus
STEMI	ST elevated myocardial infarction
SVC	superior vena cava
SVT	supraventricular tachycardia
T3	triiodothyronine
T4	thyroxine
TB	tuberculosis
tds	*ter die sumendus* (to be taken 3 times a day)
TFT	thyroid function test
TSH	thyroid stimulating hormone
TURP	transurethral resection of prostate
U&E	urea and electrolytes
UMN	upper motor neurone
URT	upper respiratory tract
URTI	upper respiratory tract infection
USS	ultrasound scan
V/Q	ventilation/perfusion
VSD	ventriculoseptal defect
WBC	white blood cell
WCC	white cell count
WHO	World Health Organization
wt	weight
ZN	Ziehl–Neelsen

History taking skills and imagination

History taking with imagination

The aim of the diagnostic process is to build up an imaginative picture of what is happening to the patient. 'Diagnosis' is derived from the Greek 'to see through' (i.e. the history, physical examination, special investigations and response to treatment). 'The diagnosis' must not imply that there is only some single hidden process that needs to be discovered. The diagnosis (or diagnostic formulation) may have to include various causes, consequences, interactions and other independent processes. As well as internal medical processes, it has to include external factors such as circumstances at home and the effects on self care, employment and leisure. Clearly, the most informative part of this broad diagnostic process will be the history. The history also allows patients and supporters to identify the issues that they want addressed in terms of discomfort, loss of function and difficulties with day to day existence. 'Gold standards for final diagnoses are best based on the outcome of patients' symptoms combined with the result of histology, biochemistry or some other measurements. So, final diagnoses are often based on initial history taking skills from which outcomes can be assessed.

Observe normal social conventions. Introduce yourself politely and invite the patient and any accompanying persons to do the same. Check details such as the patient's date of birth, address etc. It is then important to establish very clearly why the patient has sought help. This is known as the presenting complaint. Ask the patient about its severity and duration and always record this. Be prepared to act immediately to give symptomatic relief (e.g. for pain) if the patient is distressed. In some cases, the presenting complaint may not explain the decision to seek help. The patient may be too ill, shy, guilty or embarrassed to describe what is happening accurately. In other cases, it may be someone else who is unduly worried (e.g. the wife of a lethargic husband, parents of a child or carers of an elderly person who can no longer cope). Be alert and explore the real reason if there is doubt.

Having established the presenting complaint(s), establish the factual details of 'place and time'. It is the ability to give a place and time that establish the complaints as 'facts'. (Medicine shares this convention with pure science and law.) Listen to what the patient says without prompting first, but if necessary ask where they were and what they were doing when the problem was first noticed. This will help the patient to recall what happened and will also stimulate your own diagnostic imagination. Establish the speed of initial onset and subsequent change in severity with time. This helps you to imagine the kind of pathological process that is taking place. Thus an onset within seconds suggests a fit or heart rhythm abnormality, over minutes a bleed or clotting process, hours to days an acute infection, days to weeks a chronic infection, weeks to months a tumour, and months to years a degenerative process. The site may be anatomical e.g. abdominal pain, or systemic e.g. a cough. By convention, 'facts' are details which include a time and place that can be checked.

If there are other complaints, note the same details (the time courses of other new symptoms are often the same however). Ask about other associated, aggravating and relieving factors especially as a result of the patient's own actions, and those of others. Ask what the patient thinks is going on. You will have to continue with cycles of evidence, diagnosis, action, more evidence, revised diagnoses, further action etc. Establish not only what the patient's 'complaints' are and document them, but also the patient's own fears and actions. This will be the starting point for your own explanation and suggestions to the patient later about what is to be done. Write out your history in a systematic way, for example as shown in the next section and go over it with the patient, if possible, to check that it is right.

The case history: an example

Miss AM   Aged 31 (DOB: 28/2/74)
23, Smith Square, Old Town.
Emergency admission
16th October 2005 at 7.00pm

PC: *Severe sore throat, sweats and severe malaise for 2 days.*

HPC: *The patient was well until last Thursday afternoon the 14th October when she developed a sore throat at work as a secretary at an insurance company. It was relieved that day by warm drinks and paracetamol but when she woke the following morning it was very severe. It was no longer relieved by paracetamol (she found swallowing very painful) and she was too unwell to get up. There had been no previous sore throats. She thought that her neck was getting stiff. Her friend had died of meningococcal meningitis a few years previously and this worried her. She called her GP and the deputising service responded. The visiting doctor was concerned that she lived alone and looked very unwell and he referred her to hospital.*

The most striking symptom is the severe sore throat that is getting worse. This is an example of a feature with a short list of causes: a good 'lead'. Most readers will have experienced a sore throat and will be aware that it is usually due to a viral pharyngitis, tonsillitis (due to a haemolytic streptococcus), glandular fever or something else in a relatively small proportion of cases (see p134). Very rarely, these causes include the beginning of a meningococcal infection. This loomed large in the patient's mind because of the fate of her friend. The history is compatible with all these possibilities.

If a better 'lead' with an even shorter differential diagnosis turns up later, you may use that. Use the other findings to try to confirm one cause of the shortest 'lead' (and thus 'eliminate' the others). Think if the remaining abnormal findings could resolve if the confirmed diagnosis were treated. If not, look for another co-existing diagnosis. This handbook contains a selection of findings with short differential diagnoses. Single and small combinations of findings of this kind form the foundation of the process of arriving at working diagnosis (i.e. until the diagnosis is 'final' and no further tests or treatment changes are contemplated). With growing experience you will learn to recognise more combinations that usually point to a single or a few diagnoses and have to resort less often to working through the possibilities in a conscious way using the concepts described in this book. However, you will continue to be faced with new or strange situations throughout your career; this is what makes medical practice such a challenge. So, the approaches that you develop early in your career to deal with new situations will stand you in good stead for the remainder of your career.

The next step is the past medical history (PMH).

The past medical history

PMH: Thyrotoxicosis discovered 6 months ago. (Anxiety, weight loss, abnormal thyroid function tests in Osler Hospital.) Taking Carbimazole, 5mg daily.

The past medical history in this case has three components: the diagnosis, the evidence and the management. 'Thyrotoxicosis' is the diagnosis, which summarises what is imagined to have happened. 'Anxiety, weight loss, abnormal thyroid function tests' summarises the evidence for imaging what had happened. The management was 'Taking Carbimazole 5mg daily'. In many cases, the patient would not be able to provide these details and they would have to be extracted from the hospital or primary care records, in which case it is helpful to name the hospital (the fictitious Osler Hospital in this case) or primary care centre or doctor responsible. It is important to note however, that a comprehensive past medical history in this format can be written immediately after any consultation, in hospital or primary care with results and dates. It can be included with any communication so that the recipient does not have to hunt for the details. It is very helpful for those that follow (and this may include you). So, from time to time in the hand-written follow up notes, you may wish to 'take stock' and write down a 'current' past medical history which sets out the numbered list of diagnoses with the evidence and management in parentheses.

In this case, the past history also raises the possibility of recurrence of thyroid disease causing the sore throat, but the only thyroid condition to do this would be acute thyroiditis (viral or auto-immune); this is rare and not included in lists of common causes of a sore throat. The message to be taken away from this is that if the patient has had a condition in the past medical history, possible links should be recalled or looked up to see if any of these could explain the presenting problem. In this sense, a history of chronic or recurrent conditions can be used as a 'lead'. So, any type of 'lead' with a short list of possible associations should be considered.

The drug history

The drug history is often placed at the very end of the history before the examination findings; it is a matter of personal choice. However, if the patient is on medication, then it indicates that there is an active medical condition as opposed to a past medical history. Therefore, there is something to be said for documenting the drug history immediately after the past medical history so that past and current conditions can be thought about together.

Drug history: Paracetamol 1g 6 hourly (for?? Viral pharyngitis: sore throat for 2 days with fever, and general malaise) with Carbimazole 5mg daily for thyrotoxicosis (see PMH for evidence)

Alcohol 10 units per week

Non-smoker

No other recreational drugs

Diagnostic significance of the drug history

Note that the indication for paracetamol is given in the form of one possible diagnosis (other differentials could have been included) and the evidence for the diagnosis. This is good practice (not often followed). The evidence for thyrotoxicosis has been given already in the past medical history. Recreational drugs have also been covered in this drug history, but they are often included with the social history.

If the side effects of carbimazole are looked up, they will be seen to include agranulocytosis, which could explain the sore throat. If this were known when the HPC was being written out, then it could be included as a possible causal factor in the HPC.

Risk factors for future or current illnesses (such as smoking) can exist in the drug history, past medical history, family history (e.g. of diabetes) or social history.

The family history

FH:

Father aged 56	*Hypertension*
Mother aged 55	*Diabetes (onset at 50)*
siblings male:	*aged 34—alive and well*
	aged 26—alive and well
female:	*aged 30—alive and well*
Children—none	

The family history rarely contains features that form powerful leads. In general there will be risk factors in the family history. For example, the fact that the patient's mother had type 2 diabetes means that there is an increased risk of the patient developing type 2 diabetes mellitus. This may have no immediate bearing on the current problems (but she should be checked for diabetes if only to exclude its presence so far) but the patient could be advised to adopt a healthy diet and lifestyle.

The social history

The social history (SH) is always relevant. The activities of daily living can be considered under the heading of domestic, work and leisure. Imagine what any person has to do from waking up in the morning to going to sleep at night and consider whether the patient needs support with any of these activities. Fit young adults who are expected to recover completely may miss school, college or work and the timing of their return will have to be considered. Patients who are more dependent on others such as children and the elderly may need special provisions. Patients with permanent disabilities may need help with most if not all activities of daily living.

SH: Alone in a flat at present (flatmate on holiday for another week)
Parents live 200 miles away
Works as secretary for insurance firm

The systems enquiry

The systems enquiry may take place at various points in the history. Some include it after the history of presenting complaint or the past medical history or at the very end. In terms of the diagnostic thought process, putting it at the very end allows it to be used to draw together the conclusions reached at the end of the history in terms of diagnoses and risk factors. The social history will be fresh in your mind in terms of the patient's ability to deal with day to day living. You can sum up with a 'sieve' to remind you of what is happening in structural and functional terms in the different systems:

- Social and domestic issues
- Locomotor structure and function
- Skin, temperature regulation and endocrine
- Cardiovascular structure and circulation
- Respiratory structure and blood gases
- Alimentary tract and metabolism
- Genitourinary and renal function
- Neurological and psychiatric

If a direct question turns up a positive response, it has to be treated with caution. It may be a 'false positive' response to a leading question. A positive response has to be treated as an extra presenting complaint and added to the original list.

However, if there is a negative response to a direct question, this is more reliable (unless the patient is very forgetful or is purposely withholding information). The absence of *all* symptoms under a heading indicates that there is no symptomatic evidence of an abnormality in that system. If there is a normal physical examination for that system too, then there will be no clinical evidence at all of an abnormality in that system. This does not indicate with certainty that there is no abnormality. A later clinical assessment or test (e.g. a chest X-ray) might discover something.

Systems enquiry

Locomotor symptoms

- *No pain and stiffness in the neck, shoulder, elbow, wrist, hand or back*
- *No pain and stiffness in the hip, knee or foot*
- *No pain or stiffness in any joints and muscles*

Negative responses make locomotor abnormalities unlikely. If any are positive, then a 'GALS' examination screen is performed under the headings of Gait, Arms, Legs, Spine. This should be done after the general examination but before the neurological examination so that care can be taken with painfully inflamed or damaged joints.

Skin lymph nodes and endocrine

- *No heat or cold intolerance (e.g. wanting to open or close windows when others are comfortable)*
- *No sweats and shivering*
- *No drenching night sweats*
- *No episodes of rigors*
- *No rashes and itching*
- *No skin lumps or lumps elsewhere*

Negative responses make abnormal thyroid metabolism, and some skin, lymphoid and immune reactions unlikely.

Cardiovascular

- *No tiredness and breathlessness on exertion (non-specific)*
- *No syncope and dizziness*
- *No leg pain on walking*

Negative responses make cardiac output and peripheral vascular disease unlikely.

- *No ankle swelling*

A negative response makes a right sided venous return abnormality unlikely.

- *No exertional dyspnoea*
- *No orthopnoea*
- *No paroxysmal nocturnal dyspnoea*

Negative responses make left heart venous return abnormality unlikely.

- *No palpitations*
- *No central chest pain on exertion or at rest*

Negative responses make a cardiac abnormality less likely

Respiratory symptoms

- *No chronic breathlessness*
- *No acute breathlessness*

Negative responses make abnormality of overall respiratory and blood gas abnormality unlikely.

- *No hoarseness*
- *No cough, sputum, haemoptysis*
- *No wheeze*

Negative responses make airway disease unlikely.

- *No pleuritic chest pain*

A negative response makes acute pleural reactions and chest wall disease unlikely.

Alimentary symptoms

- *No loss of appetite (non-specific)*
- *No weight loss (non-specific)*
- *No jaundice, dark urine, pale stools*

Negative responses make metabolic gut and liver disease unlikely.

- *No nausea or vomiting (non-specific)*
- *No haematemesis or melaena*
- *No dysphagia*
- *No indigestion*
- *No abdominal pain*
- *No diarrhoea or constipation*
- *No recent change in bowel habit*
- *No rectal bleeding ± mucus*

Negative responses make gastrointestinal disease unlikely.

The systems enquiry (continued)

Genitourinary symptoms
- *Menstrual history—date of menarche, duration of cycle and flow normal*
- *Volume of flow and associated pain normal*
- *Any pregnancy outcomes normal*
- *No dyspareunia and vaginal bleeding*
- *No vaginal discharge*

Negative responses make gynaecological disease unlikely.
- *No haematuria or other odd colour*
- *No urgency or incontinence*
- *No dysuria*
- *No loin pain or lower abdominal pain*

Negative responses make urological disease unlikely.
- *No impotence or loss of libido*
- *No urethral discharge*

Negative responses make male urological disease unlikely.

Nervous system symptoms
- *No loss or disturbance of:*
  - *Vision (loss, blurring or double vision)*
  - *Hearing (loss or tinnitus)*
  - *Smell and taste*
- *No numbness, pins and needles or other disturbance of sensation*
- *No disturbance of speech*
- *No weakness of limbs*
- *No imbalance*
- *No headache*
- *No sudden headache and loss of consciousness*
- *No dizziness and blackouts*
- *No vertigo*
- *No 'fit'*
- *No transient neurological deficit*

Negative responses make neurological disease unlikely.

Psychiatric symptoms
- *No fatigue, not tired all the time*
- *No mood change*
- *No odd voices or odd visual effects*
- *No anxiety and sleep disturbance*
- *No loss of self confidence*
- *No new strong beliefs*
- *No phobias, no compulsions or avoidance of actions*
- *No use of recreational drugs*

Patients may of course hide or forget many symptoms. There is a school of thought that regards symptom reviews as being of little value, and that only symptoms that are volunteered are worthwhile investigating. Many doctors do not conduct systemic reviews and only ask these questions if other symptoms have been volunteered already in that system. By drawing together all the findings in the history it would look as follows:

Miss AM   Aged 31 (DOB: 28/2/74)
23 Smith Square, Old Town.
Emergency admission— 16th October 2005 at 7.00pm

PC: Severe sore throat, sweats and severe malaise for 2 days.
HPC: The patient was well until last Thursday afternoon the 14th October when she developed a sore throat at work as a secretary at an insurance company. It was relieved that day by warm drinks and paracetamol but when she woke the following morning it was very severe. It was no longer relieved by paracetamol (she found swallowing very painful) and she was too unwell to get up. There had been no previous sore throats. She thought that her neck was getting stiff. Her friend had died of meningococcal meningitis a few years previously and this worried her. She called her GP and the deputising service responded. The visiting doctor was concerned that she lived alone and looked very unwell and he referred her to hospital.
PMH: Thyrotoxicosis discovered 6 months ago. (Anxiety, weight loss, abnormal thyroid function tests in Osler Hospital.) Taking Carbimazole, 50mg daily.
DH:
Paracetamol 1g 6 hourly for?? (Viral pharyngitis: sore throat for 2 days with fever, and severe malaise)
Carbimazole 5mg for thyrotoxicosis   (see PMH)
Alcohol 10 units per week.
Non-smoker
No other recreational drugs

FH:
Father aged 56   Hypertension
Mother aged 55   Diabetes (onset at 50)
Siblings male: aged 34—alive and well
                             aged 26—alive and well
        female: aged 30—alive and well
Children—none

The systems enquiry (continued)

SH:
Alone in a flat at present (flatmate on holiday for another week)
Parents live 200 miles away
Works as secretary for insurance firm
Systems enquiry
NAD.

NAD

NAD is an abbreviation for 'no abnormality detected'. However, it is often regarded with suspicion and many readers of the notes will assume cynically that NAD means 'not actually done'. If direct questions were asked, then all the answers should be documented. If none were asked then write 'Systems enquiry not done'.

The preliminary diagnosis

Most of the diagnostic information is contained in the history. Much of the physical examination is directed at looking for information to help to confirm or exclude the diagnostic possibilities raised by the history. It is therefore worth pausing at the end of the history to think about the diagnostic possibilities so far. In some professional examinations, the candidate is asked only to take a history and to give diagnostic conclusions and a management plan of investigations and treatment options.

In this patient's case, a reasonable differential for the main diagnosis might be:

- **?Viral pharyngitis** (? means a 'reasonable' probability e.g. 20–80%)
- **?Glandular fever**
- **?Acute follicular tonsillitis**
- **?Agranulocytosis due to Carbimazole.**
- **??Meningococcal meningitis** (?? means a low probability e.g. <20%)

Other diagnoses might be:

- **Inadequate domestic support currently for acute illness**
- **??Undiscovered type 2 diabetes mellitus**

The part of the physical examination to concentrate on would be the appearance of the pharynx and tonsils to see if the latter resembled 'strawberries and cream' suggestive of acute follicular tonsillitis or simple redness with no pus, suggestive of a pharyngitis possibly of viral origin. Enlarged lymph nodes should be looked for in the neck to support a brisk response to infection and neck stiffness that would support meningitis.

The special investigations would include an urgent white cell count to see if there were absent or low white cells confirming agranulocytosis; raised neutrophil white cells suggesting bacterial infection; or raised lymphocytes suggesting viral infection. Urine should be tested for sugar and a fasting blood sugar done.

The immediate treatment options would be to continue the paracetamol for pain relief and offer additional analgesia such as codeine phosphate.

You will hear of many different approaches to history taking. Make up your own mind and write out your approach on the blank pages provided near here or inside the front cover of the book. Write out your own plan like the one in the following section.

Although there are obvious benefits to taking a systematic approach, especially if you are a student or a doctor faced with an unfamiliar problem, consultations may have to be very rapid with short cuts. The circumstances may also disrupt any attempt to be systematic, for example, when examining a fractious child, or if you are surrounded by a number of injured or very sick patients. However, to be effective, you should think in an orderly way by identifying the most urgent issue first then running through in your mind the other issues that have to be considered. For each issue keep thinking: What are the facts (symptoms, signs and test results)? What do I imagine is going on (the diagnoses)? What should I do (tests, treatments, and advice)? When you write down an account later, do so in response to the same questions. Within each of these questions, consider what is happening in each system. You can do this using 'sieves'.

Medical diagnostic sieves

The diagnostic possibilities discovered so far were triggered by the findings in the history. It might be helpful to reflect in case some other possibilities have been temporarily forgotten, or in case some other conditions are present which might be caused or complicated by the diagnostic possibilities thrown up already. This is where sieves can be useful. Reflect if there is something else that you should have considered in each system from a structural or functional point of view.

- Social system (home, work or environment) and locomotor
- Nervous system (psychiatry or neurological)
- Cardiovascular system (physiologically or structurally)
- Respiratory system (blood gas regulation or structurally)
- Alimentary system (metabolic or GI tract)
- Genitourinary system (reproductive or metabolic)
- Skin and reticulo-endothelial system
- Endocrine and autonomic system

Surgical diagnostic sieves

If there is a structural abnormality, use the surgical sieve.

- Congenital
- Infective
- Traumatic
- Neoplastic
- Degenerative

There are many variations of these sieves. They are merely self-propelling memory joggers that enhance recall where we stimulate our minds to recognise something that we may be about to forget.

Management sieves

Consider if there is a test or treatment that you may have forgotten to undertake. Think 'big' first by considering the environmental level and then work down via the whole patient to 'small' methods by considering electromagnetic radiation. Tests produce results and treatments have outcomes. Therapeutic tests are useful and legitimate. So, the distinction between a test and a treatment can be a fine one and the same sieve can be applied to both. Look at each possibility thrown up by the diagnostic sieve and consider if there is a test or treatment that you have forgotten by considering the following 'action sieve'. This may take a few minutes of reflection but the patient will be grateful. You will learn more if you do this before looking up what you have forgotten in a book.

Have I forgotten to decide about something at the:
- Environmental level e.g. social services assessment and intervention?
- 'Whole patient' level e.g. explanation from the doctor or assessment, treatment or advice from nurses, occupational therapists, physiotherapists, dietetics, speech therapy, etc?
- Organ level e.g. surgical and endoscopic?
- Cellular level e.g. cytology, haematology, transfusion, transplantation?
- Molecular level e.g. biochemical tests and drug therapy?
- Electronic level e.g. ECG, EEG, ECT and DC cardioversion?
- Radiation level e.g. radiology and radiotherapy?

Use a plan for writing out the history

Write out your history in the same way each time and it will act as a checklist to ensure that you have not forgotten something that you will later wish to rely on as evidence for your diagnosis and decisions. The following is an example; write down your own version inside the front or back cover—best with a pencil so that you can change it later.

History taker's name: *Date of assessment:*

Patient's name: *DOB:*   *Age*   *Occupation*
Patient's address:

Admitted as an emergency/from the waiting list on (date) at (time)

Presenting complaints (PC)
1st symptom—duration
2nd symptom—duration
etc

History of each presenting complaint (HPC)
1. *Nature of complaint (e.g. pain in chest), circumstances & speed of onset, progression (change with time—picture a graph), aggravating and relieving factors, associated symptoms (describe under 2 etc below)*
2. *Next associated symptom, etc. described as in (1).*

Add response to direct questions from chasing up some diagnostic possibilities that come to mind as the history is taken (some think that this should not be done as the responses may contain too many 'false positives')

Past medical history (PMH)
1st Diagnosis & when—Evidence—Treatment—Name of doctor
2nd

Drug history (DH)
Name, dose & frequency—diagnostic indication—evidence—prescriber
Next drug etc
Alcohol and tobacco consumption   Drug sensitivities and allergies

Developmental history
(in paediatrics and psychiatry): pregnancy, infancy, childhood, puberty, adulthood

Family history (FH)

	Age	Illnesses
(Arrange around 'family tree' if preferred)		*Mention especially:*
Parents		*tuberculosis*
Siblings		*asthma, eczema*
Children		*diabetes, epilepsy*
Spouse		*hypertension*

Social history (SH)
Home and domestic activity support—job and financial security—travel and leisure. (Consider the effect of all these on the illness and the effect of the illness on these.)

Physical examination skills and leads

Physical examination skills

At the end of the history in the previous chapter the patient was thought to have:

- ?Viral pharyngitis
- ?Glandular fever
- ?Acute follicular tonsillitis
- ?Agranulocytosis due to carbimazole
- ??Meningococcal meningitis
- Inadequate domestic support currently for acute illness
- ??Undiscovered type 2 diabetes mellitus

Recall what you imagined after the history. Give a subjective impression of how well the patient appears to be on a spectrum from being completely fit and well, being unwell to some degree, to moribund. Be prepared to respond appropriately.

An ability to make a subjective 'diagnosis' of degrees of well-being and imminent outcome depends on experience of observing a large number of patients and knowing what happened to them. There are early warning scores that you may be expected to use in some centres based on pulse, respiratory rate etc.

When you are being assessed by an examiner, do things deliberately so that you can be clearly seen to be doing the right thing. Students and many doctors are being assessed continuously during their day to day work and so there is much to be said for doing everything in a deliberate and transparent way at all times.

The techniques of the physical examination are not covered in detail in this *Oxford Handbook of Clinical Diagnosis*. However, the sequences of examination and documentation are described here. The skills themselves are best learnt by watching experts, copying them and practising as much as possible. There are books that already specialise in describing practical examination techniques in detail.

Watch others, read other books and choose your own sequences. Write out your chosen sequence on the blank pages provided here and inside the front cover of this book if you wish. Write out your findings in the patient's record in the same order, to reduce the chance of forgetting something. However, in some centres you will be provided with a 'clerking proforma', which you will be expected to use.

The general examination

Before examining the patient, look out for other clues e.g. state of attire, nebuliser masks, sputum pots, medication packets etc. The general examination is directed mainly at assessing the skin and reticulo-endothelial system (lymph nodes) and the related matters of temperature control and metabolic rate. During the history, the order of questioning could be decided entirely by thought processes (for example, probing indirectly for a symptom to chase up a diagnostic possibility that comes to mind) but the physical examination is different. It is more efficient to adopt a routine that is smooth and quick and not to jump about looking for physical signs that might support the diagnostic idea of that moment.

You have already been looking at the patient's face, general appearance and immediate vicinity (e.g. walking stick, medication packets etc.) when taking the history, so for the general examination, begin with the hands and work your way up by inspecting (and, when appropriate, palpating) the arms to the shoulders, examine the scalp, ears, eyes, cheeks, nose, lips, take the temperature, examine inside the mouth, then the neck, breasts, axillae, and then the skin of the abdomen, legs and feet.

Plan of the general physical examination

Hands, arms, and shoulders
- *Fingernails*
- *Clubbing*
- *Finger nodules*
- *Finger joints deformity*
- *Rashes*
- *Pain and stiffness in the elbow, shoulder, neck*

Head and neck
- *Neck stiffness*
- *Patchy hair loss*
- *Ear drum redness*
- *Perforated ear drum*

Eyes, face, and neck
- *Facial redness, general appearance*
- *Red eye*
- *Iritis*
- *Conjunctival pallor*
- *Temperature—high or low*
- *Mouth lesions*
- *Lumps in the:*
  - *Face*
  - *Submandibular region*
  - *Anterior neck*
  - *Anterior triangle of neck*
  - *Posterior triangle*
  - *Supraclavicular region*

Trunk
- *Breast discharge*
- *Nipple eczema*
- *Breast lumps*
- *Gynaecomastia in male*
- *Axillary lymphadenopathy*
- *Sparse body hair*
- *Hirsutism*
- *Scar pigmentation*
- *Abdominal striae*

Legs
- *Inguinal and generalised lymphadenopathy*
- *Sacral, leg and heel sores*

Cardiovascular system

Think first of cardiac output and inspect and feel the hands for warmth or coldness. Feel the radial pulse, take the blood pressure and check the other pulses in the arms and neck. Next think of venous return and look at the JVP. Then examine the heart itself (palpate, percuss and then listen to it). Finally examine output and venous return in the legs by feeling skin temperature, the pulses and looking for oedema of the legs, liver and lungs.

Cardiac output
- *Peripheral cyanosis*
- *Radial pulse*
  - *Rate*
  - *Rhythm (compare cardiac apex rate if irregular)*
  - *Amplitude*
  - *Vessel wall*
- *Compare pulses for volume and synchrony*
  - *Radial, brachial, carotid, (femoral, popliteal, posterior and anterior tibials after the examining the heart)*
- *Blood pressure standing and lying in right arm, repeat on left*

Venous return
- *Jugular venous pressure*

The heart
- *Trachea displaced?*
- *Apex beat displaced?*
- *Parasternal heave*
- *Palpable thrill*
- *Auscultation*
  - *Extra heart sounds*
    —Systolic murmurs
    —Diastolic murmurs

Cardiac output and venous return in the legs
- *Skin temperature*
- *Posterior and anterior tibials, popliteal, femoral*
- *Venous skin changes*
- *Vein abnormalities*
- *Calf swelling*
- *Leg oedema*
- *Sacral oedema*
- *Liver enlargement*
- *Basal lung crackles*

Respiratory system

Think of general respiratory structure and function. *Inspect* and think of oxygen and carbon dioxide levels, then the ventilation process, which depends on the chest wall and its movement. *Palpate* by feeling for tactile vocal fremitus. *Percuss* and then *auscultate*. Finally listen for wheezes thus assessing airways from small (high pitched) to large (low pitched).

General inspection
- *Tremor and muscle twitching*
- *Cyanosis of the tongue and lips*
- *Clubbing*

Chest inspection
- *Respiratory rate*
- *Distorted chest wall*
- *Poor expansion*
- *Paradoxical movement*

Palpation
- *Mediastinum*
  - *Position of trachea*
  - *Position of apex beat*

Tactile vocal fremitus
- *Present or absent (or increased)*

Percussion
- *Hyper-resonant, resonant, normal, dull or stony dull*

Auscultation
- *Diminished breath sounds*
- *Bronchial breathing*
- *Crackles*
- *Rubs*
- *Wheezes, high or low pitched or polyphonic during inspiration and expiration*

Alimentary and genitourinary systems

Think first of metabolic issues related to general nutrition (obese, normal, thin, cachexia) and ensure that the patient is weighed. Check the mucous membranes e.g. for signs of vitamin deficiency. Look for skin and eye signs of low fluid volume and then liver disease. Next turn your mind to anatomical aspects of the gastrointestinal and genitourinary systems together by inspecting, palpating and auscultating. Finally perform examinations (when indicated) that need special equipment. Finally, do the urine tests.

Inspection

- Obesity
- Cachexia
- Oral lesions
- Jaundice
- Hepatic skin stigmata
- Loss of skin turgor
- Low eye tension

Palpation

- Supraclavicular nodes

Inspection of the abdomen

- Abdominal scars
- Veins
- General distension
- Visible peristalsis
- Poor movement

Palpation

- General tenderness
- Localised tenderness
- Hepatic enlargement
- Splenic enlargement
- Renal enlargement
- Abdominal masses

Percussion

- Dull or resonant
- Shifting dullness

Auscultation

- Silent abdomen
- Tinkling bowel sounds
- Bruits

Inspection and palpation again

- Groin lumps (lymph nodes?)
- Scrotal masses
- Rectal abnormalities
- Melaena, fresh blood
- Vaginal and pelvic abnormalities
- Urine abnormalities

Nervous system

If there are no neurological symptoms or signs detected up to this point, then it is customary to perform an abbreviated examination. This is done by commenting on the fact that the patient was conscious and alert, speech was normal and that there were no cranial nerve abnormalities noted when looking at the face during the history and general examination. Also, you will have been able to note the patient's gait and movements around the hospital bed or consultation room. According to the GALS system note and record the *G*ait, appearance and movement of the *A*rms, *L*egs and *S*pine.

If the patient was not conscious and alert, then the level of consciousness has to be addressed with the Glasgow Coma Scale.

The brief neurological examination consists of checking coordination and reflexes (because this tests the sensory and motor function of the nerves and central connections involved). The findings may be recorded as follows:

Short CNS examination

- Conscious and alert
- Speech normal
- Facial appearance and movement normal
- Finger—nose pointing normal
- Hand tapping and rotating normal
- Heel—toe test normal (ran heel from opposite knee to toe and back)
- Foot tapping (examiner's hand) normal

Reflexes	Right	Left
Biceps normal	+	+
Supinators normal	+	+
Triceps normal	+	+
Knees normal	+	+
Ankles normal	+	+
Plantars normally flexor	↓	↓

The full neurological assessment

The system of examination described here is typical. The blank pages are there for you to write your comments and amendments. The general approach is to assess the conscious level (if the patient is not conscious and alert, then it will not be possible to conduct a full neurological examination, which needs the patient's cooperation).

The cranial nerve sequence follows in their numbered sequence. Motor function can be assessed next, beginning with inspection for wasting and involuntary movements and then 'palpation' by testing tone and power. The upper limbs are examined first and then the lower limbs. Sensation is then tested in the upper, then lower limbs and finally coordination, reflexes and gait. The order can be changed by addressing the area of abnormality suggested by the history. For example, if the patient complains of difficulty in walking, then it would be sensible to examine gait, then motor function and sensory function and cranial nerves last.

Nervous system
- *Conscious level*
- *Glasgow Coma Score*
- *Speech*

Cranial nerves
- *Absent sense smell*
- *Visual field defects*
- *Decreased acuity*

Opthalmoscopy:
- *Corneal opacity*
- *Lens opacity*
- *Papilloedema*
- *Pale optic disc*
- *Cupped disc*
- *Hypertensive retinopathy*
- *Dot and blot heamorrhages*
- *New vessel formation*
- *Pale/black retinal patches*

- *Ptosis*
- *Pupil*
  - *Constriction*
  - *Irregularities*
  - *Dilatation*
- *Diplopia*
- *Nystagmus*
- *Absent corneal reflex*
- *Loss of facial sensation*
- *Deviation of Jaw*
- *Jaw jerk*

- *Facial weakness*
- *Deafness*
- *Loss of taste*
- *Palatal weakness*
- *Neck or shoulder weakness*
- *Paresis of tongue*

Motor function
Upper limbs
- *Arm posture*
- *Hand tremor*
- *Wasting of hand*
- *Wasting of arm*
- *Tone abnormalities*

Weakness of
- *Shoulder abduction*
- *Elbow flexion*
- *Elbow extension*
- *Wrist extension*
- *Handgrip*
- *Finger adduction and abduction*
- *Thumb abduction and opposition*
- *Arm incoordination*

Lower limbs
- *Limitation of movement*
- *Wasting*
- *Fasciculation*
- *Tone abnormalities*

Weakness of
- *Hip flexion*
- *Knee extension and flexion*
- *Foot*
  - *Plantar flexion*
  - *Dorsiflexion*
  - *Eversion*
- *Bilateral spastic paraparesis*
- *Spastic hemiparesis*

The full neurological assessment (continued)

Sensation

Upper limb sensation

- Hypoaesthesia of
  - Palm
  - Dorsum hand
  - Lateral arm
  - Ulnar border arm
- Dissociated sensory loss
- Progressive sensory loss
- Cortical sensory loss

Lower limb

- Hypoaesthesia of
  - Inguinal area
  - Anterior thigh
  - Shin
  - Lateral foot
- Progressive downward loss
- Dissociated sensory loss
- Multiple areas of loss

Reflexes

- Brisk or
- Diminished, in biceps, supinator, triceps, knee, ankle and plantars
- Gait abnormalities

Mental state examination

Think of the sequence of perception, 'affect', drive and arousal, cognitive processes (check memory of different duration, ability to reason with that memory and then the nature of beliefs arrived at with such reasoning) and then actions in response to these:

- *Perception*: attentiveness and any hallucination, visual or auditory
- *Mood*: depression or elation
- *Mental*: *drive* rate of speech, anxiety
- *Cognition*: (6/10 or less correct implies impairment)
- *Orientation*: time to nearest hour, year, address of hospital
- *Short term memory*: repeat a given name and address, name 2 staff
- *Long term memory*: own age, date of birth, current monarch, dates of wars
- *Concentration*: count backwards from 20 to 1
- *Beliefs*: patient's perception and insight of health, self-confidence, any extreme convictions
- *Activity*: physical and social activity, employment, physical signs of drug use

Basic blood and urine test results

First check the patient's name, gender, age, and address to make sure whose sample you are handling and whose result you are interpreting. The following are interpreted in Chapter 13.

Urine testing
- *Asymptomatic microscopic haematuria*
- *Asymptomatic proteinuria*
- *Glycosuria*
- *Raised urine or plasma bilirubin*
  - *Hepatocellular jaundice*
  - *Obstructive jaundice*

Biochemistry
- *Hypernatraemia*
- *Hyponatraemia*
- *Hyperkalaemia*
- *Hypokalaemia*
- *Hypercalcaemia*
- *Hypocalcaemia*
- *Raised alkaline phosphatase*

Haematology
- *Low haemoglobin*
- *Microcytic anaemia*
- *Macrocytic anaemia*
- *Normocytic anaemia*
- *Very high ESR or CRP*

The general approach

1. Use good viewing conditions—preferably a light box in a dark area.
2. Check the patient's name, gender, age and address to ensure correct identity.
3. Check if the film is marked P-A (X-rays passing from posterior to anterior in a standard way) or A-P (X-rays passing from anterior to posterior). A-P views are done when the patient is ill, using a portable X-ray tube—these will often be semi-erect films with suboptimal exposure factors. This projection magnifies the mediastinum so A-P films should not be used to assess cardiac size or hilar configuration.
4. Check which sides are marked left and right and whether the cardiac apex is on the left if not, the patient may have dextrocardia.
5. Check the patient's positioning. Are the sterno-clavicular joints equidistant from the spinous processes of the vertebral column? If not then the patient was rotated. Rotation causes asymmetry of shoulder girdle muscles projected over the lung fields. The side which has the less space between the end of the clavicle and spinous process has more muscle projected over the lung fields and should be whiter than the other side. Be cautious in the interpretation of a rotated chest radiograph.
6. Can you see the vertebral column through the heart shadow? If not, then it is 'under-penetrated' (the X-ray beam was too weak). This means that normal lung tissue will look abnormally opaque (white).
7. If the lungs appear dark, the vertebral column can be seen very clearly and the heart shadow is vague, it was over-penetrated and abnormalities may be missed.
8. Is the diaphragm between the 5th/6th anterior rib ends? If it is higher, then the patient did not take a deep breath, and interpretation of the appearance of the lungs and mediastinum will be suboptimal. If the diaphragm is flattened then emphysematous changes are likely.
9. Having considered the technical issues, is there anything that strikes you immediately? Check for foreign bodies, e.g. endotracheal tubes, chest drains, etc. A striking radio-opaque (white) or lucent (dark) area is likely to be a good lead.
10. After noting the obvious finding, or if there is nothing dramatic, assess the X-ray systematically, as there could well be more subtle abnormalities.
11. Compare the lung fields in the lower zones, mid zones and upper zones and check 'behind' the heart.
12. Look at the superior mediastinum, the hilum, the heart, the cardio-phrenic angles, the diaphragms and the costo-phrenic angles.
13. Lastly, look at the ribs, the shoulders, the overlying soft tissue from the neck down to the upper abdomen. Note artefacts from skin folds, hair and clothing, especially braids and buttons.
14. Initially, try to look at the film without considering the clinical setting (otherwise there is a tendency to miss obvious things which do not fit in with your differential diagnosis), then look again with the clinical setting in mind.

15. Remember to compare any chest film with an abnormality with any previous X-rays. Progression over time will often hold the key to the correct diagnosis.

This brief account only includes some common X-ray features of some common diagnoses. Get the X-rays formally reported by a radiologist urgently if you do not recognise a sign and the patient is unwell. Remember that all radiation exposures have to be justified by clinical benefit to comply with IR(ME)R (Ionising Radiation Medical Exposure) Regulations.

Abnormal chest X-ray appearances

Many chest X-ray appearances may be recognisable immediately as indicating a specific diagnosis but if not, classify an appearance into one of the leads on the following pages and then approach the lead systematically.

Abnormal chest X-ray appearances

Many chest X-ray appearances may be recognisable immediately as
indicating a specific diagnosis but if not, the appearances below are
considered in Chapter 14.

• Area of uniform opacification with a well defined border
• Rounded opacity (or opacities)
• Multiple 'nodular' shadows and 'miliary mottling'
• Diffuse, poorly defined hazy opacification
• Increased linear markings
• Dark lung/lungs
• Abnormal hilar shadowing
• Upper mediastinal widening
• Abnormal cardiac shadow

Writing out the examination findings

At the end of the history in the previous chapter the patient was thought to have:

- ?Viral pharyngitis
- ?Glandular fever
- ?Acute follicular tonsillitis
- ?Agranulocytosis due to carbimazole
- ??Meningococcal meningitis
- Inadequate domestic support currently for acute illness
- ??Undiscovered type 2 diabetes mellitus

The physical examination in such a patient would focus on findings that may occur in any of the possible diagnoses brought to mind by the history. If they are absent, this absence is specified, together with all positive findings. The positive and negative findings may be written out as follows.

Looks unwell, flushed.

Wt not recorded

Temperature 38.5°C

Bilaterally swollen tonsils, large red with small white patches

Bilateral tender multiple lymph node enlargement in neck. No lymph node swelling in axillae or groins

CVS

Pulse 110/min regular low volume

BP 100/60

Heart sounds normal

No murmurs

RS

Chest shape and movement normal

Breath sounds normal

AS

Not jaundiced

Liver 1 finger breadths below costal margin

Spleen not palpable

CNS

Conscious and alert

No neck stiffness

Hand and leg coordination normal

Reflexes all normal and symmetrical

Near patient tests

Some tests can be done quickly and are available before the clinical assessment has been written up or shortly afterwards. They can then be interpreted with the symptoms and physical signs. They might be added as follows.

Investigations

Urine testing: + glucose, no protein, no blood
ECG: Sinus tachycardia and normal complexes
Random BM glucose = 9mmol/L
CXR normal
FBC: Hb 12.4gr/dL
      WCC 18.3 × 10⁹/L, Neutrophils 90%
      No atypical lymphocytes present
Lab blood glucose 8.4mmol/L
Na 134, K 4.3, Urea 4.7, Creatinine 67mmol/L
Throat swab sent—result awaited
TSH, T4 sent

The problem list and positive finding summary

It is customary to summarise the history and examination by listing the positive findings or presenting them in a brief summary. This is how clinical problems are posed in journals and examinations. If negative findings are added, then they give an indication of what the writer was thinking. There is a place for this in a case presentation (as done previously) but the problem list or positive finding summary is a preliminary device.

Problem list

- Severe sore throat for 2 days
- Sweats for 2 days
- Severe malaise for 2 days
- Thyrotoxic 2 months ago (now on carbimazole)
- Lives alone in a flat
- Unwell, flushed
- Temperature 38.5°C
- *Bilaterally swollen tonsils, large red with small white patches*
- Bilateral tender multiple lymph node enlargement in neck.
- *Urine testing: + glycosuria*
- WCC 18.3 × 10^9/L, neutrophils 90%

A clear differential diagnosis may well have occurred to the writer by now (some were already being considered at the end of the history). If this were not the case, then the next step is to look at this problem list and consider which feature(s) will be associated with the shortest list of possible causes—the best 'leads'. These are shown in bold italics.

Looking up the lead

A glance at the following extract from p272 will suggest immediately that the patient probably has acute follicular tonsillitis, but this may be associated with agranulocytosis. The neutrophil cell count is an important deciding factor. It is high, which by definition excludes agranulocytosis and makes a viral infection and glandular fever unlikely (where there is usually a lymphocytosis). However, in some cases, no streptococcus is found on the swab culture leaving a question over the definitive diagnosis.

Red pharynx and tonsils

Some differential diagnoses and typical outline evidence

Viral tonsillitis	*Suggested by:* enlarged red mass(es) lateral to back of tongue without white patches.
	Confirmed by: clinical appearance, fever and ↓WBC and relative lymphocytosis.
Acute follicular tonsillitis complicated by quinsy, scarlet fever retropharyngeal abscess	*Suggested by:* enlarged red mass(es) lateral to back of tongue with small white patches ('strawberries and cream').
	Confirmed by: clinical appearance and fever (usually high). ↑↑ WBC. Bacterial culture of streptococcus.
Infectious mononucleosis (glandular fever) due to Epstein–Barr virus	*Suggested by:* very severe throat pain with enlarged tonsils covered with creamy or grey membrane. Petechiae on palate. Profound malaise. Generalised lymphadenopathy, splenomegally. Lymphocytosis.
	Confirmed by: Paul–Bunnel test positive. Viral titres.
Agranulo-cytosis (e.g. caused by carbimazole)	*Suggested by:* sore throat, background history of taking a drug or contact with noxious substance.
	Confirmed by: low or absent neutrophil count.
Meningococcal meningitis	*Suggested by:* sore throat, red fauces without purulent patches, neck stiffness and +ve Kernig's sign. High blood neutrophil count.
	Confirmed by: lumbar puncture showing pus or neutrophil count and organisms on microscopy or culture.

The working diagnoses

The white patches on red tonsils occurs commonly in acute follicular tonsillitis but less commonly in glandular fever or anything else, including viral pharyngitis, thus making other conditions improbable. Despite all this, it is still possible that there could be agranulocytosis due to carbimazole sensitivity. However, the raised leucocyte count with 90% neutrophils excludes this diagnosis because a low or absent WBC is obviously a necessary condition for the diagnosis of agranulocytosis. There is no need therefore to stop the carbimazole immediately.

The glycosuria and random blood sugar of 8.4mmol/L makes the diagnosis of diabetes mellitus probable. If the patient has no symptoms of diabetes and an active inter-current illness (as in this case) two fasting sugars greater than 7.0mmol/L would be needed to satisfy the WHO criteria so that the diagnosis would be acceptable to other doctors. This patient's diagnosis and care will be discussed again under 'Thinking about diagnosis' (see p656).

Look at the other positive findings and also consider if they would all resolve if the acute follicular tonsillitis resolved. Use commonsense, experience and imagination from your knowledge of physiology. The only remaining problems would be the glycosuria, prior thyrotoxicosis and living alone when very unwell.

The main *working diagnosis* therefore is:
• Acute follicular tonsillitis
The other diagnoses are
• Probable type II diabetes mellitus
• Controlled thyrotoxicosis
• Inadequate home care
The plan is
• Start
  · Penicillin V 500mg qds
  · Paracetamol 1g qds
• Continue
  · Carbimazole 5mg od
• Help patient to contact family

Cardiorespiratory symptoms

Chest pain—alarming and increasing over minutes to hours

This refers to chest pain that is not sharp and is not an easily recognised pattern by the patient (e.g. as predicable familiar angina). Ideally, the detailed history is taken where resuscitation facilities are available. Early non-specific ECG changes will suggest an acute coronary syndrome, a blanket term that includes angina or infarction (MI) but serial ECG or enzyme changes may be needed to distinguish between them.

- Normal troponin 12 hours after pain: probability of MI <0.3%.
- ↑ Troponin indicates episode of muscle necrosis up to 2 weeks before.
- ↑ ST segments indicate current ischaemia (or rarely ventricular aneurysm).

Some differential diagnoses and typical outline evidence

Angina (new or unstable)	*Suggested by:* central pain ± radiating to jaw and either arm (left usually). Intermittent, relieved by rest or nitrates and lasting less than 30 minutes.
	Confirmed by: no ↑ of **troponin** after 12 hours and no ↑ of ST segments on **ECG**.
	Management: OHCM p784.
ST elevated myocardial infarction (STEMI)	*Suggested by:* central chest pain ± radiating to jaw and either arm (left usually). Continuous, usually over 30 minutes, not relieved by rest or nitrates.
	Confirmed by: ST ↑1mm in limb leads or ↑2mm in chest leads on **serial ECGs** (this is regarded as sufficient evidence to treat with thrombolysis). ↑ **Troponin** indicates episode of muscle necrosis up to 2 weeks before.
	Management: OHCM pp120–4, 782.
Non-ST elevation myocardial infarction (NSTEMI)	*Suggested by:* central chest pain ± radiating to jaw and either arm (left usually). Continuous, usually over 30 minutes, not relieved by rest or nitrates.
	Confirmed by: elevated **troponins** after 12 hours. T wave and ST segment changes but no ST ↑ on **serial ECGs**.
	Management: OHCM pp120–4, 782.
Oesophagitis and oesophageal spasm	*Suggested by:* past episodes of pain when supine, after food. Relieved by antacids.
	Confirmed by: no ↑ of **troponins** after 12 hours and no ↑ of ST segments on **ECG**. Improvement with antacids. Oesophagitis on **endoscopy**.
	Management: OHCM p216.

Pulmonary embolus arising from leg deep vein thrombosis, silent pelvic vein thrombosis, right atrial thrombosis	*Suggested by:* central chest pain, also abrupt shortness of breath, cyanosis, tachycardia, loud second sound in pulmonary area, associated DVT or risk factors of silent DVT.
	Confirmed by: **V/Q scan** mismatch between ventilation and perfusion, **CT pulmonary angiogram** shows clot in artery.
	Management: OHCM pp96, 194, 802.
Pneumothorax	*Suggested by:* abrupt pain in centre or side of chest with abrupt breathlessness. Resonance to percussion over site.
	Confirmed by: **expiration CXR** showing dark field with loss of lung markings outside sharp line containing lung tissue.
	Management: OHCM pp194, 750, 798.
Dissecting thoracic aortic aneurysm	*Suggested by:* 'tearing' pain often radiating to back, abnormal or absent peripheral pulses, early diastolic murmur, low BP and wide mediastinum on *CXR*.
	Confirmed by: loss of single clear lumen on **CT scan** or **MRI**.
	Management: OHCM pp92, 480.
Chest wall pain e.g. Tietze's syndrome	*Suggested by:* chest pain and tenderness of chest wall on twisting of neck or thoracic cage.
	Confirmed by: no ↑ of **troponins** after 12 hours, no ↑ of **CK-MB** and no ↑ of ST segments or T wave changes serially on **ECG**. Response to rest and analgesics.
	Management: OHCM p736.

Chest pain—sharp and aggravated by breathing or movement

This is a common symptom that is experienced in mild or transient forms by many in the population and resolves with no cause being discovered. It frightens a patient into seeking advice when it is severe or accompanied by other symptoms, such as breathlessness, when a specific cause is more likely to be found.

Some differential diagnoses and typical outline evidence

Pleurisy due to pneumonia	*Suggested by:* being worse on inspiration, shallow breaths, pleural rub, evidence of infection (fever, cough, consolidation etc.).
	Confirmed by: opacification in lung periphery on CXR and sputum/blood culture.
	Management: OHCM pp173–6.
Pulmonary infarct due to embolus arising from DVT in leg, silent pelvic vein thrombosis, silent right atrial thrombosis	*Suggested by:* sudden shortness of breath, pleural rub, cyanosis, tachycardia, loud P2, associated DVT or risk factors such as recent surgery, childbirth, immobility, etc.
	Confirmed by: **V/Q scan** mismatch, **CT pulmonary angiogram** shows clot in artery.
	Management: OHCM pp194, 802.
Pneumothorax	*Suggested by:* pain in centre or side of chest with abrupt breathlessness. Diminished breath sounds resonance to percussion over site.
	Confirmed by: **expiration CXR** showing loss of lung markings outside sharp line.
	Management: OHCM pp194, 750, 798.
Pericarditis caused by MI, infection especially viral, malignancy, uraemia, connective tissue diseases	*Suggested by:* sharp pain worse lying flat or trunk movement, relieved by leaning forward. Pericardial rub.
	Confirmed by: **ECG:** concave ↑ST. **CXR** globular heart shadow and relief with pericardial drainage (if hypotensive).
	Management: OHCM pp158, 159.
Musculoskeletal injury or inflammation (often Borholm's disease—Cocksackie B infection)	*Suggested by:* associated focal tenderness. Often history of trauma.
	Confirmed by: excluding other explanations. Normal troponin.
	Management: OHCM pp156, 158, 720.

Chest wall pain e.g. Tietze's syndrome	*Suggested by:* chest pain and tenderness of chest wall on twisting of neck or thoracic cage.
	Confirmed by: no ↑ of **troponins** after 12 hours, no ↑ of **CK-MB** and no ↑ of ST segments or T wave changes serially on **ECG**. Response to rest and analgesics.
	Management: OHCM p736.
Referred cervical root pain	*Suggested by:* previous minor episodes exacerbation by neck movement (producing closure of nerve root foraminae related to area of pain).
	Confirmed by: clinical features and MRI scan.
	Management: OHCS p660.
Shingles	*Suggested by:* pain (often burning in nature) in a dermatomal distribution, recent exposure to chicken pox or previous shingles attacks.
	Confirmed by: vesicles appearing within days.
	Management: OHCM p568.

Severe lower chest or upper abdominal pain

Upper abdominal pain may also be difficult for the patient to separate from lower chest pain, so the causes of chest pain also have to be borne in mind.

Some differential diagnoses and typical outline evidence

Gastro-oesophageal reflux/gastritis	*Suggested by:* central or epigastric burning pain, onset over hours, dyspepsia, worse lying flat, worsened by food, alcohol, NSAIDs.
	Confirmed by: **OGD** showing inflamed mucosa.
	Management: OHCM pp215, 217.
Biliary colic	*Suggested by:* post-prandial chest pain, severe and 'griping' or colicky, usually in right upper quadrant and that can radiate to right scapula. Onset over hours.
	Confirmed by: **USS** showing gallstones and biliary dilatation and also on **ERCP**.
	Management: OHCM p484.
Pancreatitis (often due to gallstone impacted in common bile duct)	*Suggested by:* mid-epigastric pain radiating to back, associated with nausea and vomiting, gallstones. Onset over hours.
	Confirmed by: ↑*serum amylase* to 5 times normal.
	Management: OHCM p478.
Myocardial infarction (often inferior)	*Suggested by:* continuous pain, usually over 30 minutes, not relieved by rest or (anti-anginal) medication. Onset over minutes to hours.
	Confirmed by: T waves inversion ± ST ↑ of 1mm in limb leads or 2mm in chest leads on **serial ECGs** or ↑*CK-MB* or ↑*troponin*.
	Management: OHCM pp120–4, 782.

Sudden breathlessness, onset over seconds

This situation may be life-threatening; the severity of the underlying condition often creates helpful diagnostic information.

Some differential diagnoses and typical outline evidence

Pulmonary embolus arising from DVT in leg, pelvic vein or right atrium	*Suggested by:* central chest pain also with abrupt shortness of breath, cyanosis, tachycardia, loud second sound in pulmonary area, associated DVT or risk factors of silent DVT. PO_2 low, CO_2 normal or low.
	Confirmed by: **V/Q scan** ventilation/perfusion mismatch. **Spiral CT scan:** clot in artery, pulmonary angiogram shows filling defect (see above).
	Management: OHCM pp96, 194, 802.
Pneumothorax	*Suggested by:* pain in centre or side of chest with abrupt breathlessness. Resonance to percussion over same side especially lung apex.
	Confirmed by: **expiration CXR** showing loss of lung markings outside sharp line.
	Management: OHCM pp194, 750, 798.
Anaphylaxis	*Suggested by:* dramatic onset over minutes, history of prior allergen exposure, acute bronchospasm with wheeze and dyspnoea, flushing, sweating and a feeling of dread, facial oedema, urticaria and warm but clammy extremities. Tachycardia and hypotension.
	Confirmed by: clinical presentation and by controlled allergen exposure and examination. Response to adrenaline IM.
	Management: OHCM p780, OHCS p237.
Inhalation foreign body	*Suggested by:* history of putting an object in mouth e.g. peanut. Sudden stridor, severe cough, low pitched, monophonic wheeze.
	Confirmed by: relief in extremis by performing Heimlich manoeuvre etc. or if not in extremis, foreign body seen on **CXR/CT** or **bronchoscopy**.
	Management: OHCS p795.

Orthopnoea and paroxysmal nocturnal dyspnoea (PND)

Orthopnoea is shortness of breath when lying flat. (Try to confirm by observing what happens when patient lies flat.) This can be explained by oedema gathering along the posterior length of the lungs or less efficient lung movement when the abdominal contents press against the diaphragm. PND can happen when the patient slides down in bed at night or by bronchospasm due to night-time asthma.

Some differential diagnoses and typical outline evidence

Pulmonary oedema	*Suggested by:* displaced apex beat, 3rd heart sound, bilateral basal fine crackles.
due to congestive (chronic) left ventricular failure (due to ischaemic heart disease, mitral stenosis)	*Confirmed by:* **CXR** appearances. Impaired LV function on **echocardiogram**. Abnormal **ECG** reflecting underlying heart disease.
	Management: OHCM pp136–9.
COPD	*Suggested by:* dry cough/white sputum, wheeze. Smoking history of ≥10 pack-years. Chest hyperinflation, pursed lips. Reduced breath sounds, accessory muscles of respiration used. Reduced peak flow rate.
	Confirmed by: **CXR:** radiolucent lungs. **Spirometry:** <15% reversibility, reduced FEV$_1$ and FVC (also reduced FEV$_1$/FVC ratio), hypoxia ± ↑ arterial CO_2. ± Reduced *α-1 antitrypsin* levels.
	Management: OHCM pp188, 189, 796.
Asthma	*Suggested by:* wheeze or dry cough. Other specific triggers to breathlessness. Other allergies. Past history of similar attacks unless 1st presentation.
	Confirmed by: reduced **peak flows**, FEV$_1$ that improve >15% with treatment and symptomatic response to treatment.
	Management: OHCM pp184–6, 794.

Palpitations

Very subjective and non-specific unless forceful, fast and associated with dizziness or loss of consciousness.

Some differential diagnoses and typical outline evidence

Runs of SVT ?due to IHD	*Suggested by:* abrupt onset, sweats and dizziness.
	Confirmed by: baseline *ECG* or *24 hour ECG* showing premature normal QRS complexes with absent or abnormal P waves >140/min. *Exercise ECG* to see if precipitated by exercise (and due to IHD).
	Management: OHCM p128.
Episodic heart block	*Suggested by:* onset over minutes or hours, slow and forceful beats. Loss of consciousness, pallor if significant loss of cardiac output.
	Confirmed by: fixed or progressive prolonged PR interval, P–R dissociation and slow QRS rate on baseline or *24 hour ECG*.
	Management: OHCM p103.
Sinus tachycardia (multitude of causes, anxiety, caffeine, febrile illness, hypovolaemia, pulmonary embolism, hyper-ventilation, etc.)	*Suggested by:* gradual onset over minutes of regular palpitations and pulse. History of precipitating cause usually.
	Confirmed by: basal *ECG* and resolution by stopping precipitating factors or resolution of potential cause.
	Management: OHCM p96.
Atrial fibrillation	*Suggested by:* onset over seconds, irregularly irregular radial and apex pulse, apical–radial pulse deficit and variable BP.
	Confirmed by: *ECG* showing no P waves and irregularly irregular QRS complexes.
	Management: OHCM p130.
Ventricular ectopics unifocal (benign) or multifocal (may have underlying pathology)	*Suggested by:* history palpitations, noted over hours or days, associated anxiety.
	Confirmed by: premature wide QRS complexes on *baseline ECG* or *24 hour ECG*.
	Management: OHCM p132.

Menopause	*Suggested by:* sweats, mood changes, irregular or no more periods, getting worse over weeks or months.
	Confirmed by: ↓*serum oestrogen*, ↑*FSH/LH* and response to hormone replacement.
Thyrotoxicosis	*Suggested by:* anxiety, irritability, weight loss, sweating, loose frequent stools, lid retraction and lag, brisk reflexes. Onset over weeks or months.
	Confirmed by: ↑*FT4*, and/or ↑*FT3* and ↓*TSH*.
	Management: OHCM p304, *OHCS* p256.
Phaeochromocytoma (rare)	*Suggested by:* abrupt episodes of anxiety, fear, chest tightness, sweating, headaches, and marked rises in BP.
	Confirmed by: catecholamines *(VMA, HMMA)* or *free metadrenaline* ↑ in urine and blood soon after episode.
	Management: OHCM pp314, 822.

Acute breathlessness, wheeze ± cough

This symptom suggests airway narrowing due to a foreign body, spasm, inflammation or hydrostatic oedema.

Some differential diagnoses and typical outline evidence

Asthma	*Suggested by:* wheeze with exacerbations over hours (silent chest if very severe) and prolonged expiration. Anxiety, tachypnoea, tachycardia and use of accessory muscles. Usually known asthmatic.
	Confirmed by: reduced peak flows, FEV_1 that improve by >15% with treatment.
	Management: OHCM pp184–6, 794.
COPD	*Suggested by:* wheeze with exacerbations over hours to days often with pursed lips. Long history of cough, breathlessness and wheeze.
	Confirmed by: response to hydration and bronchodilators and in new doubtful cases by little reversibility on lung function (FEV_1 that improves by <15% with treatment).
	Management: OHCM pp188, 189, 796.
Acute viral or bacterial bronchitis	*Suggested by:* onset of wheeze over days. No dramatic progression. Fever, mucopurulent sputum, dyspnoea.
	Confirmed by: **sputum culture** and sensitivities, response to antibiotics (if bacterial).
	Management: OHCM pp188, 189, 796.
Acute left ventricular failure	*Suggested by:* onset over minutes or hours of breathlessness and wheeze, displaced tapping apex beat, 3rd heart sound, bilateral basal late fine inspiratory crackles and wheeze.
	Confirmed by: **CXR:** fluffy opacification greatest around the hilum, horizontal linear opacities peripherally, large heart. Impaired LV function on **echocardiogram**.
	Management: OHCM pp136–8, 786.
Anaphylaxis	*Suggested by:* dramatic onset over minutes, acute bronchospasm with wheeze and dyspnoea, flushing, sweating and a feeling of dread, facial oedema, urticaria and warm but clammy extremities. Tachycardia and hypotension.
	Confirmed by: clinical presentation and later by controlled allergen exposure and examination. Response to adrenaline IM.
	Management: OHCM p780, *OHCS* p237.

Cough and pink frothy sputum

This is due to a combination of frothy sputum of pulmonary oedema mixed with blood from haemoptysis.

Some differential diagnoses and typical outline evidence

Acute pulmonary oedema	*Suggested by:* onset over minutes or hours of short-ness of breath, orthopnoea, displaced apex, loud 3rd heart sound, fine crackles at lung base.

Acute pulmonary oedema — *Suggested by:* onset over minutes or hours of shortness of breath, orthopnoea, displaced apex, loud 3rd heart sound, fine crackles at lung base.

Confirmed by: CXR appearance (see p640) poor LV function on echocardiogram.

Management: OHCM pp136–8, 786.

Mitral stenosis — *Suggested by:* months or years of orthopnoea, mitral facies, tapping, displaced apex, loud 1st heart sound, diastolic murmur, fine crackles at lung base. Enlarged left atrial shadow (behind heart) and splayed carina on CXR.

Confirmed by: large left atrium and mitral stenosis on echocardiogram.

Management: OHCM p146.

Frank haemoptysis (or sputum streaking)

This may have a sinister causes that needs urgent diagnosis and treatment.

Some differential diagnoses and typical outline evidence

Acute viral or bacterial bronchitis	*Suggested by:* days of fever, mucopurulent sputum, dyspnoea.
	Confirmed by: **sputum culture** and sensitivities, response to appropriate antibiotics.
	Management: OHCM p188.
Pulmonary infarction due to embolus from DVT in leg, pelvis or right atrium	*Suggested by:* sudden shortness of breath, pleural rub, cyanosis, tachycardia, loud P2, associated DVT or risk factors such as recent surgery, childbirth, immobility, etc.
	Confirmed by: **V/Q scan** mismatch, **spiral CT scan** showing clot in artery, **pulmonary angiogram** showing filling defect.
	Management: OHCM pp194, 802.
Carcinoma of lung	*Suggested by:* weeks or months of weight loss, smoking history, new or worsening cough.
	Confirmed by: opacity on **CXR** and/or **CT**. Tumour cells on **sputum cytology** or on biopsy.
	Management: OHCM p182.
Pulmonary tuberculosis	*Suggested by:* weeks or months of fever, malaise, weight loss and a contact history. CXR: opacification especially in apical segments.
	Confirmed by: AFB on **smear sputum, culture** and or response to treatment (when cultures negative and no other explanation for symptoms).
	Management: OHCM pp564–6.
URTI abnormalities and bleeding e.g. nasal polyps, laryngeal carcinoma, pharyngeal tumours	*Suggested by:* days of purulent rhinorrhoea (blood from URTI swallowed or inhaled and coughed back up).
	Confirmed by: **nasendoscopy, CT/MRI,** surgery and biopsy.
	Management: OHCS p560.

Lung abscess	*Suggested by:* days or weeks of copious and foul smelling sputum, fevers, chest pain.
	Confirmed by: **CXR:** circular opacity with fluid level, **sputum culture**.
	Management: OHCM pp176, 618.
Bronchiectasis	*Suggested by:* months of cupful(s) of pus-like sputum per day. Coarse late inspiratory crepitations and finger clubbing.
	Confirmed by: **CXR:** cystic shadowing; **high resolution CT chest:** honeycombing and thickened dilated bronchi.
	Management: OHCM pp178,179.
Wegener's granulomatosis	*Suggested by:* months of cough, breathless, haematuria. Classic triad of URT, LRT and renal abnormalities. Multisystem vasculitis e.g. arthritis, myalgia, skin rashes and nasal bridge collapse.
	Confirmed by: ↑titres of **cANCA** antibody and microscopic arteritis on biopsy.
	Management: OHCM p738.
Goodpastures' syndrome (very rare)	*Suggested by:* profuse haemoptysis, months or years of ill health, renal failure, ↑BP and chest pain.
	Confirmed by: glomerular basement antibody on **renal biopsy**.
	Management: OHCM p724.
Pulmonary arteriovenous malformation	*Suggested by:* haemoptysis alone. No other symptoms. CXR normal.
	Confirmed by: vascular red-blue lesion on **bronchoscopy**, enhancing lesion **CT chest** with contrast, **pulmonary arteriogram**, also showing feeding blood vessels.

Cough with sputum

The majority of patients presenting with a productive cough will have a short history of days or weeks but many will have a background of a chronic cough.

Some differential diagnoses and typical outline evidence

Chronic bronchitis	*Suggested by:* grey sputum, slow progression over years and a smoker (nearly always).
	Confirmed by: grey sputum >3 months over two consecutive years.
	Management: OHCM p188.
Acute viral bronchitis	*Suggested by:* onset over hours or days. Fever, white/yellow sputum.
	Confirmed by: no consolidation on **CXR**, quick spontaneous resolution.
Acute bacterial bronchitis	*Suggested by:* onset over hours or days. Fever, mucopurulent sputum, dyspnoea.
	Confirmed by: **sputum culture** and sensitivities, response to appropriate antibiotics.
	Management: OHCM p188.
Pneumonia	*Suggested by:* onset over hours or days. Rusty brown sputum (i.e. purulent sputum tinged with blood). Sharp chest pain worse on inspiration, pleural rub, fever, cough, consolidation etc.
	Confirmed by: patchy shadowing on **CXR** and sputum/blood culture.
	Management: OHCM pp173–6.
Bronchiectasis	*Suggested by:* progression over months or years. Finger clubbing, cupful(s) of pus-like sputum per day. Coarse late inspiratory crepitations.
	Confirmed by: **CXR**: cystic shadowing; high resolution **CT chest**: honeycombing and thickened dilated bronchi.
	Management: OHCM pp178, 179.
Lung abscess	*Suggested by:* copious amount of foul smelling pus/brown sputum, haemoptysis, high swinging fever, chest pain over weeks, usually preceded by a prior significant respiratory infection (e.g. pneumonia).
	Confirmed by: fluid level in cavity on **CXR**, **CT chest**, response to physiotherapy, antibiotics and aspiration.
	Management: OHCM pp176, 618.

Persistent dry cough with no sputum

The duration of symptoms, severity and progression will affect the causes of a dry cough.

Some differential diagnoses and typical outline evidence

Viral infection with slow recovery	*Suggested by:* original onset over days, fever, sore throat, generalised aches.
	Confirmed by: natural history of spontaneous improvement.
Chronic asthma	*Suggested by:* progression or static over months or years. Worse at night/early am. Assoc. wheeze, exacerbations with exercise or atopic exposure.
	Confirmed by: spirometry (reduced **FEV₁**), PEFR chart—classical diurnal dipping and variability. >15% improvement in **spirometry** with treatment.
	Management: OHCM pp184–6.
COPD	*Suggested by:* chronic breathlessness, little variation, a history of smoking. Signs of hyperinflation, reduced breath sounds, hyper-resonance and poor chest expansion.
	Confirmed by: CXR showing generalised loss of lung markings and flat diaphragms. spirometry (reduced **FEV₁**). **Spirometry:** FEV₁<70% with <15% improvement with beta-agonists. ↓ α-1 antitrypsin levels in those with genetic component.
	Management: OHCM pp188–9.
Bronchogenic carcinoma	*Suggested by:* weight loss, chest pain, haemoptysis. Smoker. Opacity with irregular outline on **CXR** or **CT chest**.
	Confirmed by: tumour cells in sputum or on biopsy at **bronchoscopy**.
	Management: OHCM p182.
Tuberculosis	*Suggested by:* fever, malaise, weight loss, contact history.
	Confirmed by: **CXR**, AFB on smear, **culture of sputum** or biopsy or response to trial of therapy.
	Management: OHCM pp564–6.

Hoarseness

Hoarseness of some weeks' or months' duration may have some sinister causes that need urgent attention.

Some differential diagnoses and typical outline evidence

Laryngeal carcinoma	*Suggested by:* progressive hoarseness over weeks to months. Smoker, including cannabis. Dysphagia, haemoptysis, ear pain.
	Confirmed by: **laryngoscopy** and biopsy of glottic, supra-glottic or sub-glottic tumour and staging.
	Management: OHCS pp570–6.
Chronic laryngitis	*Suggested by:* onset over months or years. History of recurrent acute laryngitis.
	Confirmed by: inflamed cords at **laryngoscopy** and no other pathology.
	Management: OHCS p568.
Singer's nodes	*Suggested by:* onset over months. Long history often occupational in teachers or singers due to voice strain, singing, alcohol, fumes etc.
	Confirmed by: nodules on cord at **laryngoscopy**. Resolution with speech therapy or after **surgical removal**.
	Management: OHCS p568.
Functional hoarseness	*Suggested by:* recurrence at times of stress. Able to cough normally.
	Confirmed by: no other pathology at **laryngoscopy**.
	Management: OHCS p568.
Vocal cord paresis due to vagal nerve trauma, cancer (thyroid, oesophagus, pharynx, bronchus) or TB, MS, polio, syringomyelia, (no cause in 15%)	*Suggested by:* onset after surgery or otherwise over weeks and months. Bovine cough. Symptoms of cause.
	Confirmed by: paresis or abnormal movement of cords on **laryngoscopy** and **CXR, Barium swallow, MRI**.
	Management: OHCS p569.

Myxoedema	*Suggested by:* onset over months or years. Fatigue, puffy face, obesity cold intolerance, bradycardia, slow relaxing reflexes. *Confirmed by:* swollen vocal cords at **laryngoscopy**. ↑*TSH*, ↓*FT4*. *Management:* OHCM pp304, 306, 820 (Myx); pp291, 324 (Acromeg).
Acromegaly	*Suggested by:* swollen vocal cords at **laryngoscopy**. Large wide face, embossed forehead, jutting jaw (prognathism), widely spaced teeth and large tongue. *Confirmed by:* **IGF** ↑, failure to suppress GH to <2mU/L with **oral GTT**. **Skull X-ray** confirm bony abnormalities. **Hand X-ray** showing typical tufts on terminal phalanges. **MRI or CT scan**, showing enlarged pituitary fossa. *Management:* OHCM p324.
Sicca syndrome	*Suggested by:* onset over months to years. Dry mouth and eyes. *Confirmed by:* clinical presentation and inflamed cords at **laryngoscopy** and no other pathology. *Management:* OHCM pp426, 734.
Granulomas due to syphilis, TB, sarcoid, Wegener's	*Suggested by:* onset over months with symptoms and signs in other systems. *Confirmed by:* granulomata on cords at **laryngoscopy**. Biopsy of cord or other affected tissues. *Management:* OHCM pp199, 738.

Syncope

This is sudden loss of consciousness over seconds. Think of abnormal 'electrical' activity in the CNS or a temporary drop in cardiac output and BP that improves as soon as the patient is in a prone position. Fits can occur due to a profound fall in BP so they are not specific of epilepsy.

Some differential diagnoses and typical outline evidence

Vasovagal attack—simple faint	*Suggested by:* seconds or minutes of preceding emotion, pain, fear, or prolonged standing—with nausea, sweating and darkening of vision. Recovery within minutes. Incontinence rare.
	Confirmed by: history. No abnormal physical signs.
	Management: OHCM p344.
Postural hypotension often due to BP-lowering drugs, dehydration, anaemia or blood loss	*Suggested by:* sudden loss of consciousness after getting up from sitting or lying position.
	Confirmed by: Fall in BP from reclining to standing, confirmation of a causal diagnosis.
	Management: OHCM p80.
Stokes–Adams attack	*Suggested by:* sudden loss of consciousness with no warning. Pallor, then recovery within seconds or minutes.
	Confirmed by: **24 hour ECG** showing episodes of asystole or heart block, SVT or VT.
	Management: OHCM p344.
Aortic stenosis	*Suggested by:* syncope on exercise. Cool extremities, slow rising pulse, low BP and pulse pressure and heaving apex. Mid systolic murmur.
	Confirmed by: **ECG** (tall R waves and left axis deviation). **Echocardiogram** and **cardiac catheter:** stenosed valve.
	Management: OHCM p148.
Hypertrophic cardiomyopathy	*Suggested by:* syncope on exercise. FH of sudden death or HOCM. Angina, breathless, jerky pulse, high JVP with 'a' wave, double apex beat, thrill and murmur best at left sternal edge.
	Confirmed by: **echocardiogram** showing hypertrophied septum and ventricular walls with small ventricular cavities esp. on left.
	Management: OHCM p156.

Micturition syncope	*Suggested by:* sudden loss of consciousness after micturating, usually in a man at night. Often history of prostatism.
	Confirmed by: history and examination not indicative of associated condition.
	Management: OHCM p344.
Cough syncope	*Suggested by:* sudden loss of consciousness after severe bout of coughing.
	Confirmed by: history and examination not indicative of associated condition.
	Management: OHCM p344.
Carotid sinus syncope	*Suggested by:* sudden loss of consciousness after turning head e.g. while shaving.
	Confirmed by: history and onset of symptoms on careful repeat of movement.
	Management: OHCM p344.
Hypoglycaemia	*Suggested by:* preceded by seconds or minutes by hunger, sweating and darkening of vision. Usually in diabetic, usually on insulin.
	Confirmed by: **blood sugar** <2mmol/L and exclusion of associated cardiac condition.
	Management: OHCM p820.
Epilepsy (may be due to profound fall in BP)	*Suggested by:* preceding aura for few minutes then tonic phase with cyanosis, clonic jerks of limbs, incontinence of urine and or faeces.
	Confirmed by: history from witness. *EEG* changes e.g. 'spike and wave'.
	Management: OHCM pp370–80.

Leg pain on walking—intermittent claudication

This is analogous to the more familiar angina but pain comes on in the legs instead of the chest on exercise. Quantify the effect on daily activity (esp. distance walked) and ability to cope at home, work, recreation and rest.

Some differential diagnoses and typical outline evidence

Arterial disease in legs associated impotence = Leriche's syndrome	*Suggested by:* predictable leg, calf, thigh or buttock pain (worse on hills, better downhill) better with rest (if also present at rest, this implies incipient gangrene). Sleeps with leg hanging down e.g. over edge of bed or in chair. Abnormal pulses, poor perfusion of skin and toes.
	Confirmed by: **Doppler ultrasound** or **arteriogram** showing stenosis and poor flow.
	Management: OHCM p490.
Spinal claudication	*Suggested by:* weakness and pain in leg, calf, thigh or buttock and pain improving slowly with rest but variable. Worse downhill. No cold toes, normal pulses.
	Confirmed by: **MRI** showing canal stenosis or disc compression of cord or cauda equina.
	Management: OHCS p674.

Leg pain on standing—relieved by lying down

Think of something relieved by reducing 'pressure' on lying down. Two possibilities are relief of the pressure transmitted down to leg tissues by incompetent venous valves or relief of pressure by the spinal column on a damaged disc, aggravating its protrusion and pressure on adjacent nerve roots.

Some differential diagnoses and typical outline evidence

Peripheral venous disease and varicose veins	*Suggested by:* generalised ache, assoc. itching, varicose veins and venous eczema ± ulcers. Cough impulse felt and Trendelenberg test shows filling down along extent of communicating valve leaks.
	Confirmed by: clinical findings or **Doppler ultrasound** probe to confirm if incompetence is present or not in the sapheno-femoral junction or the short saphenous vein.
	Management: OHCM p528.
Disc protrusion ('slipped disc')	*Suggested by:* severe referred ache or shooting pains, affected by position. Neurological deficit in root distribution.
	Confirmed by: **MRI** sacral and dorsal spine showing disc impinging on nerve roots (but may be less obvious as patient lies down in scanner).
	Management: OHCM p410, *OHCS* p674.

Unilateral calf or leg swelling

Swelling is explained as fluid gathering in the extravascular space. Think of this possibly being due to ↑ pressure within the veins or lymphatic vessels. It can also be due to unilateral damage to the local small veins and capillaries due to local inflammation. Unilateral swelling thus implies local inflammation, damage or obstruction to a vein or lymphatic duct. The speed of onset allows one to imagine what process might be taking place—traumatic, thrombotic or infective.

Some differential diagnoses and typical outline evidence

Deep venous thrombosis	*Suggested by:* onset over hours, presence of risk factors e.g. obesity, immobility, carcinoma, contraceptive. Associated pulmonary embolus. Leg(s) firm, warm, tender.
	Confirmed by: poor flow on **Doppler ultrasound scan**, filling defect on **venogram**.
	Management: OHCM pp446, 456, 457.
Ruptured Baker's cyst (leaking synovial fluid, sometimes no cyst)	*Suggested by:* onset sudden over seconds e.g. when walking up a step. Usually known to have an arthritic knee.
	Confirmed by: normal flow on **Doppler ultrasound scan**, no filling defect on **venogram**. Leakage of contrast from joint capsule if **arthrogram** done soon after the event.
Cellulitis	*Suggested by:* firm, warm, tender erythema, tracking (red lines), fever, very tender over vein, ↑**WBC**, with onset over days.
	Confirmed by: skin swabs if discharge from skin, blood cultures, response to antibiotics.
	Management: OHCM pp298, 456, 486, 548.
Abnormal lymphatic drainage caused by lymphoma or malignant infiltration (or trypsomoniasis in tropics). Rarely a hereditary condition affecting young women.	*Suggested by:* onset over years, firm, non-tender non-pitting oedema of gradual onset over years.
	Confirmed by: obstruction to flow on **lymphangiogram**.
	Management: OHCM p730.
Congenital oedema (Milroy's syndrome)	*Suggested by:* presence since childhood.
	Confirmed by: history and **lymphangiogram**.
	Management: OHCM p730.

Bilateral ankle swelling

Think of ↑ pressure within the veins or lymphatic vessels or low albumin in the vascular space, bilateral damage to veins, lymphatics or capillaries due to local inflammation.

Some differential diagnoses and typical outline evidence

Right ventricular failure due to pulmonary hypertension or congestive cardiac failure	*Suggested by:* ↑JVP, liver enlargement and pulsation, RV heave. Onset over months usually.
	Confirmed by: dilated RV on **echocardiogram**.
	Management: OHCM pp136–9.
Poor venous return due to abdominal or pelvic masses, post-phlebitic or thrombotic venous damage	*Suggested by:* onset over months. Worse on prolonged standing or sitting, varicosities, venous eczema, pigmentation or ulceration. Non-pitting oedema if chronic.
	Confirmed by: clinically with Trendelenberg test showing filling along extent of communicating valve leaks or on venous **Doppler ultrasound**.
Low albumin states caused by liver failure, nephrotic syndrome, malnutrition, etc.	*Suggested by:* generalised oedema often including face after lying down. Onset usually over months.
	Confirmed by: low **serum albumin**.
	OHCD p694.
Bilateral cellulitis often associated with diabetes mellitus	*Suggested by:* warm, red and tender legs, thrombophlebitis and tracking, ulcers etc. Onset over days.
	Confirmed by: positive *blood cultures* (usually streptococcal or staphylococcal). (**Blood sugar** ↑ in diabetes.)
	Management: OHCM pp298, 456, 486, 548.
Inferior vena cava obstruction due to prolonged immobility, carcinoma, and oral combined contraceptive use)	*Suggested by:* bilateral leg swelling onset over hours, assoc. risk factors (obesity, smoker, FH). Symptoms of PE.
	Confirmed by: **CT abdomen**, low flow on **Doppler ultrasound scan** or filling defect on **venogram**.
	Management: OHCM p194.

Bilateral thromboses	*Suggested by:* onset over hours, risk factor of obesity, history of immobility, carcinoma, contraceptive. Assoc. PE. Leg(s) firm, warm, tender.
	Confirmed by: no flow on **Doppler ultrasound scan** or filling defect on **venogram**.
	Management: OHCM pp446, 456, 457.
Impaired lymphatic drainage	*Suggested by:* firm non-tender, non-pitting oedema of gradual onset over months to years.
	Confirmed by: obstruction to flow **lymphangiogram**.

GI **and** GU **symptoms**

Severe weight loss over weeks or months

The degree and speed of weight loss is relevant; the more severe, the more likely is it to be due to a demonstrable cause.

Some differential diagnoses and typical outline evidence

Any advanced malignancy	*Suggested by:* progressive onset over weeks or months of specific symptoms e.g. neurological deficit, haemoptysis, rectal bleeding, change of bowel habit, etc.
	Confirmed by: metastases on **CXR**, metastases on **ultrasound scan of liver** or leukaemic changes on **FBC** or tumour on **bronchoscopy**, or **GI endoscopy**, etc.
Depression	*Suggested by:* sleep disorders, poor concentration, social withdrawal, lack of interest in usual activities etc.
	Confirmed by: response to antidepressants. Psychotherapy.
	Management: OHCS pp336–41.
Thyrotoxicosis	*Suggested by:* heat intolerance, tremor, nervousness, palpitation, frequency of bowel movements, goitre, fine tremor, warm and moist palm.
	Confirmed by: **TSH↓, ↑FT4, ↑FT3.**
	Management: OHCM p304.
Uncontrolled diabetes mellitus	*Suggested by:* thirst, polydipsia, polyuria.
	Confirmed by: **Fasting blood glucose** ≥7.0 mmol/L (on two occasions) OR fasting, random or **GTT** glucose ≥ 11.1mmol/L once only in the presence of symptoms.
	Management: OHCM pp292–6.
Infection e.g. tuberculosis	*Suggested by:* night sweats, fever, malaise, cough.
	Confirmed by: **CXR** showing opacification of pneumonia and presence of **AFB in sputum** on microscopy and culture.
	Management: OHCM pp564–6.
Addison's disease	*Suggested by:* lethargy, weakness, dizziness, pigmentation (buccal, scar), hypotension.
	Confirmed by: 9 a.m. plasma cortisol ↓ and impaired response to short ACTH stimulation test (**short Synacthen test**).
	Management: OHCM p312.

Vomiting

Vomiting is not only a feature of GI disorders, but is also associated with a wide variety of local and systemic disorders. Therefore, more leads are needed. Ask about the amount, frequency and nature of vomitus—red blood, 'coffee-ground', timing of vomit i.e. in relation to meals, AND ask about weight loss, fever, headache and abdominal pain.

Try subdividing into:
- Vomiting *with* weight loss
- Vomiting *without* weight loss
- Vomiting *(within hours)* of food
- Vomiting unrelated to food but *with abdominal pain AND fever*
- Vomiting unrelated to food, *with abdominal pain but NO fever* (non-metabolic)
- Vomiting unrelated to food, *with abdominal pain but NO fever* (metabolic)
- Vomiting unrelated to food *without* abdominal pain *but with headaches*
- Vomiting *unrelated* to food and *without* abdominal pain or headaches

Vomiting with weight loss

Some differential diagnoses and typical outline evidence

Oesophageal carcinoma	*Suggested by:* dysphagia to solid food first, then semisolid and finally fluid.
	Confirmed by: **barium swallow** showing filling defect, **fibreoptic gastroscopy** with mucosal biopsy of visible tumour.
	Management: OHCM pp508, 718.
Gastric carcinoma	*Suggested by:* satiety after small meal.
	Confirmed by: **oesophagogastroscopy** showing and allowing biopsy of visible tumour, **barium meal** showing filling defect.
	Management: OHCM p508.
Achalasia	*Suggested by:* vomiting after large meals, undigested solid food and fluid, dysphagia to fluid, nocturnal regurgitation.
	Confirmed by: **barium swallow** demonstrating the absence of peristaltic contractions, **oesophagogastroscopy** showing dilatation.
	Management: OHCM p212.
Oesophageal stricture	*Suggested by:* undigested solid food and fluid in vomitus.
	Confirmed by: **barium swallow, oesophagogastroscopy** showing food residue and fixed narrowing.
	Management: OHCM p212.
Small intestinal tumour e.g. lymphoma	*Suggested by:* abdominal pain, anorexia.
	Confirmed by: **small bowel follow-through, CT abdomen, flexible enteroscopy with biopsy**.

Vomiting without weight loss

Some differential diagnoses and typical outline evidence

Pharyngeal pouch	*Suggested by:* no pain, regurgitation of undigested food.
	Confirmed by: **barium swallow** showing saccular opacification outside pharynx.
	Management: OHCS p572.
Achalasia	*Suggested by:* vomiting after large meals, undigested solid food and fluid, dysphagia to fluid, nocturnal regurgitation.
	Confirmed by: **barium swallow** demonstrating the absence of peristaltic contractions, **oesophagogastroscopy** showing dilatation.
	Management: OHCM p212, OHCS p572.
Oesophagitis and ulceration	*Suggested by:* retrosternal pain, heartburn, dyspepsia, 'waterbrash'.
	Confirmed by: **oesophagogastroscopy** showing inflammation and/or ulceration.
	Management: OHCM p216.

Vomiting shortly after food

Some differential diagnoses and typical outline evidence

Gastritis/peptic ulcer disease	*Suggested by:* epigastric pain, dull or burning discomfort, (gastric ulcer pain typically exacerbated by food and duodenal ulcer pain relieved by it), 'waterbrash'.
	Confirmed by: **oesophagogastroscopy, barium meal and pH study.**
Gastroparesis due to diabetes mellitus	*Suggested by:* intermittent vomiting, abdominal fullness or bloating, distended upper abdomen, succussion splash, history of diabetes.
	Confirmed by: **oesophagogastroscopy, double contrast barium meal** showing normal mucosa but dilatation.
Gastric outlet obstruction e.g. carcinoma, lymphoma, chronic scarring, congenital pyloric stenosis in newborn	*Suggested by:* intermittent vomiting, abdominal fullness or bloating, distended upper abdomen, succussion splash.
	Confirmed by: **oesophagogastroscopy, double contrast barium meal** shows structural abnormality.
Small intestinal tumour e.g. lymphoma	*Suggested by:* abdominal pain, anorexia, weight loss.
	Confirmed by: **small bowel barium meal and follow-through** showing filling defect, **CT abdomen** showing abnormal tumour in wall, **flexible enteroscopy** with biopsy showing abnormal histology.
Acute cholecystitis due to cholelithiasis	*Suggested by:* symptoms after fatty food with colicky abdominal pain.
	Confirmed by: ↑**serum amylase, ultrasound scan** of biliary tree/gallbladder.
	Management: OHCM pp484–5.
Acute pancreatitis	*Suggested by:* severe epigastric/central abdominal pain, jaundice, tachycardia, Cullen's sign (periumbilical discolouration) or Grey Turner's sign (discolouration at the flank).
	Confirmed by: ↑↑**serum amylase**, ↓Ca^{2+}.
	Management: OHCM p478.

Vomiting with abdominal pain and fever

The vomiting is usually unrelated to eating.

Some differential diagnoses and typical outline evidence

Gastroenteritis	*Suggested by:* diarrhoea, ↑bowel sounds.
	Confirmed by: **stools for WBC and culture**.
	Management: OHCM p556.
Food poisoning	*Suggested by:* associated with diarrhoea, eating companions affected.
	Confirmed by: **stools for WBC and culture, cultures of vomitus, food and blood**.
	Management: OHCM p556.
Urinary tract infection	*Suggested by:* dysuria, frequency, abnormal dipstix.
	Confirmed by: **MSU microscopy and culture**. (US scan for possible anatomical abnormality.)
	Management: OHCM p262.
Acute appendicitis, mesenteric adenitis	*Suggested by:* **RLQ** pain anorexia, low grade fever.
	Confirmed by: RLQ guarding or right sided rectal tenderness.
	Management: OHCM p476.
Hepatitis A or B	*Suggested by:* **RUQ** pain, jaundice.
	Confirmed by: ALT ↑↑ and bilirubin ↑, **hepatitis serology**.
	Management: OHCM p576.
Toxic shock syndrome	*Suggested by:* use of tampons, high fever, vomiting and profuse watery diarrhoea, confusion, skin rash, hypotension, myalgia.
	Confirmed by: **cultures of blood, stool, vaginal swab** for Staphylococcus and toxin. Thrombocytopenia on **FBC**. ↑**CPK**.
	Management: OHCM p590.
Pneumonia (lower lobe)	*Suggested by:* cough, dyspnoea, fever.
	Confirmed by: **CXR** shows consolidation. **Sputum and blood cultures**. **Serology** if atypical.
	Management: OHCM p172.
Pelvic inflammatory disease	*Suggested by:* lower abdominal pain, fever, vaginal discharge.
	Confirmed by: high vaginal swab, elevated **ESR** and **CRP**. **FBC**: leucocytosis, **pelvic ultrasound**, ± **laparoscopy**.
	Management: OHCS p286.

Haemolytic uraemic syndrome	*Suggested by:* haematuria, fever, confusion.
	Confirmed by: **FBC:** thrombocytopaenia, fragmented RBCs on **blood film**, renal failure on **U&E**.
	Management: OHCM p282.
Malaria	*Suggested by:* recent travel to malaria zone, periodic paroxysms of rigors, fever, sweating, nausea.
	Confirmed by: Plasmodium in **blood smear**.
	Management: OHCM pp560–2.

Vomiting with abdominal pain alone (unrelated to food and no fever)— non-metabolic causes

This is associated with a wide variety of GI and systemic disorders it is non-specific.

Some differential diagnoses and typical outline evidence

Large bowel obstruction e.g. malignancy, strangulated hernia	*Suggested by:* faecal vomiting, abdominal distension.
	Confirmed by: **AXR showing bowel dilation, barium enema, colonoscopy**.
	Management: OHCM p492.
Hepatic carcinoma, primary or secondary	*Suggested by:* RUQ pain and mass, jaundice.
	Confirmed by: **weight loss over weeks to months, ultrasound/CT of liver** showing hepatic mass.
	Management: OHCM pp242–3.
Mesenteric artery occlusion	*Suggested by:* periumbilical pain, diarrhoea, melaena.
	Confirmed by: **mesenteric angiography** showing filling defect.
	Management: OHCM p488.
Intussusception	*Suggested by:* child, usually between 6–18 months of life, acute onset of colicky intermittent abdominal pain, red currant 'jelly' PR bleed, ± a sausage shape mass in upper abdomen.
	Confirmed by: **barium enema**, may reduce with appropriate hydrostatic pressure.
	Management: OHCM p494.
Ectopic pregnancy, miscarriage	*Suggested by:* cramping pain, spotting, PV bleeding.
	Confirmed by: positive pregnancy test, **USS of pelvis**.
	Management: OHCS pp262–3.
Renal calculi	*Suggested by:* colicky loin pain, haematuria.
	Confirmed by: **plain abd X-ray, ultrasound, IVU**.
	Management: OHCM p264.
Acute inferior myocardial infarction	*Suggested by:* retrosternal chest pain, sweating, nausea.
	Confirmed by: ↑ST on **ECG**, ↑**cardiac enzymes** e.g. **CK-MB or troponin**.
	Management: OHCM pp120–4.

Congestive cardiac failure (and liver congestion)	*Suggested by:* dyspnoea, orthopnoea, PND, liver enlargement and tenderness, leg oedema.
	Confirmed by: **CXR and echocardiogram**.
	Management: OHCM pp136–9.

Vomiting with abdominal pain alone (unrelated to food and no fever)— metabolic causes

This is associated with a wide variety of GI and systemic disorders. It is non-specific.

Some differential diagnoses and typical outline evidence

Drugs overdose e.g. digoxin	*Suggested by:* drug history.
	Confirmed by: **serum drug levels**.
	Management: OHCM p830.
Diabetic ketoacidosis	*Suggested by:* polyuria, dehydration, ± Kussmaul respiration.
	Confirmed by: ↑**blood glucose, ↓pH, ketonuria** or **plasma bicarbonate** <15mmol/L.
	Management: OHCM p818.
Hypercalcaemia	*Suggested by:* lethargy, confusion, constipation, muscle weakness, polydipsia and polyuria.
	Confirmed by: ↑**serum Ca^{2+}**.
	Management: OHCM p696.
Acute intermittent-porphyria	*Suggested by:* family history, constipation, peripheral neuropathy, hypertension, psychoses, urine darkens on standing.
	Confirmed by: Elevated **urinary-aminolevulinic acid and porphobilinogen, plasma porphyrins**.
	Management: OHCM p708.
Lead poisoning	*Suggested by:* anorexia, personality changes, head-aches, metallic taste.
	Confirmed by: elevated whole **blood lead concentration** >2.4µmol/L.
	Management: OHCM pp210, 628.
Vitamin A intoxication	*Suggested by:* ↑intracranial pressure, headache, irritability.
	Confirmed by: symptoms and signs disappearing within 1–4 weeks after stopping vitamin A ingestion.

Phaeochromo-cytoma	*Suggested by:* headache, sweating, palpitations, pallor, nausea, hypertension (intermittent or persistent), tachycardia.
	Confirmed by: **24 hour urinary metanephrines ↑, serum catecholamines ↑ (adrenaline, noradrenaline), CT abdomen, MRI scan.**
	Management: OHCM pp314, 822.

Vomiting with headache alone (unrelated to food and no abdominal pain)

Some differential diagnoses and typical outline evidence

Migraine	*Suggested by:* throbbing headache with preceding visual auras or other transient sensory symptoms and 'trigger' factors e.g. pre-menstrual, stress, particular foods.
	Confirmed by: history, but if in doubt **MRI scan** to exclude anatomical abnormalities.
	Management: OHCM p342.
Raised intracranial pressure	*Suggested by:* being worse in morning, on coughing and leaning forward, papilloedema.
	Confirmed by: **CT scan head** showing flattening of sulci and darkening of brain tissue.
	Management: OHCM p816.
Meningitis (viral or bacterial)	*Suggested by:* photophobia, fever, neck stiffness.
	Confirmed by: **CT scan:** no signs of ↑intracranial. pressure and **LP:** ↑lymphocytes in viral, ↑neutrophils in bacterial with organisms on staining and culture.
	Management: OHCM pp370–1.
Haemorrhagic stroke	*Suggested by:* sudden onset of headache, hemiparesis, sparing of upper face, dysarthia ± dysphasia, extensor plantar response.
	Confirmed by: **CT brain scan:** high attenuation area representing haemorrhage.
	Management: OHCM pp354–8.
Severe hypertension	*Suggested by:* continuous throbbing headache (non-severe hypertension is usually asymptomatic) but headache ± visual disturbance in malignant hypertension.
	Confirmed by: **serial BP measurement:** usually >140mmHg diastolic and/or >240mmHg systolic.
	Management: OHCM pp140–2.
Epilepsy	*Suggested by:* aura, altered consciousness, abnormal movements.
	Confirmed by: **EEG** result: spikes and waves over focus.
	Management: OHCM p380.

Acute glaucoma	*Suggested by:* blurred vision, painful red eye, coloured haloes.
	Confirmed by: ↑**intraocular pressure** on measurement.
	Management: OHCM p430.
Addison's disease	*Suggested by:* lethargy, weakness, dizziness, pigmentation (buccal, scar), hypotension.
	Confirmed by: 9 a.m. plasma cortisol ↓ and impaired response to short ACTH stimulation test (**short Synacthen test**).
	Management: OHCM p312.

Vomiting alone (unrelated to food and without abdominal pain or headaches)

Some differential diagnoses and typical outline evidence

Gastroenteritis	*Suggested by:* diarrhoea, decreased bowel sounds.
	Confirmed by: **stools for WBC and culture**.
	Management: OHCM p556.
Sliding hiatus hernia	*Suggested by:* occasional chest pain precipitated by heavy meals, lying flat.
	Confirmed by: **barium meal** showing reflux.
	Management: OHCM p216.
Acute viral labyrinthitis	*Suggested by:* vertigo, nystagmus.
	Confirmed by: being self-limiting over days.
	Management: OHCM p346–7.
Ménière's disease	*Suggested by:* vertigo, tinnitus, deafness.
	Confirmed by: **audiometry**: sensory hearing loss.
	Management: OHCM p346, OHCS p554.
Pregnancy	*Suggested by:* being worse soon after waking, amenorrhoea.
	Confirmed by: pregnancy test +ve.
Anaphylaxis	*Suggested by:* bronchospasm, laryngeal oedema, flushing, urticaria, angioedema.
	Confirmed by: relief with antihistamines or steroids.
	Management: OHCM p780, OHCS p237.
Renal failure (CRF)	*Suggested by:* fatigue, pruritus, anorexia, nausea, 'lemon-tinge' skin.
	Confirmed by: **↑serum creatinine, ↓creatinine clearance**. If chronic CRF: Hb low, and small kidneys on **renal ultrasound**.
	Management: OHCM pp272–4.

Addison's disease	*Suggested by:* lethargy, weakness, dizziness, pigmentation (buccal, scar), hypotension.
	Confirmed by: 9 a.m. plasma cortisol low ↓ and impaired response to short ACTH stimulation test (**short Synacthen test**).
	Management: OHCM p312.
Drugs e.g. antibiotics, cytotoxics, any overdose, excessive alcohol ingestion etc.	*Suggested by:* history of drug ingestion.
	Confirmed by: response of symptoms to avoidance of drug.
Functional	*Suggested by:* vomiting during or soon after a meal ± other psychological disturbance and no symptoms and physical signs of organic disease.
	Confirmed by: response to psychotherapy.

Jaundice

This can be a symptom reported by the patient or a physical sign. It is confirmed by ↑bilirubin in the plasma. Yellow sclerae and skin usually becomes visible when serum bilirubin level is >35μmol/L, so urine tests may provide the first clue. First subdivide into the 5 leads below. Remember that haemolysis causes ↑urinary urobilinogen and ↓serum haptoglobin. Hepatic failure causes ↑serum unconjugated bilirubin but intrahepatic or extra hepatic biliary obstruction results in ↑serum conjugated bilirubin.

Some differential diagnoses and typical outline evidence

Carotinaemia	*Suggested by:* onset over months. Skin yellow with white sclerae, normal stools and normal urine. Diet rich in yellow vegetables/fruits).
	Confirmed by: no bilirubin, no *urobilinogen* in the urine and normal **serum bilirubin**. Normal *liver function tests*. Response to diet change.
'Pre-hepatic' jaundice due to haemolysis	*Suggested by:* jaundice and anaemia (the combination seen as 'lemon' or pale yellow). Normal dark stools and normal looking urine.
	Confirmed by: ↑ (unconjugated and thus insoluble) **serum bilirubin** but normal (conjugated and soluble) bilirubin and thus no ↑bilirubin in urine. ↑*urobilinogen in urine* and ↓*serum haptoglobin*. Normal liver function tests. ↑***Reticulocyte count, Hb↓***.
	Management: OHCM pp222–3.
'Hepatic' jaundice due to congenital enzyme defect	*Suggested by:* Normal looking stools and normal looking urine.
	Confirmed by: ↑**serum bilirubin** (unconjugated), but no (conjugated) bilirubin in urine. No *urobilinogen in urine* and *normal haptoglobin*. Normal *liver function tests*.
	Management: OHCM pp222–3.
'Hepatocellular' jaundice ('hepatic' with element of 'obstructive' jaundice)	*Suggested by:* onset of jaundice over days or weeks, stools pale or normal but *dark* urine.
	Confirmed by: ↑serum (conjugated) **bilirubin** and thus ↑**urine bilirubin**. Normal urine urobilinogen. Liver function tests all abnormal esp. ↑↑**ALT**.
	Management: OHCM pp222–3.

'Obstructive' jaundice	*Suggested by:* onset of jaundice over days or weeks with *pale* stools and *dark* urine. Bilirubin ↑ (i.e. conjugated and thus soluble) in urine.
	Confirmed by: ↑**serum conjugated bilirubin** and thus ↑ **urine bilirubin** but no ↑urobilinogen in urine. Markedly (↑↑) **alkaline phosphatase**, but less abnormal liver function tests and ↑γGT.
	Management: OHCM p484.

Pre-hepatic jaundice due to haemolysis

Suggested by: jaundice and anaemia (the combination often seen as 'lemon' or pale yellow). Normal dark stools and normal looking urine.

Confirmed by: ↑(unconjugated and thus insoluble) **serum bilirubin** but normal (conjugated and thus soluble) bilirubin and in turn no bilirubin in urine. Evidence of haemolysis as: ↑**urinary urobilinogen** and ↓**serum haptoglobin**. ↑**Reticulocyte count**. Normal **liver function tests, Hb↓**.

Some differential diagnoses and typical outline evidence

Hereditary haemolytic anaemia	*Suggested by:* family history, anaemia, splenomegaly, leg ulcers.
	Confirmed by: above evidence of haemolysis, ↑*osmotic fragility*; enzyme deficiency e.g. **G6PD, pyruvate kinase**.
	Management: OHCM pp624, 636, 638.
Acquired haemolytic anaemia	*Suggested by:* sudden onset, in later life, and on medication.
	Confirmed by: above evidence of haemolysis, **blood film**, +ve **Coombs' test** in autoimmune type.
	Management: OHCM pp624, 636, 638.
Septicaemic haemolysis due to pneumonia, UTI, etc	*Suggested by:* fever, ± shock symptoms and signs of infection.
	Confirmed by: evidence of haemolysis, **blood culture** positive.
	Management: OHCM pp624, 636, 638.
Malaria	*Suggested by:* recent travel to malaria zone, periodic paroxysms of rigors, fever, sweating, nausea.
	Confirmed by: Plasmodium in **blood smear**.
	Management: OHCM pp549, 560–3.

Hepatic jaundice due to congenital enzyme defect

Suggested by: jaundice. Normal looking stools and normal looking urine.

Confirmed by: ↑**serum bilirubin** (unconjugated), but no (conjugated) bilirubin in urine. No **urobilinogen in urine** and **normal haptoglobin**. Normal **liver function tests**.

Some differential diagnoses and typical outline evidence

Gilbert's syndrome (Normal lifespan)	*Suggested by:* above evidence of impaired conjugation, asymptomatic.
	Confirmed by: demonstration of unconjugated hyper-bilirubinaemia with normal *LFT*, no haemolysis. Rise in **bilirubin when fasting and after nicotinic acid**.
	Management: OHCM p724.
Crigler–Najjar syndrome (Type I: Severe, neonatal and often fatal Type II: Normal lifespan)	*Suggested by:* above evidence of impaired conjugation.
	Confirmed by: unconjugated hyperbilirubinaemia with otherwise normal *LFT*, no haemolysis. No rise in **bilirubin when fasting or after nicotinic acid**.
	Management: OHCM pp222, 720.

Hepatocellular jaundice (due to hepatitis or very severe liver failure)

Suggested by: onset of jaundice over days or weeks, stools and urine pale or dark but *dark* urine.

Confirmed by: ↑serum (conjugated) *bilirubin* and thus ↑*urine bilirubin*. Normal urine urobilinogen. Liver function tests all increasingly abnormal esp. ↑↑*ALT*.

Some differential diagnoses and typical outline evidence

Acute (viral) hepatitis A	*Suggested by:* tender hepatomegaly.
	Confirmed by: presence of **hepatitis A IgM antibody** suggests acute infection.
	Management: OHCM p576.
Acute hepatitis B	*Suggested by:* history of iv drug user, blood transfusion, needle punctures, tattoos, tender hepatomegaly.
	Confirmed by: presence of **HBsAg in serum**.
	Management: OHCM p576.
Acute hepatitis C	*Suggested by:* history of iv drug user, blood transfusion, tender hepatomegaly.
	Confirmed by: presence of **anti-HCV antibody, HCV-PCR**.
	Management: OHCM p576.
Alcoholic hepatitis	*Suggested by:* history of drinking, presence of spider naevi and other signs of chronic liver disease. *AST:ALT* ratio >2.
	Confirmed by: resolution with abstinence.
	Management: OHCM p223.
Drug-induced hepatitis e.g. paracetamol halothane	*Suggested by:* drug history, recent surgery.
	Confirmed by: drug levels improvement after stopping the offending drug.
	Management: OHCM p223.
Primary hepatoma	*Suggested by:* weight loss, abdominal pain, RUQ mass.
	Confirmed by: ultrasound/CT liver, liver biopsy, ↑alpha-fetoprotein.
	Management: OHCM pp242, 243.

Right heart failure	*Suggested by:* ↑*JVP*, hepatomegaly, ankle oedema.
	Confirmed by: **CXR:** large heart. **Echocardiogram:** dilated right ventricle.
	Management: OHCM pp136–9.
Glandular fever (infectious mononucleosis)	*Suggested by:* cervical lymphadenopathy, sharp edge, ± Splenomegaly, ± jaundice.
	Confirmed by: **Paul-Bunnell, +ve heterophil antibody** test.
	Management: OHCM p570.

Obstructive jaundice

Suggested by: jaundice with *pale* stools and *dark* urine. Bilirubin in urine (i.e. conjugated and thus soluble).

Confirmed by: ↑*serum conjugated bilirubin* and thus **urine bilirubin** but no ↑urobilinogen in urine. Markedly (↑↑) **alkaline phosphatase**, but less abnormal (↑) liver function tests and ↑γGT.

Management: OHCM p484.

Some differential diagnoses and typical outline evidence

Common bile duct stones	*Suggested by:* pain in RUQ ± Murphy's sign.
	Confirmed by: **ultrasound liver**: dilatation of biliary ducts.
	Management: OHCM pp484, 485.
Cancer of head of pancreas	*Suggested by:* progressive painless jaundice, palpable gall-bladder (*Courvoisier's law*), weight loss.
	Confirmed by: **ultrasound liver**: dilatation of biliary ducts. **CT pancreas, ERCP** or **MRCP**: obstruction within head of pancreas.
	Management: OHCM p248.
Sclerosing cholangitis	*Suggested by:* progressive fatigue, pruritus.
	Confirmed by: ↑**ALP. Ultrasound liver:** no gallstones. **ERCP:** (beading of the intra- and extra-hepatic biliary ducts).
	Management: OHCM p238.
Primary biliary cirrhosis	*Suggested by:* scratch marks, non-tender hepatomegaly, ± splenomegaly, xanthelasmata and xanthomas, arthralgia.
	Confirmed by: +ve **anti-mitochondrial antibody,** ↑↑**serum IgM**: infiltrate around hepatic bile ducts and cirrhosis on **liver biopsy**.
	Management: OHCM p238.
Drug-induced	*Suggested by:* drug history of oral contraceptive pill, phenothiazines, anabolic steroids, erythromycin, etc.
	Confirmed by: symptoms receding when drug discontinued.
	Management: OHCM p223.

Pregnancy (last trimester)	*Suggested by:* jaundice during pregnancy.
	Confirmed by: resolution following delivery.
	Management: OHCS p26.
Alcoholic hepatitis or cirrhosis	*Suggested by:* history of excess alcohol intake, presence of spider naevi and other signs of chronic liver disease.
	Confirmed by: **ultrasound** or CT **liver, liver biopsy**, improvement if abstinence.
	Management: OHCM p254.
Dubin–Johnson syndrome (decreased excretion of conjugated bilirubin, see OHCM p722)	*Suggested by:* intermittent jaundice, and associated pain in the right hypochondrium. No hepatomegaly.
	Confirmed by: normal **ALP**, normal **LFT**. ↑**urinary bilirubin**. Pigment granules on **liver biopsy**.

Dysphagia for solids which stick

The patient is often able to point to a specific point where the food sticks.

Some differential diagnoses and typical outline evidence

Oesophageal stricture	*Suggested by:* history of gastrooesophageal reflux, ingestion of corrosives, radiation or trauma.
	Confirmed by: **barium swallow and meal, fibreoptic endoscopy** show necrotic mucosa ± ulceration.
	Management: OHCS p572.
Carcinoma of oesophagus	*Suggested by:* progressive dysphagia, weight loss.
	Confirmed by: **barium swallow**, shows filling defect, **fibreoptic endoscopy** with biopsy of mass.
	Management: OHCM pp508, 718, OHCS p572.
Carcinoma of cardia of stomach	*Suggested by:* weight loss, epigastric pain, vomiting.
	Confirmed by: **barium swallow** shows filling defect, **fibreoptic endoscopy** with biopsy of mass.
	Management: OHCM pp508, 718.
External oesophageal compression	*Suggested by:* few other GI symptoms.
	Confirmed by: **barium swallow** shows filling defect, **endoscopy** shows normal mucosa, **CT thorax** shows extrinsic mass from retrosternal goitre, neoplasms (lung or mediastinal tumours, lymphoma); aortic aneurysm.

Dysphagia for solids (which do not stick) > fluids

It is important to distinguish from odynophagia—painful swallowing.

Some differential diagnoses and typical outline evidence

Pharyngeal pouch (pharyngo-oesophageal diverticulum)	*Suggested by:* regurgitation of undigested food, a sensation of a lump in the throat, halitosis, neck bulge on drinking, aspiration into lungs.
	Confirmed by: **barium swallow** shows extra luminal collection (oesophagoscopy avoided).
	Management: OHCS p564.
Xerostomia	*Suggested by:* dryness of mouth, elderly, especially females.
	Confirmed by: clinical appearance of atrophic, dry oral mucosa.
	Management: OHCM pp210, 734, *OHCS* p579.
Post-cricoid web congenital or Plummer–Vincent or Paterson–Kelly Syndrome	*Suggested by:* untreated severe iron deficiency anaemia.
	Confirmed by: **barium swallow** shows a thin, horizontal shelf; **endoscopy** to exclude malignancy.
	Management: OHCM p626, *OHCS* p570.
Globus pharyngeus	*Suggested by:* feeling of a lump in the throat which needs to be swallowed, may be associated with anxiety.
	Confirmed by: normal **barium swallow/endoscopy resolution** with reassurance and/or **psychotheraphy**.
	Management: OHCS p572.

Sore throat

With odynophagia—painful swallowing.

Some differential diagnoses and typical outline evidence

Viral pharyngitis	*Suggested by:* sore throat, pain on swallowing, fever, cervical lymphadenopathy and injected fauces. ↑ lymphocytes, leucocytes normal in WBC.
	Confirmed by: negative **throat swab** for bacterial culture, self-limiting: resolution within days.
Acute follicular tonsillitis (streptococcal)	*Suggested by:* severe sore throat, pain on swallowing, fever, enlarged tonsils with white patches (like strawberries and cream). Cervical lymphadenopathy especially in angle of jaw. Fever, ↑ leucocytes in WBC.
	Confirmed by: **throat swab** for culture and sensitivities of organisms.
	Management: OHCS p564.
Infectious mononucleosis (glandular fever) due to Epstein–Barr virus	*Suggested by:* very severe throat pain with enlarged tonsils covered with creamy membrane. Petechiae on palate. Profound malaise. Generalised lymphadenopathy, splenomegaly.
	Confirmed by: ↑ atypical lymphocytes in **WBC**. **Paul–Bunnel test** positive. **Viral titres**.
	Management: OHCM p570.
Candidiasis of buccal or oesophageal mucosa	*Suggested by:* painful dysphagia, white plaque, history of immunosuppression/diabetes/recent antibiotics.
	Confirmed by: **oesophagoscopy** showing erythema and plaques, **brush cytology ± biopsy** shows spores and hyphae.
	Management: OHCM p210.
Agranulocytosis	*Suggested by:* sore throat, background history of taking a drug or contact with noxious substance.
	Confirmed by: low or absent neutrophil count.
	Management: OHCM p662.
Meningococcal meningitis	*Suggested by:* headache, photophobia, vomiting, sore throat, red fauces without purulent patches, neck stiffness. High blood neutrophil count.
	Confirmed by: lumbar puncture showing pus or neutrophil count and organisms on microscopy or culture.
	Management: OHCM p370.

Dysphagia for fluids > solids

This implies that there is a neuromuscular as opposed to an obstructive cause.

Some differential diagnoses and typical outline evidence

Myasthenia gravis	*Suggested by:* difficult start to swallowing movement, cough (inhalation) precipitated by swallowing.
	Confirmed by: inhalation on **Gastrografin swallow**. Response to **Tensilon test, ↑anti-acetylcholine receptor antibody**.
	Management: OHCM p400.
Pseudobulbar palsy	*Suggested by:* nasal, 'Donald Duck'-like speech, small spastic tongue.
due to brain stem stroke, multiple sclerosis, motor neurone disease, etc.	*Confirmed by:* inhalation of **Gastrografin**, clinical features of brain stem stroke, multiple sclerosis, motor neurone disease, etc.
	Management: OHCM p394.
Bulbar palsy	*Suggested by:* nasal, quiet or hoarse speech, flaccid, fasciculating tongue.
	Confirmed by: clinical features of motor neurone disease/Guillain–Barré syndrome/brain stem tumour/syringobulbia/pontine demyelination.
	Management: OHCM p394.
Motor neurone disease	*Suggested by:* combination of upper and lower motor neurone signs.
	Confirmed by: **EMG** and **nerve conduction studies**.
	Management: OHCM p331.
Achalasia (progressive)	*Suggested by:* dysphagia with almost every meal, regurgitation (postural and effortless, contains undigested food).
	Confirmed by: **barium swallow, oesophageal manometry, oesophagoscopy** demonstrate absence of progressive peristalsis.
	Management: OHCM p212.
Diffuse oesophageal spasm (intermittent)	*Suggested by:* intermittent crushing retrosternal pain.
	Confirmed by: **barium swallow**—sometimes 'corkscrew oesophagus', **oesophageal manometry** show abnormal pressure profiles.
	Management: OHCM p212.

Scleroderma

Suggested by: reflux symptoms: cough and inhalation of fluids, tight skin, hooked nose, mouth rugae.

Confirmed by: **barium swallow**—diminished or absent peristalsis, **oesophageal manometry**—subnormal or absent lower oesophageal sphincter tone.

Management: OHCM p420.

Acute pain in the upper abdomen

Trying to localise pain in the upper abdomen to the right, left or middle may be difficult for the patient.

Some differential diagnoses and typical outline evidence

Oesophagitis	*Suggested by:* retrosternal pain, heartburn.
	Confirmed by: **oesophagogastroscopy**.
	Management: OHCM p216.
Acute coronary syndrome (unstable angina or infarction)	*Suggested by:* chest tightness or pain on exertion.
	Confirmed by: **exercise ECG ± coronary angiography** if troponin normal, or later if troponin ↑.
	Management: OHCM pp120–4, 782.
Hiatus hernia	*Suggested by:* heartburn, worsens with stooping or lying, relieved by antacids.
	Confirmed by: **oesophagogastroscopy, barium meal**.
	Management: OHCM p532.
Gastritis	*Suggested by:* epigastric pain, dull or burning discomfort, nocturnal pain
	Confirmed by: **oesophagogastroscopy, barium meal and pH study**.
	Management: OHCM p214.
Gallstone colic (with no acute inflammation or infection)	*Suggested by:* jaundice, biliary colic, pain in epigastrium or RUQ radiating to right lower scapula. No fever or ↑WBC.
	Confirmed by: **ultrasound of gallbladder and biliary ducts**.
	Management: OHCM pp484, 485.
Acute cholecystitis	*Suggested by:* fever, guarding and positive Murphy's sign (abrupt stopping of inspiration when the palpating hand meets the inflamed gall bladder descending with the liver from behind the sub-costal margin on the right side—but not on the left side). ↑WBC.
	Confirmed by: **ultrasound gallbladder and biliary ducts**.
	Management: OHCM p484.

Duodenal ulcer	*Suggested by:* epigastric pain, dull or burning discomfort, typically relieved by food, nocturnal pain.
	Confirmed by: **oesophagogastroscopy, barium meal and pH study:** (*Helicobacter pylori* often present in mucosa or serology).
	Management: OHCM p214.
Gastric ulcer	*Suggested by:* epigastric pain, dull or burning discomfort, typically exacerbated by food, nocturnal pain.
	Confirmed by: **oesophagogastroscopy, barium meal and pH study**.
	Management: OHCM p214.
Gastric carcinoma	*Suggested by:* marked anorexia, fullness, pain, Troisier's sign (a 'Virchow's' node i.e. large lymph node in the left supraclavicular fossa).
	Confirmed by: **upper GI endoscopy with biopsy**.
	Management: OHCM p508.
Pancreatitis	*Suggested by:* pain radiating straight through to the back, better on sitting up or leaning forward.
	Confirmed by: **↑serum amylase, CT pancreas**.
	Management: OHCD p478.

Acute central abdominal pain

Some differential diagnoses and typical outline evidence

Small bowel obstruction	*Suggested by:* vomiting, constipation with complete obstruction.
	Confirmed by: **AXR** shows small bowel loops and fluid levels.
	Management: OHCM p492.
Crohn's disease	*Suggested by:* chronic diarrhoea with abdominal pain, weight loss, palpable RLQ mass or fullness, mouth ulcers.
	Confirmed by: **colonoscopy with biopsy, barium studies** showing 'skip lesions', string sign in advanced cases.
	Management: OHCM p246.
Mesenteric artery occlusion	*Suggested by:* vomiting, bowel urgency, melaena, diarrhoea.
	Confirmed by: **mesenteric angiography, exploratory laparotomy**.
	Management: OHCM p488.
Abdominal aortic dissection	*Suggested by:* tearing pain ± shock ± hypotension and peripheral cyanosis.
	Confirmed by: **ultrasound or CT abdomen**.
	Management: OHCM p480.

Acute lateral abdominal pain

Some differential diagnoses and typical outline evidence

Pyelonephritis	*Suggested by:* pain in loin (upper lateral), rigors, fever, vomiting, frequency of micturition, renal angle tenderness
	Confirmed by: **FBC:** leucocytosis. **MSU:** pyuria, urine culture and sensitivities.
	Management: OHCM pp258, 262, 276.
Renal calculus	*Suggested by:* renal colic mainly in loin (upper lateral), haematuria.
	Confirmed by: **urinalysis, renal ultrasound, IVU, CT/MRI.**
	Management: OHCM p264.
Ureteric calculus	*Suggested by:* renal colic, moving from loin (upper lateral) down to *RLQ*, haematuria.
	Confirmed by: **urinalysis, renal ultrasound, IVU, CT/MRI.**
	Management: OHCM p264.
Appendicitis	*Suggested by:* pain initially central, then radiating to *right* lower quadrant, anorexia, low grade fever, constipation. *RLQ* tenderness and guarding.
	Confirmed by: Inflamed appendix at laparotomy
	Management: OHCM p476.
Salpingitis	*Suggested by:* fever, nausea, vomiting, muco-purulent cervical discharge, irregular menses. Bilateral lower abdominal tenderness and guarding.
	Confirmed by: **FBC:** leucocytosis. **High vaginal swab, laparoscopy.**

Acute lower central (hypogastric) abdominal pain

Some differential diagnoses and typical outline evidence

Infective or ulcerative colitis	*Suggested by:* abdominal pain, diarrhoea with blood and mucus.
	Confirmed by: **stool microscopy and culture, colonoscopy**.
	Management: OHCM pp218–19, 244–5.
Large bowel obstruction	*Suggested by:* severe distension, late vomiting, visible peristalsis, resonant percussion, increased bowel sounds. Supine **AXR** showing peripheral abdominal large bowel shadow (with haustra partly crossing the lumen). Fluid levels on erect film.
	Confirmed by: **abdominal ultrasound and laparotomy findings**.
	Management: OHCM p492.
Cystitis	*Suggested by:* frequency, urgency, dysuria, ± haematuria.
	Confirmed by: **MSU** for microscopy and culture.
	Management: OHCS p262.
Pelvic inflammatory disease	*Suggested by:* vaginal discharge, dysuria, dyspareunia, pelvic tenderness on moving cervix, ↑ ESR and CRP. WBC: leucocytosis.
	Confirmed by: **High vaginal swab, pelvic ultrasound, ± laparoscopy**.
	Management: OHCS p286.
Pelvic endometriosis	*Suggested by:* dysmenorrhoea, ovulation pain, dyspareunia, infertility, pelvic mass.
	Confirmed by: **laparoscopy**.
	Management: OHCS p288.
Ectopic pregnancy	*Suggested by:* constant unilateral pain ± referred shoulder pain, amenorrhoea, vaginal bleeding (usually less than normal period), faintness with an acute rupture.
	Confirmed by: pregnancy test +ve, bimanual examination reveals slightly enlarged uterus, **pelvic ultrasound** shows empty uterus with thickened decidua.
	Management: OHCS p262–3.

Sudden diarrhoea, fever and vomiting

Sudden diarrhoea with fever, ± malaise, colicky abdominal pain, vomiting.

Some differential diagnoses and typical outline evidence

Antibiotic induced bacterial opportunist: **Clostridium difficile**	*Suggested by:* diarrhoea with a history of recent antibiotic therapy, ↑ WBC. *Confirmed by: Cl. difficile* toxin in *stool culture*. *Management: OHCM* pp218, 219.
Viral gastroenteritis: **Rotavirus**	*Suggested by:* diarrhoea in children <5 years, symptoms resolve in a week. *Management: OHCM* p540.
Norwalk virus	*Suggested by:* diarrhoea in older children and adults, symptoms resolve in 2 weeks.
Food poisoning/ toxins **Staphylococcus aureus**	*Suggested by:* eating 'doubtful' meat, incubation period <6 hours, marked vomiting. *Confirmed by:* isolation of Staph. aureus from ***examination of suspected food***. *Management: OHCM* p556.
Bacillus cereus	*Suggested by:* eating 'doubtful' rice, incubation period <6 hours, marked vomiting. *Confirmed by: **stool microscopy** and culture. *Management: OHCM* pp556, 221.
Vibrio para haemolyticus	*Suggested by:* 'doubtful' seafood, incubation period 16–72 hours. *Confirmed by: **stool microscopy and culture***. *Management: OHCM* pp596, 621.
Clostridium perfringens	*Suggested by:* eating 'doubtful' meat, incubation period 8–16 hours, abdominal cramps, little vomiting. *Confirmed by:* organism ***isolation from faeces or suspected food***.

Botulism	*Suggested by:* eating 'doubtful' canned food, incubation period 18–36 hours, but may vary from 4 hours to 8 days, abdominal cramps, dry mouth, diplopia, progressive paralysis.
	Confirmed by: C. botulinum **toxin in serum or faeces;** *C. botulinum* toxin **isolation from suspected food.**
	Management: OHCM pp591, 830.
Salmonella typhimurium	*Suggested by:* eating 'doubtful' meat, egg, poultry. Fever (with relative bradycardia), headache, dry cough.
	Confirmed by: **stool microscopy and culture.**
	Management: OHCM p596.

Recurrent diarrhoea with blood ± mucus—bloody flux

Recurrent diarrhoea with blood-stained stools ± mucus or fever.

Some differential diagnoses and typical outline evidence

Crohn's disease	*Suggested by:* chronic diarrhoea with abdominal pain, weight loss, RLQ mass or fullness, mouth ulcers.
	Confirmed by: **colonoscopy with biopsy, barium studies** showing 'skip lesions', string sign (in advanced cases).
	Management: OHCM p246.
Ulcerative colitis	*Suggested by:* lower abdominal cramps, ↑urgency to defaecate, severe diarrhoea, ↑fever in acute attack. **FBC** showing ↑WBC, U&E; ↑urea and creatinine in dehydration.
	Confirmed by: **colonoscopy with biopsy, barium studies** show loss of haustration, mucosal oedema, ulceration.
	Management: OHCM p244.
Colonic carcinoma	*Suggested by:* alternate diarrhoea and constipation.
	Confirmed by: **barium enema** showing filling defect, **colonoscopy with biopsy** shows mass and malignant histology.
	Management: OHCM pp506, 507.
Colorectal carcinoma	*Suggested by:* sensation of incomplete evacuation.
	Confirmed by: **sigmoidoscopy with biopsy** showing mass and malignant histology, **barium enema** shows filling defect.
Diverticular disease/ diverticulitis	*Suggested by:* middle-aged or elderly, diarrhoea, LIF pain, abdominal and rectal mass.
	Confirmed by: **barium enema** showing opaque filling diverticula, **colonoscopy** showing inflammatory foci.

Acute bloody diarrhoea ± mucus— 'dysentery'

Some differential diagnoses and typical outline evidence

Shigella (bacillary) dysentery	*Suggested by:* blood and mucus, fever, abdominal pain.
	Confirmed by: **stool microscopy** revealing red cells, pus cells and appearance of organism.
	Management: OHCM p596.
Campylobacter enteritis	*Suggested by:* associated severe abdominal pain.
	Confirmed by: **stool microscopy** and **culture** of organism.
	Management: OHCM p556.
Enteroinvasive *Escherichia coli*	*Suggested by:* fever, watery diarrhoea.
	Confirmed by: **stool microscopy** and **culture** of organism.
	Management: OHCM pp218, 556.
Enterohaemorrhagic type 0157 *E. coli*	*Suggested by:* bloody diarrhoea ± haemolytic-uraemic syndrome.
	Confirmed by: **stool microscopy and culture** of organism.
	Management: OHCM pp282, 556.
Entamoeba histolytica (amoebic) dysentery	*Suggested by:* abdominal discomfort, flatulence, frequent watery, bloody diarrhoea.
	Confirmed by: **stool microscopy** and **culture** of organism.
	Management: OHCM p606.
First episode of cause of recurrent 'bloody flux' (see p148)	*Suggested by:* no specific features.
	Confirmed by: **barium enema** and **colonoscopy** showing evidence chronic cause after acute episode.

Watery diarrhoea

Note that diarrhoea can result in severe dehydration.

Some differential diagnoses and typical outline evidence

Traveller's diarrhoea	*Suggested by:* recent travel, no obvious ingestion of contaminated water or food.
	Confirmed by: rapid resolution or response to ciprofloxacin.
	Management: OHCM pp541, 554.
Enterotoxigenic *E. coli* (commonest)	*Suggested by:* incubation period 12–72 hours in relation to contact to others with similar features.
	Confirmed by: **stool microscopy and culture**.
	Management: OHCM pp218, 556.
Vibrio cholera	*Suggested by:* incubation period from a few hours to 5 days, profuse watery diarrhoea, fever, vomiting.
	Confirmed by: **stool microscopy and culture**.
	Management: OHCM p596.
Rotavirus	*Suggested by:* diarrhoea in children <5 years and symptoms resolve in a week.
	Management: OHCM pp540–1.
Norwalk virus	*Suggested by:* diarrhoea in older children and adults and symptoms resolve in 2 weeks.

Recurrent diarrhoea with no blood in the stools, no fever

Some differential diagnoses and typical outline evidence

Irritable bowel syndrome	*Suggested by:* no weight loss, intermittent daytime diarrhoea, pain relieved by defaecation, abdominal distension, mucus but no blood in the stool.
	Confirmed by: normal **colonoscopy and barium studies**.
	Management: OHCM p249.
HIV infection	*Suggested by:* weight loss, other opportunistic infection, lympadenopathy, Kaposi's sarcoma.
	Confirmed by: **HIV serology, stool microscopy and cultures** showing *Cryptosporidium*, microsporidia, *Isospora belli*, enteropathy, etc.
	Management: OHCM p580.
Malabsorption due to coeliac disease, lactose intolerance, pancreatic disease, Whipple's disease	*Suggested by:* pale, bulky offensive stools, weight loss, signs of nutritional deficiencies.
	Confirmed by: **coeliac screen, small bowel biopsy; or lactose tolerance test; intestinal biopsy** shows foamy macrophages containing PAS positive glycoprotein in Whipple's.
	Management: OHCM p252.
Drug-induced	*Suggested by:* history of laxative abuse, magnesium alkalis, antibiotics, hypotensive agents, alcohol.
	Confirmed by: resolution on withdrawing drug.
Faecal impaction with overflow	*Suggested by:* elderly patient and hard faeces on rectal examination.
	Confirmed by: **AXR** may show faecal impaction. Response to suppositories/removal of faeces.
Diabetic autonomic neuropathy	*Suggested by:* intermittent diarrhoea, postural hypotension, impotence, urinary retention, history of diabetes.
	Confirmed by: lying and standing BP, loss of **beat to beat variation** during slow deep breathing.
Thyrotoxicosis	*Suggested by:* heat intolerance, tremor, nervousness, palpitation, frequent bowel movements, goitre.
	Confirmed by: ↓↓**TSH**, ↑**FT4** or ↑**FT3**.
	Management: OHCM p304.
Carcinoid syndrome	*Suggested by:* facial flushing ± wheeze, abdominal pain
	Confirmed by: ↑24 hour **urinary 5-HIAA**.
	Management: OHCM p250.

Change in bowel habit

This may be an increase in constipation or diarrhoea or both alternating.

Some differential diagnoses and typical outline evidence

Colonic carcinoma	*Suggested by:* alternate diarrhoea and constipation, anaemia or weight loss.
	Confirmed by: **colonoscopy with biopsy, barium enema**.
	Management: OHCM pp506, 507.
Change in diet	*Suggested by:* history of ↓diet fibre, ↓fluid intake.
	Confirmed by: normal **endoscopy** and response to diet change.
Drug-induced	*Suggested by:* constipating drugs (opioids, hypotensive agents, aluminium alkalis etc.), purgative dependence.
	Confirmed by: normal **endoscopy** and response to withdrawal of suspected agent.
Depression	*Suggested by:* sleep disorders, social withdrawal, lack of interest in usual activities etc.
	Confirmed by: normal **endoscopy** and response to lifting of depression.
	Management: OHCM pp336, 340.
Immobility	*Suggested by:* history.
	Confirmed by: normal **endoscopy** and history.
Cerebral or spinal cord lesion	*Suggested by:* neurological symptoms and signs ± abnormal sphincter tone and anal sensation.
	Confirmed by: **CT or MRI**.
	Management: OHCM p350.
Metabolic disturbances: hypothyroidism, hyperthyroidism, hypercalcaemia, hypokalaemia	*Suggested by:* symptoms of metabolic disturbance or absence of anatomical abnormality.
	Confirmed by: **TFT, serum calcium, potassium**, etc.
	Management: OHCM pp306, 692, 696.

Haematemesis ± melaena

Vomiting of bright red blood and/or passage of black tarry motions. This implies bleeding usually from the upper GI tract: oesophagus, stomach and duodenum.

Some differential diagnoses and typical outline evidence

Bleeding duodenal ulcer	*Suggested by:* epigastric pain and tenderness, nausea.
	Confirmed by: **oesophagogastroscopy** showing bleeding ulcer.
	Management: OHCM p214.
Gastric erosion	*Suggested by:* history of NSAIDs or alcohol ingestion, epigastric pain, dull or burning discomfort, nocturnal pain.
	Confirmed by: appearance of erosion on **oesophagogastroscopy** and **pH study** showing hyperacidity.
	Management: OHCM pp214, 216.
Gastric ulcer	*Suggested by:* epigastric pain, dull or burning discomfort, nocturnal pain.
	Confirmed by: appearance of ulcer on **oesophagogastroscopy** and **pH study** showing hyperacidity.
	Management: OHCM p214.
Mallory–Weiss tear	*Suggested by:* preceding marked vomiting, later bright red blood.
	Confirmed by: **oesophagogastroscopy** showing tear.
	Management: OHCM p728.
Gastro-oesophageal reflux	*Suggested by:* heartburn worse when lying flat, anorexia, nausea, ± regurgitation of gastric content.
	Confirmed by: appearance of erosion on **oesophagoscopy, barium meal** and **pH study** showing hyperacidity.
	Management: OHCM pp216, 217.
Hiatus hernia	*Suggested by:* heartburn, worse with stooping, relieved by antacids.
	Confirmed by: herniation of stomach into chest on plain (X-ray or Ba meal), appearance of erosion on **oesophagoscopy** and **pH study** showing hyperacidity.
	Management: OHCM p532.

False haematemesis	*Suggested by:* swallowed nose bleed or haemoptysis.
	Confirmed by: normal **oesophagogastroscopy** and **bleeding** source identified in nose.
Oesophageal carcinoma	*Suggested by:* progressive dysphagia with solids, which sticks, weight loss.
	Confirmed by: **barium swallow, fibreoptic gastroscopy with mucosal biopsy** showing malignant tissue.
	Management: OHCM pp508, 718.
Gastric carcinoma	*Suggested by:* marked anorexia, fullness, pain, Troissier's sign (enlarged left supraclavicular lymph (Virchow's) node).
	Confirmed by: **oesophagogastroscopy with biopsy** showing malignant tissue.
	Management: OHCM p508.
Ingestion of corrosives	*Suggested by:* history of ingestion etc.
	Confirmed by: **oesophagogastroscopy** showing severe erosions.
Oesophageal varices	*Suggested by:* liver cirrhosis, splenomegaly, prominent upper abdominal veins.
	Confirmed by: **oesophagogastroscopy** showing varicose mucosa and blood distally and in stomach.
	Management: OHCM p226.
Meckel's diverticulum	*Suggested by:* no haematemesis, usually asymptomatic, anaemia, rectal bleeding.
	Confirmed by: **technetium-labelled red blood cell scan**, showing isotopes in gut lumen and laparotomy.
	Management: OHCM p246.
Other causes: angiodysplasia, bleeding disorders	

Passage of blood per rectum

May only be discovered on rectal examination.

Some differential diagnoses and typical outline evidence

Bleeding haemorrhoids	*Suggested by:* pain, discharge, pruritus, staining of toilet paper following defaecation.
	Confirmed by: physical and digital rectal examination, proctoscopy.
	Management: OHCM pp458, 522.
Anal fissure	*Suggested by:* skin tag, pain on defaecation, staining of toilet paper following defaecation, exquisite anal tenderness.
	Confirmed by: history and clinical examination.
	Management: OHCM p520.
Diverticulitis	*Suggested by:* bloody 'splash in the pan', abdominal pain, usually LIF, diarrhoea and constipation.
	Confirmed by: **colonoscopy, barium enema**.
	Management: OHCM p482.
Carcinoma rectum	*Suggested by:* rectal bleeding with defaecation.
	Confirmed by: **sigmoidoscopy with biopsy**.
	Management: OHCM pp506, 507.
Colonic carcinoma	*Suggested by:* red blood mixed with stool and alternate diarrhoea and constipation.
	Confirmed by: **flexible colonoscopy with biopsy**.
	Management: OHCM pp506, 507.
Ulcerative colitis	*Suggested by:* lower abdominal pain, ↑urgency to defaecate, severe bloody diarrhoea, ↑fever in acute attack.
	Confirmed by: **colonoscopy with biopsy, barium studies** show loss of haustration, mucosal oedema, ulceration.
	Management: OHCM p244.
Meckel's diverticulum	*Suggested by:* usually asymptomatic, anaemia, rectal bleeding.
	Confirmed by: **technetium-labelled red blood cell scan, laparotomy**.
	Management: OHCM p730.

Crohn's disease	*Suggested by:* chronic diarrhoea with abdominal pain, weight loss, palpable RLQ mass or fullness, mouth ulcers.
	Confirmed by: **colonoscopy with biopsy, barium studies** show 'skip lesions', string sign in advanced cases.
	Management: OHCM p246.
Massive upper GI bleed	*Suggested by:* bright or dark red 'maroon' coloured stool.
	Confirmed by: **upper GI endoscopy**.
	Management: OHCM pp224, 226.
Trauma (in children, possible non-accidental injury)	*Suggested by:* fresh blood, sometimes external signs of trauma.
	Confirmed by: sensitive and careful history, possible surveillance etc.
Intussusception	*Suggested by:* child in first 6–18 months of life, acute onset of colicky intermittent abdominal pain, red currant 'jelly' PR bleed, ± a sausage shape mass in upper abdomen.
	Confirmed by: **barium enema**, ± reduction of intussusception with appropriate hydrostatic pressure.
	Management: OHCM p494.

Tenesmus

Intense desire to defaecate but no stool.

Some differential diagnoses and typical outline evidence

Rectal inflammation (proctitis)	*Suggested by:* rectal bleeding, mucus discharge.
	Confirmed by: proctoscopy or *sigmoidoscopy reveals* inflamed rectal mucosa.
	Management: OHCM pp244, 588.
Rectal tumour	*Suggested by:* rectal bleeding with defaecation, blood limited to surface of stool.
	Confirmed by: *sigmoidoscopy with rectal biopsy*.
	Management: OHCM pp506, 507.
Tumour of descending colon	*Suggested by:* alternate diarrhoea and constipation.
	Confirmed by: *colonoscopy with biopsy, barium enema*.
	Management: OHCM pp506, 507.
Pelvic inflammatory disease	*Suggested by:* lower abdominal pain, fever, vaginal discharge, dysuria, elevated ESR and CRP, leucocytosis.
	Confirmed by: *high vaginal swab, pelvic ultrasound, ± laparoscopy*.
	Management: OHCS p286.

Anorectal pain

Some differential diagnoses and typical outline evidence

Anal fissure	*Suggested by:* skin tag, pain on defaecation, staining of toilet paper following defaecation.
	Confirmed by: physical examination of anal region.
	Management: OHCM pp520, 522.
Haemorrhoids (thrombotic pile)	*Suggested by:* rectal bleeding following defaecation, perianal protrusion with pain.
	Confirmed by: digital rectal examination.
	Management: OHCM pp458, 522.
Perianal abscess	*Suggested by:* tender lump, redness.
	Confirmed by: digital rectal examination.
	Management: OHCM p246.
Proctitis	*Suggested by:* rectal bleeding, mucus discharge.
	Confirmed by: proctoscopy or **sigmoidoscopy** revealing inflamed rectal mucosa.
	Management: OHCM pp244, 588.
Prostatitis	*Suggested by:* rigor, ↑fever, urinary frequency and urgency, dysuria, haemospermia.
	Confirmed by: tender prostate gland on PR examination, **urine microscopy**.
	Management: OHCM pp262, 588.
Proctalgia fugax, coccydynia	*Suggested by:* fleeting pain in rectum or coccyx which may be related to sitting, but not defaecation.
	Confirmed by: physical examination, tenderness of levator muscle.

Urinary frequency ± dysuria

Some differential diagnoses and typical outline evidence

Urinary tract infection	*Suggested by:* vomiting, fever, abdominal pain, ↑nitirites, white cells and blood on urine 'dipstick'.
	Confirmed by: MSU microscopy and culture. US scan for possible anatomical abnormality.
	Management: OHCM pp172–6.
Bladder or urethral calculus	*Suggested by:* suprapubic pain, macroscopic or microscopic haematuria.
	Confirmed by: ultrasound of bladder, plain X-ray, IVU.
	Management: OHCM pp264–5.
Uterine prolapse	*Suggested by:* incontinent of urine, cervix observed in lower vagina.
	Confirmed by: pelvic examination.
	Management: OHCM p500, OHCS p296.
Prostatic hypertrophy	*Suggested by:* hesitancy, poor stream, large prostate on rectal examination.
	Confirmed by: PSA↑, ultrasound of prostate gland and response to TURP.
	Management: OHCM pp496, 497.
'Spastic' bladder due to upper motor neurone lesion	*Suggested by:* weakness, increased tone and reflexes in lower limbs.
	Confirmed by: small bladder on ultrasound.
	Management: OHCM pp500–1.

Incontinence of urine alone (not faeces)

Some differential diagnoses and typical outline evidence

Prostatism	*Suggested by:* hesitancy, dribbling, poor stream, frequency.
	Confirmed by: ↑PSA, ultrasound of prostate gland.
	Management: OHCM p500.
Uterine prolapse	*Suggested by:* low volume urinary frequency.
	Confirmed by: pelvic examination.
	Management: OHCM p500; *OHCS* p290.
Urinary tract infection	*Suggested by:* dysuria, frequency, fever, vomiting, ↑nitrites, white cells and blood on 'dipstick'.
	Confirmed by: MSU microscopy and culture. US scan for possible anatomical abnormality.
	Management: OHCM pp172–6.
Weakness of pelvic floor muscles	*Suggested by:* incontinence during coughing, sneezing, laughing.
	Confirmed by: **Urodynamic studies**.
	Management: OHCM p500; *OHCS* p306.

Incontinence of urine and faeces

Some differential diagnoses and typical outline evidence

'Neurogenic' bladder	*Suggested by:* paresis, low tone and diminished reflexes in lower limbs, sensory loss in anal region.
	Confirmed by: small and spastic bladder (upper motor neurone) or large and hypotonic bladder (lower motor neurone) on *US scan*.
	Management: OHCM p500.
Epileptic fits	*Suggested by:* history of loss of consciousness, tongue biting, jerking movements.
	Confirmed by: clinical history, EEG.
	Management: OHCM pp378–81.
Dementia	*Suggested by:* chronic worsening confusion, elderly, previous strokes.
	Confirmed by: low mental scores, cerebral atrophy on **CT head scan**.
	Management: OHCM p374–7.
Severe depression	*Suggested by:* severe lack of motivation.
	Confirmed by: response to treatment of depression.
	Management: OHCM pp15, 60; *OHCS* p336–41.
Faecal impaction with 'overflow'	*Suggested by:* hard rock-like faeces in rectum.
	Confirmed by: response to evacuation of faeces.
	Management: OHCM pp72, 73.

Painful haematuria (with dysuria)

Some differential diagnoses and typical outline evidence

Urinary tract infection	*Suggested by:* dysuria, frequency, ± low grade fever ±abdominal pain, ↑nitrites, white cells and blood on urine 'dipstick'.
	Confirmed by: MSU microscopy and culture. US scan for possible anatomical abnormality.
	Management: OHCM pp172–6.
Renal calculus	*Suggested by:* dysuria spasmodic loin to groin pain, no fever.
	Confirmed by: urinalysis, renal ultrasound, IVU.
	Management: OHCM pp264–5.
Trauma	*Suggested by:* dysuria, urethral catheterisation, or recent painful sexual intercourse ('honeymoon cystitis').
	Confirmed by: history, normal MSU renal ultrasound, IVU.

Painless haematuria

False positives—vaginal or anorectal bleeding.

Some differential diagnoses and typical outline evidence

Renal tumour	*Suggested by:* palpable mass, fever (often previously of unknown origin).
	Confirmed by: ultrasound or CT of abdomen/kidney, IVU.
	Management: OHCM p498.
Ureteric tumour	*Suggested by:* colicky pain if obstructed.
	Confirmed by: ultrasound or CT abdomen/kidney, IVU.
	Management: OHCM p498.
Bladder tumour	*Suggested by:* pelvic pain, pelvic mass.
	Confirmed by: cystoscopy, IVU shows filling defects of bladder.
	Management: OHCM p502.
Bleeding diathesis	*Suggested by:* anticoagulant therapy, easy bruising, or other bleeding sites.
	Confirmed by: abnormal clotting screen ± low platelets.
	Management: OHCM p644–9.
Urinary tract infection	*Suggested by:* frequency, ± low grade fever, ↑nitrites, white cells, blood on 'dipstick'.
	Confirmed by: MSU microscopy and culture. US scan for possible anatomical abnormality.
	Management: OHCM pp172–4.

Secondary amenorrhoea

Absence of menstruation for ≥ 3 months.

Some differential diagnoses and typical outline evidence

Pregnancy	*Suggested by:* presentation during child bearing age.
	Confirmed by: pregnancy test +ve, pelvic ultrasound.
	Management: OHCS p8.
Normal menopause	*Suggested by:* >40 years of age, hot flushes.
	Confirmed by: FSH high.
	Management: OHCS p256.
Premature ovarian failure	*Suggested by:* hot flushes <40 years of age and no signs of other endocrine disease (adrenal failure, hypothyroidism, etc.).
	Confirmed by: LH, FSH ↑, estradiol ↓, ovarian biopsy: atrophic.
	Management: OHCS p256.
Polycystic ovary syndrome	*Suggested by:* oligo-/amenorrhoea, hirsutism, obesity.
	Confirmed by: ↓ sex hormone binding globulin, ↑ testosterone, ↑ LH, cystic ovaries on pelvic ultrasound.
	Management: OHCM p316; OHCS p252.
Hyperprolactin-aemia	*Suggested by:* galactorrhoea, ± headache or bitemporal visual field defect (if due to large prolactinoma).
	Confirmed by: ↑serum prolactin. Appearance of pituitary fossa on skull X-ray or CT scan.
	Management: OHCM p322.
Thyrotoxicosis	*Suggested by:* heat intolerance, tremor, nervousness, palpitation, frequent bowel movements, goitre.
	Confirmed by: ↓ TSH, ↑ FT4, (± ↑ FT3).
	Management: OHCM p304.

Excessive menstrual loss: menorrhagia

Menorrhagia can be due to uterine or systemic disorders.

Some differential diagnoses and typical outline evidence

Fibroids	*Suggested by:* (sometimes) urinary frequency, constipation, recurrent abortion, infertility.
	Confirmed by: pelvic examination, ultrasound or CT.
	Management: OHCS pp276–7.
Endometrial carcinoma	*Suggested by:* abnormal uterine bleeding, blood-stained vaginal discharge, postmenopausal bleeding.
	Confirmed by: pelvic ultrasound, tissue sampling of endometrium, hysteroscopy.
	Management: OHCS pp278–9.
Pelvic endometriosis	*Suggested by:* dysmenorrhoea, dyspareunia, infertility, pelvic mass.
	Confirmed by: laparoscopy.
	Management: OHCS p288.
Chronic pelvic inflammatory disease	*Suggested by:* lower abdominal pain, fever, vaginal discharge, dysuria, ↑ ESR and ↑ CRP, leucocytosis.
	Confirmed by: high vaginal swab, pelvic ultrasound, ± laparoscopy.
	Management: OHCS p286.
Intrauterine contraceptive device	*Suggested by:* history of its insertion ± painful periods.
	Confirmed by: symptoms subside after removal of IUCD.
Primary hypothyroidism	*Suggested by:* cold intolerance, tiredness, constipation, bradycardia.
	Confirmed by: ↑ TSH, ↓ FT4.
	Management: OHCM p306.
Bleeding diathesis	*Suggested by:* family history, tendency to bleed, easy bruising.
	Confirmed by: abnormal clotting screen.
	Management: OHCM pp644–9.

Intermenstrual or post coital bleeding

Expert pelvic examination is required.

Some differential diagnoses and typical outline evidence

Carcinoma of uterus	*Suggested by:* abnormal/intermenstrual uterine bleeding, blood-stained discharge, postmenopausal bleeding.
	Confirmed by: pelvic ultrasound, tissue sampling of endometrium, hysteroscopy.
	Management: OHCS pp278–9.
Carcinoma of cervix	*Suggested by:* irregular vaginal bleeding, offensive, watery or blood-stained vaginal discharge, obstructive uropathy and back pain in late stage.
	Confirmed by: appearance on vaginal speculum examination, biopsy of cervix.
	Management: OHCS p272–4.
Cervical or intrauterine polyps	*Suggested by:* intermenstrual spotting or post-menstrual staining.
	Confirmed by: appearance on vaginal speculum examination, hysteroscopy.
	Management: OHCS p270.

Chapter 5

Neurological symptoms

Headache—acute, new onset

Onset over seconds to hours.

Some differential diagnoses and typical outline evidence

Meningitis viral or bacterial	*Suggested by:* photophobia, fever, neck stiffness, vomiting, Kernig's sign. Petechial or purpuric rash (in meningococcal meningitis).
	Confirmed by: **CT brain** if neurological signs present, **Lumbar puncture**—Viral meningitis: CSF clear, ↑lymphocytes, ↑protein, normal glucose). Bacterial meningitis: CSF with ↑neutrophils, ↑protein, ↓glucose ± visible bacteria on gram stain.
	Management: OHCM pp368–71, 808.
Low CSF pressure	*Suggested by:* worsening or recurrence of headache after lumbar puncture (usually for suspected meningitis) made worse by sitting up.
	Confirmed by: spontaneous resolution after few days.
	Management: OHCM p753.
Subarachnoid haemorrhage	*Suggested by:* sudden occipital headache (often described as 'like a blow to the head'), variable degree of consciousness, ± neck stiffness, subhyaloid haemorrhage, ± focal neurological signs.
	Confirmed by: **CT or MRI brain scan. Lumbar puncture:** blood-stained CSF that does not clear in successive bottles, presence of xanthochromia in CSF (up to 2 weeks after the haemorrhage).
	Management: OHCM pp362, 363, 752.
Intracranial haemorrhage	*Suggested by:* focal neurological signs.
	Confirmed by: **CT/MRI brain scan.**
	Management: OHCM p354.
Head injury with cerebral contusion	*Suggested by:* history of trauma, cuts/bruises, reduced conscious level, lucid period, amnesia.
	Confirmed by: **skull X-ray, CT head** normal or showing oedema but no subdual haematoma or extradural haemorrhage.
	Management: OHCM p814.
Acute angle-closure glaucoma	*Suggested by:* red eyes, haloes, reduced visual acuity due to corneal clouding, pupil abnormality.
	Confirmed by: raised **intra-ocular pressure.**
	Management: OHCM pp340, 427.

Sinusitis	*Suggested by:* fever, facial pain, mucopurulent nasal discharge, tender over sinuses ± URTI.
	Confirmed by: **X-ray of sinuses or CT scan:** mucosal thickening, a fluid level or opacification.
	Management: OHCM p340; OHCS p562–3.
Tension headache	*Suggested by:* generalised or bilateral, continuous, tight bandlike, worsens as the day progresses, associated with stress or tension, ± aggravated by eye movement.
	Confirmed by: spontaneous improvement with simple analgesia.
Bilateral migraine	*Suggested by:* bilateral, throbbing, ± vomiting, aura ± visual or other neurological disturbances with precipitating factor e.g. premenstrual.
	Confirmed by: resolution over hours in dark room and analgesics, helped by sleep.
	Management: OHCM p342.

Headache—subacute onset

Onset over hours to days.

Some differential diagnoses and typical outline evidence

Raised intracranial pressure due to tumour, hydrocephalus, cerebral abscess etc.	*Suggested by:* dull headache, worse on waking, vomiting, aggravated by e.g. cough, sneezing, bending, look for papilloedema, ↑BP, ↓pulse rate, progressive focal neurological signs.
	Confirmed by: CT/MRI brain scan.
	Management: OHCM p816.
Encephalitis	*Suggested by:* fever, confusion, reduced conscious level.
	Confirmed by: CSF microscopy, serology or PCR.
	Management: *OHCM p369.*
Temporal/giant cell or cranial arteritis	*Suggested by:* scalp tenderness, jaw claudication, loss of temporal arterial pulsation, sudden loss of vision. ↑↑ESR.
	Confirmed by: **temporal artery biopsy** (may be done shortly after starting prednisolone).
	Management: OHCM pp424–5.

Headache—chronic and recurrent

Onset over weeks to months.

Some differential diagnoses and typical outline evidence

Tension headache	*Suggested by:* generalised or bilateral, continuous, tight bandlike, worsens as the day progresses, associated with stress or tension, often aggravated by eye movement.
	Confirmed by: spontaneous improvement with simple analgesia.
Migraine	*Suggested by:* typically unilateral, throbbing, ± vomiting, aura ± visual disturbances, precipitating factors.
	Confirmed by: resolution over hours in dark room and analgesics, helped by sleep.
	Management: OHCM p342.
Cluster headache	*Suggested by:* episodic, typically nightly pain in 1 eye for weeks.
	Confirmed by: episodes resolving over hours (like migraine).
	Management: OHCM p340.
Cervical root headache	*Suggested by:* occipital and back of the head, temples, vertex and frontal regions, worse on neck movement or restricted neck movements
	Confirmed by: **cervical X-ray** showing degenerative changes (or normal) and response to NSAIDs.
	Mangement: OHCS p660.
Eye strain	*Suggested by:* headaches worse after reading. Refractory error.
	Confirmed by: improvement with appropriate spectacles.
	Mangement: OHCS p426.
Drug side effect	*Suggested by:* drug history (e.g. nitrates).
	Confirmed by: improvement on drug withdrawal.

Stroke

This is a sudden onset of a neurological deficit.

Some differential diagnoses and typical outline evidence

Cerebral infarction	*Suggested by:* onset over minutes to hours of hemiaparesis or major neurological defect that lasts >24 hours.
	Confirmed by: **CT scan** appearing after days.
	Management: OHCM pp354, 356.
Transient cerebral ischaemic attack	*Suggested by:* onset over seconds to minutes of a neurological deficit that is improving already.
	Confirmed by: deficit resolving within 24 hours.
due to carotid artery stenosis etc. (see below)	*Management:* OHCM p360.
Cerebral embolus due to atheroma, atrial fibrillation, myocardial infarction	*Suggested by:* onset over seconds of hemiaparesis or other neurological defect that lasts >24 hours.
	Confirmed by: **CT scan** and **lumbar puncture** showing little change originally. Evidence of a potential source for an embolus.
	Management: OHCM p354.
Cerebral haemorrhage due to atheromatous degeneration, cerebral tumour	*Suggested by:* onset over seconds of hemiaparesis or major neurological defect that lasts >24 hours.
	Confirmed by: **CT showing** high attenuation ± 'low' (dark) 'oedema' area ± high density 'blood' in ventricles.
	Management: OHCM p354.
Subdural haemorrhage due to blunt head injury	*Suggested by:* onset over hours, days or weeks of a fluctuating hemiaparesis following history of head injury or fall especially in elderly or alcoholic.
	Confirmed by: **CT showing** low attenuation parallel to skull if chronic but high attenuation if acute.
	Management: OHCM pp366–7.
Extradural haemorrhage due to skull fracture lacerating middle meningeal artery	*Suggested by:* onset over minutes or hours of confusion, disturbed consciousness and hemiaparesis after 'lucid interval' of hours following head injury.
	Confirmed by: **CT head** showing high attenuation adjacent to skull ± hyper-density ± dark 'oedema' ± midline shift.
	Management: OHCM pp366–7.

Subarachnoid haemorrhage from berry aneurysm	*Suggested by:* sudden onset over seconds of headache ± disturbance of consciousness (usually under 45 years of age), neck stiffness.
	Confirmed by: **CT head** showing high attenuation area on surface of brain. **Lumbar puncture** showing blood.
	Management: OHCM pp360–2, 363, 752.
Cerebellar stroke	*Suggested by:* sudden onset of ataxia.
	Confirmed by: **MRI scan** (CT head poorly visualises hind brain).
Pontine stroke	*Suggested by:* sudden loss of consciousness. Cheyne–Stokes breathing (speeding up and slowing down over minutes), pin-point pupils, hemiparesis and eyes deviated towards paresis.
	Confirmed by: above clinical findings ± MRI scan.
	Management: OHCM p354.

Dizziness

Dizziness is often non-specific (nothing significant is ever found), but one of the following will be discovered in a proportion of patients. Distinguish between dizziness and vertigo (which has a sensation of movement), the latter being more 'specific' of an identifiable lesion.

Some differential diagnoses and typical outline evidence

Panic attacks and hyperventilation	*Suggested by:* associated anxiety and claustrophobia. Finger and lip paraesthesia of hyperventilation. Resting tachypnoea, no hypoxia.
	Confirmed by: **ABGs:** O_2 normal or ↑, ↓CO_2, **CXR:** normal, **spirometry** normal and **VQ scan** normal. Response to anxiolytics and physiotherapy.
Postural hypotension due to drugs to lower BP, loss of circulating volume, dehydration, diabetic autonomic neuropathy, old age + heavy meal, dopamine agonists, Addison's disease	*Suggested by:* assoc. palpitations, loss of consciousness. Supine and standing BP after 1 minute: >10mm drop.
	Confirmed by: response of BP changes to treatment of cause.
	Management: OHCM pp80, 344, 346.
Anaemia	*Suggested by:* subconjunctival pallor (± face, nail and hand pallor).
	Confirmed by: **FBC:** ↓Hb.
	Management: OHCM p624.
Hypoxic	*Suggested by:* blue hands and tongue (central cyanosis), restlessness, confused, drowsy or unconscious.
	Confirmed by: **ABG:** ↓P_aO_2 <8kPa on blood gas analysis or **pulse oximetry** of <90% saturation (mild) or <80% (severe).
	Management: OHCM p192.

Carotid sinus hypersensitivity	*Suggested by:* onset on head turning or shaving neck.
	Confirmed by: reproduction of symptoms while turning neck or pressure on carotid sinus.
	Management: OHCM p344.
Epilepsy	*Suggested by:* aura followed by other 'positive' neurological symptoms.
	*Confirmed by: **EEG:*** focal abnormality or 'spike γ wave' etc.
	Management: OHCM pp378–80.
Drug effect	*Suggested by:* history of taking sedative or hypotensive drug inc. alcohol.
	Confirmed by: resoloution of symptom after stopping drug.

Vertigo

Vertigo is a sensation of movement of self ± the environment especially rotation or oscillation.

Some differential diagnoses and typical outline evidence

Vertibrobasilar insufficiency (brain stem ischaemia)	*Suggested by:* visual disturbances, other signs of cerebral ischaemia e.g. dysarthria, faint.
	Confirmed by: **carotid doppler** evidence of arterial disease. MRA of brain and neck vessels.
	Management: OHCM pp333, 344, 346, 360.
Benign positional vertigo	*Suggested by:* attacks with duration of minutes only.
	Confirmed by: **head tilt test:** nystagmus after 5 secs, lasting a minute. Shorter duration when repeated.
	Management: OHCM pp346; OHCS p555.
Ménière's disease	*Suggested by:* attacks with duration of up to 24 hours. Progressive deafness (especially in older age groups).
	Confirmed by: **audiometry:** hearing loss with loudness recruitment.
	Management: OHCM pp346; OHCS p554.
Vestibular neuronitis	*Suggested by:* sudden single prostrating attack usually with nystagmus with resolution over weeks.
	Confirmed by: **caloric testing**.
	Management: OHCM p346; OHCS p554.
Middle ear disease	*Suggested by:* painful ear, recurrent attacks or persistent vertigo and nystagmus.
	Confirmed by: **audiometry:** conductive deafness. Otoscopic appearance of otitis media or cholesteotoma.
	Management: OHCM pp346, 387; OHCS p544.
Reversible drug toxicity	*Suggested by:* vertigo, slurring of speech and nystagmus with suggestive drug history e.g. alcohol, barbiturates, phenytoin.
	Confirmed by: resolution on withdrawal of drug. Drug levels if in doubt.
Wernicke's encephalopathy (due to thiamine deficiency usually in alcoholism)	*Suggested by:* persistence of vertigo, slurring of speech and nystagmus despite withdrawal of alcohol.
	Confirmed by: resolution or improvement on thiamine treatment.
	Management: OHCM p738.

Ototoxic drugs	*Suggested by:* recurrent attacks or persistent vertigo and little nystagmus, history of streptomycin, gentamicin, kanamycin, phenytoin, quinine or salicylates, etc.
	Confirmed by: bilateral loss of response to **caloric tests.** No signs of disease in brain stem, ears or cerebellum.
	Management: OHCM p542.
Brain stem ischaemia	*Suggested by:* sudden onset, and associated with peripheral vascular disease.
	Confirmed by: associated cranial nerve abnormalities, long tract signs.
	Management: OHCM pp346, 354.
Posterior fossa tumour	*Suggested by:* mild vertigo of onset over months and slight nystagmus. Bilateral papilloedema. Ipsilateral absent corneal reflex. Cranial nerve lesions V, VI, VII, X and XI. Ipsilateral cerebellar and contralateral pyramidal signs.
	Confirmed by: **MRI scan** showing tumour.
Multiple sclerosis	*Suggested by:* sudden onset and central type nystagmus (occurs equally in both directions and sometimes vertically) in young person, other neurological disturbances, scanning speech, optic atrophy.
	Confirmed by: other similar neurological episodes 'disseminated in time and space' and multiple, enhancing lesions in various parts of nervous system on **MRI scan.**
	Management: OHCM p385.
Migraine	*Suggested by:* associated headache (vertigo instead of visual aura).
	Confirmed by: resolution and recurrence consistent with natural history of migraine.
	Management: OHCM p342.
Temporal lobe epilepsy	*Suggested by:* associated temporal lobe symptoms, e.g. odd taste, smells, visual hallucinations.
	Confirmed by: **EEG** findings.
	Management: OHCM p378.
Ramsay Hunt syndrome	*Suggested by:* associated ear pain, lower motor neurone facial palsy.
	Confirmed by: zoster vescicles at the external auditory meatus, or fauces.
	Management: OHCM pp346, 389.

'Fit'

History of aura, loss of consciousness, tonic and clonic movements.

Some differential diagnoses and typical outline evidence

Febrile convulsion	*Suggested by:* young age, especially in childhood and associated with a febrile illness.
	Confirmed by: normal **EEG** and **CT scan** and no subsequent recurrence without febrile illness on follow up.
	Management: OHCM pp378–81.
Idiopathic epilepsy—new presentation	*Suggested by:* young age, especially in teens.
	Confirmed by: abnormal or normal **EEG** and normal **CT scan** but subsequent recurrence.
	Management: OHCM pp378–81.
Known idiopathic epilepsy	*Suggested by:* history of previous fits.
	Confirmed by: PMH of past investigations and on treatment.
	Management: OHCM pp378–81.
Brain tumour	*Suggested by:* older age (but any age), headaches, papilloedema.
	Confirmed by: **CT** or **MRI scan** showing cerebral mass.
	Management: OHCM pp386, 387.
Epilepsy due to meningitis	*Suggested by:* fever, neck stiffness.
	Confirmed by: CT scan and lumbar puncture.
	Management: OHCM pp368, 369.
Epilepsy due to old brain scar tissue	*Suggested by:* past history of serious head injury, or stroke.
	Confirmed by: abnormal **EEG, CT** or **MRI brain scan**.
	Management: OHCM pp378–81.
Alcohol withdrawal	*Suggested by:* recent heavy alcohol intake (usually super-imposed on habitually high intake).
	Confirmed by: subsequent episodes in similar circumstances.
	Management: OHCM pp245, 355.
Hypoglycaemia due too much insulin with too little food in diabetic, or Insulinoma	*Suggested by:* sweating, hunger ± known diabetic on insulin or medication.
	Confirmed by: blood sugar ↓ (<2mmol/L) during episode.
	Management: OHCM p820.

Sudden severe hypotension (especially cardiac arrest)	*Suggested by:* peripheral and central cyanosis, no pulse or BP.
	Confirmed by: **ECG** shows asystole or ineffectual fast or slow rhythm (or electro-mechanical dissociation).
Severe electrolyte disturbance due to very high or low sodium, calcium, magnesium, etc.	*Suggested by:* abnormality on serum biochemistry.
	Confirmed by: no recurrence of fits after metabolic abnormality treated.
	Management: OHCM pp245, 355.
'Functional' (pseudo-fit)	*Suggested by:* always occurring in front of audience, eyes closed during episode.
	Confirmed by: normal EEG when episode documented on video-recording. Normal CT scan.

Transient neurological deficit

Sudden dysphasia, facial or limb weakness resolving within 24 hours.

Some differential diagnoses and typical outline evidence

Transient cerebral ischaemic attack 'TIA' from platelet embolus ? due to carotid artery stenosis or vasculitic process	*Suggested by:* onset over minutes and then immediate improvement with prospect of complete resolution within 24 hours ± carotid bruit.
	Confirmed by: resolution within 24 hours, absence of previous fit, no throbbing migrainous headache, no chest pain, normal *ECG* and *Troponin* after 12 hours, normal *plasma sodium*, normal *blood sugar*, no witnessed fits and normal *CT* or *MRI scan*. *Doppler ultrasound* of carotids (to seek operable stenosis). *ESR* or *CRP* ↑ (if there is a vasculitic process e.g. cranial arteritis).
	Management: OHCM p360.
Atrial fibrillation with cerebral embolus	*Suggested by:* Irregularly irregular pulse.
	Confirmed by: irregularly irregular QRS complexes, no P wave on *ECG*.
	Management: OHCM p130.
Intracerebral space occuping lesion: tumour, aneurysm haematoma, arteriovenous malformation	*Suggested by:* associated headache.
	Confirmed by: *CT* or *MRI scan* appearance.
	Management: OHCM p388.
Transient hypotension due to arrhythmia or myocardial infarction	*Suggested by:* history of chest pain or PMH of IHD.
	Confirmed by: *ECG:* ST changes. ↑*Troponin. 24 hour ECG:* recurrence of arrhythmia.
	Management: OHCM pp120–33.
Todd's paralysis (following focal epileptic fit)	*Suggested by:* witness's history of fitting.
	Confirmed by: *EEG* changes.
	Management: OHCM pp378, 736.

Migraine	*Suggested by:* associated headache (neurological deficit instead of visual aura).
	Confirmed by: resolution consistent with other features of migraine.
	Management: OHCM p342.
Hypoglycaemic episode	*Suggested by:* a known diabetic and associated sudden hunger, sweating, confusion.
	Confirmed by: **blood sugar** <2mmol/L.
	Management: OHCM p820.
Hyponatraemia	*Suggested by:* ↓↓sodium concentration (e.g. <120mmol/l) and ↓↓serum osmolality. Associated confusion.
	Confirmed by: resolution of deficit as **sodium concentration** and **osmolality** abnormality corrected.
	Management: OHCM p463.
Multiple sclerosis	*Suggested by:* sudden onset and central type nystagmus (occurs equally in both directions and sometimes vertically) in young person, other neurological disturbances, scarring speech, optic atrophy.
	Confirmed by: other similar neurological episodes 'disseminated in time and space' and multiple, enhancing lesions in various parts of nervous system on **MRI scan**.
	Management: OHCM p385.
Psychological	*Suggested by:* past history of similar episodes from young (<30 years) age.
	Confirmed by: absence of any objective evidence of physical cause of deficit on follow-up.

Fatigue, 'tired all the time'

Generally a poor lead—but consider the following.

Some differential diagnoses and typical outline evidence

Depression	*Suggested by:* early morning wakening, fatigue worse in the morning that never goes during the day, anhedonia, poor appetite.
	Confirmed by: response to psychotherapy or antidepressants.
	Management: *OHCS* p336–461.
Sleep apnoea syndrome	*Suggested by:* frequent awakening at night, snoring and breathing pauses during sleep (history from a sleeping partner) and sleepiness during the day.
	Confirmed by: multiple dips in O_2 levels whilst asleep during home or hospital monitoring.
	Management: OHCM p204.
Drug induced	*Suggested by:* taking sedating drug, including anti-epileptic treatment.
	Confirmed by: improvement by stopping or changing drug.
Post viral fatigue	*Suggested by:* history of recent viral illness especially glandular fever.
	Confirmed by: resolution after weeks or months.
	Management: *OHCM* p72.
Diabetes mellitus	*Suggested by:* thirst, polyuria, polydipsia, family history (but all may be absent).
	Confirmed by: **fasting blood glucose** $\geq$7.0mmol/L on two occasions OR fasting, **random** or **GTT glucose** $\geq$11.1mmol/L in combination with symptoms.
	Management: *OHCM* pp292–9.
Chronic fatigue syndrome (CFS)	*Suggested by:* (1) impaired memory/concentration unrelated to drugs or alcohol use, (2) unexplained muscle pain, (3) polyarthralgia, (4) unrefreshing sleep, (5) post-exertional malaise lasting over 24h, (6) persisting sore throat not caused by glandular fever, (7) unexplained tender cervical or axillary nodes.
	Confirmed by: 4/7 or more of the above present for >6 months.

Poor sleep habit	*Suggested by:* long working hours, little sleep, insomnia.
	Confirmed by: sleep diary and improvement with better sleep habits.
Parasomnias	*Suggested by:* restless legs, cataplexy, narcolepsy and day-time somnolescence.
	Confirmed by: response of symptoms to stimulant medication.

Joint symptoms

Muscle stiffness or pain

Usually worse in the early morning often with pain and stiffness.

Some differential diagnoses and typical outline evidence

Normal response to strenuous exercise	*Suggested by:* fit healthy, unaccustomed exercise 1–2 days before. *Confirmed by:* spontaneous resolution.
Polymyalgia rheumatica	*Suggested by:* onset over weeks or months, stiff, painful, and tender proximal muscles. Fatigue, fever in elderly person. *Confirmed by:* ↑↑*ESR*. **Rheumatoid factor** –ve, prompt response to prednisolone, no other cause (e.g. infection on follow-up). *Management:* OHCM p424.
Rheumatoid arthritis	*Suggested by:* early morning stiffness. Fingers showing 'swan neck' or 'boutonnière' deformities. Thumbs show Z-deformities. MCP joints and wrists—sublux giving ulnar deviation. Knees—valgus or varus deformity and popliteal 'Baker's' cysts. Feet—subluxation of meta-tarsal heads with hallux valgus, clawed toes. *Confirmed by:* **rheumatoid factor** +ve, ↑*anti-IgG autoantibody*. *FBC:* Normochromic anaemia, ↑*ESR* when active. *Management:* OHCM p414.
Ankylosing spondylitis	*Suggested by:* onset over months or years. Stiffness and progressive loss of spinal movement. Kyphosis and spinal extension. *Confirmed by:* 'bamboo' spine on **back X-ray** and loss of sacroileal joint space. **Rheumatoid factor** –ve, **HLA-B$_{27}$** +ve. *Management:* OHCM pp410, 418.
Primary muscle disease	*Suggested by:* onset over weeks to years. Predominant weakness. *Confirmed by:* **CPK** ↑, electromyography and muscle biopsy. *Management:* OHCM p420.
Primary hypothyroidism	*Suggested by:* onset over weeks to months. Predominant fatigue. Also cold intolerance, depression. *Confirmed by:* ↑*TSH*, ↓*FT4*. *Management:* OHCM p306.

Early manifestation of occult malignancy	*Suggested by:* onset over weeks or months. Weight loss, anorexia.
	Confirmed by: subsequent appearance of malignancy, especially spinal secondary deposits.
'Fibromyalgia'	*Suggested by:* variable onset—weeks to years. Diffuse pain and stiffness but no features of specific diagnosis.
	Confirmed by: no 'subsequent' development of features of a specific diagnosis, normal ESR, Rheumatoid factor –ve, CPK normal, TSH & FT4 normal.

Monoarthritis

One joint affected by pain, swelling, overlying redness, stiffness and local heat (± fever).

Some differential diagnoses and typical outline evidence

Acute septic arthritis	*Suggested by:* extremely painful, hot red joint, high fever.
	Confirmed by: ↑↑WBC. **Joint aspiration:** synovial fluid turbid. **Culture** growing staphylococcus or streptococcus or pseudomonas or gonococci or TB, etc.
	Management: OHCM p412.
Gout	*Suggested by:* one acutely inflamed joint (usually small esp. big toe) at a time, but other joints in hands, arms, legs, and feet deformed. Tophi on ears and tendon sheaths.
	Confirmed by: **serum urate** ↑(not always). Urate crystals (negatively birefringent in plane-polarised light) present on **joint aspiration**.
	Management: OHCM p416.
Pseudogout (Ca^{2+} pyrophosphate arthropathy/ chondrocalcinosis)	*Suggested by:* one painful joint (usually knee) especially in elderly or history of hyperparathyroidism or myxoedema or osteoarthritis or haemochro-matosis or acromegaly.
	Confirmed by: **joint aspiration:** synovial crystal deposits positively bifringent in plane-polarised light.
	Management: OHCM p416.
Reiter's disease	*Suggested by:* monoarthritis, urethritis, conjunctivitis—especially in a young man—or a history of diarrhoea (dysentery). Also suggested by associated iritis, keratoderma blenorrhagica (brown, aseptic abscesses on soles and palms), mouth ulcers, circinate balanitis (painless serpiginous penile rash), plantar fasciitis, achilles tendonitis, and aortic incompetence.
	Confirmed by: **rheumatoid factor** –ve (i.e. 'seronegative'). **Urinalysis:** 1st glass of a 2-glass urine test shows debris in urethritis.
	Management: OHCM p418.
Traumatic haemarthrosis	*Suggested by:* acutely inflamed joint after trauma.
	Confirmed by: **joint aspiration:** aspiration of blood from joint.

Psoriasis	*Suggested by:* acutely inflamed terminal interphalyngeal or I-P) joint but other joints deformed especially terminal I-P joints and pitting and thickening of fingernails.
	Confirmed by: psoriatic plaques on elbows and extensor surfaces of limbs, scalp, behind ears and around navel. **Rheumatoid factor** −ve (i.e. 'seronegative').
Rheumatoid arthritis	*Suggested by:* Early morning stiffness. Fingers: 'swan neck' or 'boutonnière' deformities. Thumbs have Z-deformities. MCP joints and wrists: sublux acquiring ulnar deviation. Knees: valgus or varus deformity and popliteal 'Baker's' cysts. Feet: Subluxation of metatarsal heads with hallux valgus, clawed toes, and callouses.
	Confirmed by: **Rheumatoid factor** +ve (i.e. 'seropositive'), ↑*anti-IgG autoantibody*. *FBC:* Normochromic anaemia, ↑*ESR* when active.
	Management: OHCM p414.
Leukaemic joint deposits	*Suggested by:* acutely inflamed joint.
	Confirmed by: leukaemic picture on **peripheral film** and **bone marrow**.
Reactive arthritis (aseptic)	*Suggested by:* asymmetric mono- or oligoarthritis developing about 1 week after infection elsewhere.
	Confirmed by: Lab evidence of venereal or enteric infection, *Yersinia*, *Chlamydia trachomatis*, *Campylobacter*, *Salmonella/Shigella* and *Chl. pneumoniae*, HIV, *Vibrio parahaemolyticus*, *Borrelia burgdorferi*, *Clostridium difficile*.

Polyarthritis

Several joints affected by pain, swelling, overlying redness, stiffness and local heat (± fever).

Some differential diagnoses and typical outline evidence

Viruses	*Suggested by:* several acutely inflamed joints. History of recent rubella or mumps or Hepatitis A or Epstein–Barr viral infection, etc.
	Confirmed by: ↑*viral tires* rheumatoid factor –ve (seronegative).
Rheumatoid arthritis	*Suggested by:* History of early morning stiffness. Fingers: 'swan neck' or 'boutonnière' deformities. Thumbs have Z-deformities. MCP joints and wrists: sublux acquiring ulnar deviation. Knees: valgus or varus deformity and popliteal 'Baker's' cysts. Feet: subluxation of metatarsal heads with hallux valgus, clawed toes, and callouses.
	Confirmed by: **rheumatoid factor** +ve, ↑**anti-IgG autoantibody**. ↑*ESR* when active.
	Management: OHCM p414.
Sjögren's syndrome	*Suggested by:* several acutely inflamed joints and diminished lacrimation causing dry eyes and diminished salivation causing dry mouth.
	Confirmed by: **rheumatoid factor** +ve and **anti-Ro** (SSA) and **anti-La** (SSB) antibodies present (not always).
	Management: OHCM p733.
Rheumatic fever (reactive arthritis to earlier infection with Lancefield Group A β-haemolytic streptococci)	*Suggested by:* flitting polyarthritis (a major 'Jones criterion').
	Confirmed by: evidence of recent streptococcal infection plus 1 more major revised Jones criteria, or 2 more minor criteria. Evidence of streptococcal infection = scarlet fever or positive **throat swab** or increase in *ASOT* >200 or ↑*DNase B titre*. [Major criteria = carditis or flitting polyarthritis or subcutaneous nodules or erythema marginatum or Sydenham's chorea. Minor criteria = fever or ↑*ESR/CRP*, arthralgia (but not if arthritis is one of the major criteria), prolonged P–R interval on *ECG* (but not if carditis is major criterion), previous rheumatic fever.] **Rheumatoid factor** –ve.
	Management: OHCM p144.

Systemic lupus erythematosus	*Suggested by:* polyarthritis with periarticular and tendon involvement, muscle pain, proximal myopathy. *Confirmed by:* **double-stranded DNA antibodies** titre ↑↑. **ANA** +ve and **rheumatoid factor** +ve. *Management:* OHCM pp422–3.
Ulcerative colitis	*Suggested by:* large joint polyarthritis, sacroilitis, ankylosing spondylitis, background of gradual onset of diarrhoea with blood amd mucus and crampy abdominal discomfort. *Confirmed by:* **rheumatoid factor** –ve. Inflamed, friable mucosa on **sigmoidoscopy** and biopsy shows inflammatory infiltrate, goblet cell depletion, etc. *Management:* OHCM pp244–5.
Crohn's disease	*Suggested by:* large joint polyarthritis, sacroilitis, ankylosing spondylitis, background of gradual onset of diarrhoea, abdominal pain, weight loss. *Confirmed by:* **rheumatoid factor** –ve. **Small bowel enema** showing ileal strictures, proximal dilatation, inflammatory mass or fistula. **Barium enema:** 'cobblestoning', 'rose thorn' ulcers, colonic strictures with rectal sparing. *Management:* OHCM p246.
Drug reaction	*Suggested by:* several acutely inflamed joints. History of suspicious drug. *Confirmed by:* **rheumatoid factor** –ve and improvement on withdrawing drug.
Reiter's syndrome	*Suggested by:* polyarthritis, urethritis, conjunctivitis—especially in a young man—or a history of diarrhoea (dysentery). Also suggested by associated iritis, keratoderma blenorrhagica (brown, aseptic abscesses on soles and palms); mouth ulcers, circinate balanitis (painless serpiginous penile rash), plantar fasciitis, achilles tendonitis, and aortic incompetence. *Confirmed by:* **rheumatoid factor** –ve. **Urinalysis:** 1st glass of a 2-glass urine test shows debris in urethritis. *Management:* OHCM p418.
Psoriasis	*Suggested by:* several acutely inflamed joints (usually terminal inter-phalyngeal or I-P) and other joints deformed especially terminal I-P joints with pitting and thickening of fingernails. *Confirmed by:* psoriatic plaques on elbows and extensor surfaces of limbs, scalp, behind ears and around navel. **Rheumatoid factor** –ve.

Pain or limitation of movement in the hand

Ask patient to flex and extend fingers and then wrists. Observe opening and closing buttons. Note degree of movement, any limitation or pain.

Some differential diagnoses and typical outline evidence

Dupuytren's contracture usually familial or associated with alcohol or anti-epileptic therapy	*Suggested by:* progressive flexion deformity of base ring and little fingers mainly with palmar fibrosis. Often bilateral. Family history. *Confirmed by:* fixed flexion at metacarpo-phalyngeal joints first then inter phalyngeal joints. (Inability to place hand on flat surface = severe).
Ganglion	*Suggested by:* painless spherical swelling around wrist. *Confirmed by:* fluctuant, soft sphere. Disappears spontaneously or after blow e.g. from a book.
Rheumatoid arthritis	*Suggested by:* 'swan neck' or 'boutonnière' deformities of fingers. Thumbs have Z-deformities. MCP joints and wrists: sublux acquiring ulnar deviation. Nodules on elbows and extensor tendons. *Confirmed by:* rheumatoid factor +ve. Anti-IgG autoantibody ↑. *Management:* OHCM p414.
Psoriasis	*Suggested by:* several acutely inflamed joints (usually terminal inter-phalyngeal or I-P) and other joints deformed especially terminal I-P joints with pitting and thickening of fingernails. *Confirmed by:* psoritic plaques on extensor surfaces of limbs, scalp, behind ears and around navel. **Rheumatoid factor** –ve.
Trigger finger due to nodule sticking in tendon sheath	*Suggested by:* fixed flexion at the ring or little finger with no fibrosis in palm. Patient unable to extend finger spontaneously. *Confirmed by:* 'click' as fingers passively extended. Nodule then palpable on flexor surface of finger.

De Quervain's syndrome—stenosing tenosynovitis	*Suggested by:* pain at the wrist e.g. when lifting teapot. History of forceful hand-use e.g. wringing clothes.
	Confirmed by: pain over radial styloid process, made worse by forced adduction and flexion of thumb into palm.
Volkmann's ischaemic contracture due to ischaemia flexor muscles of thumb and fingers (supplied by brachial artery)	*Suggested by:* flexion deformity at the thumb, fingers, wrist and elbow with forearm pronation. History of trauma or surgery near to brachial artery or plaster of Paris applied too tightly to forearm.
	Confirmed by: cold, dark, ischaemic arm, no pulse at the wrist, and pain when fingers extended.
Recent trauma	*Suggested by:* history of recent impact and acute deformity.
	Confirmed by: acute pain and deformity clinically and on **elbow X-ray**.

Pain or limitation of movement at the elbow

Ask the patient to straighten arms and compare for deformity and deviation from the normal valgus angle. Ask the patient to flex elbow and to supinate and rotate normally over 90°. Note degree of movement, any limitation or pain.

Some differential diagnoses and typical outline evidence

Epicondylitis: tennis elbow (teno-periostitis)	*Suggested by:* preceding repetitive strain e.g. use of screwdriver, tennis raquet. Pain worse when patient asked to flex fingers and wrist and pronate hand.
	Confirmed by: pain when patient's extended wrist pulled. Improvement after avoidance of preceding repetitive movement.
	Management: OHCS p666.
Osteoarthritis	*Suggested by:* joint deformity, intermittent pain and swelling, past history of fracture. 'Locking' if loose bodies.
	Confirmed by: impairment of flexion and extension but rotation full. **Elbow X-ray** confirming loose bodies.
	Management: OHCS p666.
Old trauma	*Suggested by:* history of past impact or fracture and deformity.
	Confirmed by: deformity on clinical examination and **elbow X-ray**.
Recent trauma	*Suggested by:* history of recent impact and acute deformity.
	Confirmed by: acute pain and deformity clinically and on **elbow X-ray**.

Pain or limitation of movement at the shoulder

Ask patients to put their arms behind their head and note angle at which any restriction and pain occurs.

Some differential diagnoses and typical outline evidence

Rotator cuff tears of the supraspinatus tendon or adjacent subsapularis or infraspinatus tendons	*Suggested by:* limitation and/or pain on abduction at the shoulder to the first 60° range (achieved by scapular rotation). Aged >40 years.
	Confirmed by: passive movement pain-free and spontaneous above 90°. **MRI** showing communication between joint capsule and subacromial bursa.
	Management: OHCS p664.
Supraspinatus tendinopathy (due to partial tear)	*Suggested by:* limitation and/or pain on abduction at the shoulder in the final 60° to 90° range. Aged 35–60 years.
	Confirmed by: some active movement up to 90°. Movement pain-free and spontaneous above 90°.
	Management: OHCS p664.
Chronic supraspinatus inflammation ± calcification	*Suggested by:* past history of acute limitation and continued limitation and/or pain on abduction at the shoulder in the final 60° to 90° range. Aged 35–60.
	Confirmed by: clinically or calcification in muscle on **shoulder X-ray** sometimes.
	Management: OHCS p664.
Biceps tendonitis	*Suggested by:* pain in front of the shoulder aggravated by contraction of the biceps.
	Confirmed by: above clinical findings.
	Management: OHCS p664.
Rupture of long head of biceps	*Suggested by:* pain in front of the shoulder.
	Confirmed by: pain aggravated by contraction of the biceps and lump (contracting muscle belly) appears.
	Management: OHCS p664.
Frozen shoulder—adhesive capsulitis	*Suggested by:* marked reduction in active and passive movement with less than 90° abduction.
	Confirmed by: above clinical findings and normal **shoulder X-ray**.
	Management: OHCS p664.

Pain or limitation of movement at the neck

Look from the side to see if there is normal cervical (and lumbar) lordosis. Ask the patient to tilt head: move ear towards shoulder. Note angle at which any restriction and pain occurs.

Some differential diagnoses and typical outline evidence

Spasmodic torticollis/ cervical dystonia due to trapezius and sternomastoid spasm	*Suggested by:* recurrent onset of sudden painful stiff neck with torticollis from aged 10–30. Family history or minor injury.
	Confirmed by: history and absence of root compression pattern pain or paresis.
	Management: OHCS p660.
Infantile torticolis due to birth damage of steromastoid	*Suggested by:* onset early childhood (up to 3 years). Head tilted to shoulder and retarded facial growth on affected muscle side.
	Confirmed by: palpable nodule in muscle on affected side. *Biopsy of nodule*—fibrous only and no gangliocytoma.
Cervical rib with compression of lower brachial plexus affecting median and ulnar nerves and brachial artery	*Suggested by:* weakness, pain and numbness in forearm and hand, usually on ulnar side.
	Confirmed by: wasting and weakness of thenar and hypothenar muscles. Loss of sensation medial hand and arm. Arm cyanosis and absent pulse. Cervical rib may not be visible on *neck X-ray* (fibrous band instead).
	Management: OHCS p660.
Posterior prolapsed cervical disc usually C5/C6 disc and C6/C7 disc effect on nerve roots	*Suggested by:* torticollis, stiffness and pain in neck over side of disc lesion. Pain, numbness in arm and tip of little or middle finger or thumb.
	Confirmed by: loss of biceps or supinator reflexes. Loss sensation in medial or lateral borders of hand. *MRI scan* shows posterior protrusion.
	Management: OHCS p660.
Anterior prolapsed cervical disc usually C5/C6 disc and C6/C7 disc affect spinal cord	*Suggested by:* torticollis, stiffness and pain in neck over side of disc lesion. Numbness and weakness in leg.
	Confirmed by: flaccid first then spastic paresis of leg. Loss of knee, ankle reflexes, and extensor plantar response. Loss of vibration sense, touch and pain with sensory level. *MRI scan* shows protrusion.
	Management: OHCS p660.

Pain or limitation of movement of the back: with sudden onset over seconds to hours originally

Look from the side to see if there is normal lumbar lordosis. Ask patients to touch their toes and watch for movement of spine (rounded?) and hips. Ask the patient to arch backwards, bend to each side, and rotate trunk from side to side. Lie patient down and measure length of legs. Raise each straight leg for any restriction before 45°.

Some differential diagnoses and typical outline evidence

Mechanical pain	Strains, tears or crushing of ligaments, discs, vertebrae with normal healing.
	Suggested by: recent onset over minutes of pain and restriction of movement in lower back.
	Confirmed by: recovery with minimal loss of function over days or weeks.
Posterior lumbar disc prolapse	*Suggested by:* onset over seconds of severe back pain on coughing, sneezing or twisting after earlier strain. Radiation to buttock, thigh or calf if prolapse compresses posterior root.
	Confirmed by: back flexed and extension restricted. Straight leg raising stopped before 45° by pain. Loss of sensation lateral foot (L4/5). Loss of ankle jerk and sensation sole of foot (S1).
	Management: OHCS p674–6.
Anterior lumbar disc prolapse	*Suggested by:* onset over seconds of severe back pain on coughing, sneezing or twisting after earlier strain. (If large, prolapse compresses cauda equina, with leg weakness, incontinence and numbness around perineum).
	Confirmed by: flaccid paresis of leg(s). Loss of knee, ankle reflexes and extensor plantar response. Loss of vibration sense, touch and pain with sensory level. **MRI scan** shows protrusion.
	Management: OHCS p674–6.
Spondylolisthesis due to spondylolysis, congenital malformation of articular process, osteoarthritis of posterior facet joints	*Suggested by:* sudden onset over minutes of back pain with or without sciatica in adolescence.
	Confirmed by: **plain back X-ray** shows forward displacement of vertebra over one below.
	Management: OHCS p674–6.

Central disc protrusion	*Suggested by:* sudden onset over minutes or hours with bilateral sciatica, disturbance of bladder or bowel function. Saddle or perineal anaesthesia.
	Confirmed by: history and compression of cord visible on **MRI scan**.
	Management: OHCS p674–6.

Pain or limitation of movement of the back: with onset over days to months originally

Look from the side to see if there is normal lumbar lordosis. Ask the patient to touch toes and watch for movement of spine (rounded?) and hips. Ask to arch backwards, bend to each side and rotate trunk from side to side. Lie patient down and measure length of legs. Raise each straight leg for any restriction before 45°.

Some differential diagnoses and typical outline evidence

Lumbar spinal stenosis due to facet joint osteoarthrosis	*Suggested by:* onset of pain over months worse on walking with ache and weakness in one leg.
	Confirmed by: pain on extension of back. Straight leg raising normal. Few CNS signs (but may appear shortly after exercise).
	Management: OHCS p674.
Spinal tumours primary arising in spinal cord, meninges, nerve roots Secondary usually lung, breast, prostate, thyroid, kidney Lymphoma, myeloma	*Suggested by:* onset of back pain over months with progressive pain or paresis in one or both legs. (Physical signs depend on part of cord or nerve roots affected).
	Confirmed by: 'hot spot' on bone scan with erosion or sclerosis on plain X-ray of 'hot spot'. Space occupying lesion on *MRI* or *CT scan* and **histology on biopsy**.
	Management: OHCS p678.
Pyogenic spinal infection usually of disc space due to staphylococcus, *Salmonella typhi*, etc.	*Suggested by:* onset of pain over days or weeks. Little or no fever, tenderness or raised WBC. ESR raised. Background debilitation, surgery or diabetes.
	Confirmed by: bone rarefaction or erosion with joint space narrowing on **back X-ray**. 'Hot spot' on **isotope bone scan** and space occupying lesion on *MRI* or *CT scan*.
	Management: OHCS p678.
Spinal TB with abscesses and cord compression (Pott's para-plegia), Psoas abscess.	*Suggested by:* onset of weeks or months. Little fever, tenderness or ↑ WBC. ESR ↑. Background debilitation, diabetes.
	Confirmed by: bone rarefaction or erosion with joint space narrowing then wedging of vertebrae. Space occupying lesion on *MRI and CT scan*. Tubercle baccili on stains or **culture of drainage material**.
	Management: OHCS p678.

Pain or limitation of movement of the back: with onset over years

This is a notoriously poor lead. Look from the side to see if there is normal lumbar lordosis. Ask the patient to touch toes and watch for movement of spine (rounded?) and hips. Ask the patient to arch backwards, bend to each side and rotate trunk from side to side. Lie patient down and measure length of legs. Raise each straight leg for any restriction before 45°.

Some differential diagnoses and typical outline evidence

Kyphotic pain	*Suggested by:* onset over years usually, but days with wedge fracture. History of stoop for years usually, but days with wedge fracture. Spinal curvature visible from the side. Associated neuromuscular disease.
	Confirmed by: X-ray appearance suggestive of congenital deformity, Scheurmann's or Calve's osteochondritis, wedge fracture from osteoporosis or carcinoma, ankylosing spondylitis.
	Mangement: OHCS p672.
Scoliotic pain	*Suggested by:* lateral curvature visible from the back and associated rib prominence apparent from the front.
	Confirmed by: history and X-ray appearance of bony congenital anomaly, past poliomyelitis, syringomyelia, torsion dystonia, spinal tumours, spondylolisthesis, arthrogryphosis, enchondromatosis, osteogenesis imperfecta, neurofibromatosis, Chiari malformation, Duchenne muscular dystrophy, Freiderich's ataxia, Marfan's syndrome, Pompe's disease.
	Mangement: OHCS p672.
Idiopathic scoliosis of thoracic or lumbar spine	*Suggested by:* progressive loss over years of horizontal alignment of shoulders and hips with age usually in adolescent girls more than boys.
	Confirmed by: absence of evidence of specific or treatable cause. Increased scoliosis with growth.
	Mangement: OHCS p672.

Pain or limitation of movement of the hip

Assess activity. Test flexion (normal > 120°) by grasping ankle in one hand and iliac crest in the other to eliminate pelvic rotation. Test abduction (normal 30–40°) preventing pelvic tilt. Test abduction in flexion (normal > 70°) and adduction (normal > 30°) by moving one foot over the other, internal and external rotation (normal > 30°). Measure true length of legs from anterior superior iliac spines to medial malleoli. Trendelenburg test is positive if hip drops when foot on that same side is lifted from ground.

Some differential diagnoses and typical outline evidence

Osteoarthritis	*Suggested by:* onset over months or years. Pain, stiffness and limitation of movement, initially of internal rotation.
	Confirmed by: **A-P and lateral X-ray of hips** show loss of joint space, deformity of head and acetabulum with oesteophytes and sclerosis.
	Mangement: OHCS p682.
Coxa vara (angle between neck and femur <125°) caused by congenital slipped upper femoral epiphyses, fracture with malunion or non-union, osteo-malacia or Paget's disease	*Suggested by:* limp with Trendelenburg 'dip' to affected side. True shortening of leg.
	Confirmed by: angle between neck and femur <125° on **X-ray**.
	Mangement: OHCS p680.
Perthes' disease	*Suggested by:* pain in hip or knee with limp with onset over months from 3–11 years of age. Limitation of hip movement in all ranges.
	Confirmed by: **A-P and lateral X-ray** of hips show widening of joint space and ↓ in size of femoral head, patchy density and later collapse.
	Mangement: OHCS p682.
Slipped femoral epiphysis	*Suggested by:* pain in groin, front of thigh or knee and limping with onset over minutes if acute or weeks to months. Limitation of flexion, abduction and medial rotation.
	Confirmed by: displacement of growth plate visible on **lateral view of hip** (not A-P).
	Mangement: OHCS p682.

Tuberculous arthritis	*Suggested by:* pain and limp in 2–5 year old especially from poor country. Pain and spasm in all directions of movement.
	Confirmed by: rarefaction of bone on **X-ray** then fuzziness of joint margin then erosions. AFB in **biopsy ± culture of synovial membrane**.
	Mangement: OHCS p682.
Developmental dysplasia with dislocation leading to osteoarthritis	*Suggested by:* pain, stiffness and restricted movement in childhood or adolescence if undiagnosed (*or* noisy reduction of dislocation in neonatal click test).
	Confirmed by: shallow acetabulum with or without current dislocation on **A-P and lateral X-ray of hips** (or ultrasound in neonate).
	Mangement: OHCS p684.

Pain or limitation of movement of the knee

Look for quadriceps wasting ability to weight bear, deformity of the knee or swelling. Feel for swelling with palm of other hand pressing above patella. Compare flexion and extension on both sides. Abduct and adduct tibia with knee flexed at 30° to test medial and lateral ligaments. With knee flexed at 90° pull and push tibia to test anterior and posterior cruciate ligaments.

Some differential diagnoses and typical outline evidence

Osteoarthritis	*Suggested by:* onset of months or years, worse in cold and damp. Deformity (especially varus—bow legged) and swelling. Crepitus on passive movement.
	Confirmed by: above history and examination. Loss of joint space on X-ray with deformity, ostephytes and sclerosis.
	Mangement: OHCS p670.
Chondromalacia patellae	*Suggested by:* patella aching after sitting in young adults. Patellar tenderness.
	Confirmed by: above history and examination or softening or fibrillation of patellar cartilage on arthroscopy or MRI.
	Mangement: OHCS p688.
Recurrent patella subluxation	*Suggested by:* knee often giving way (especially in knocked-kneed girls).
	Confirmed by: above increased lateral movement of patella.
	Mangement: OHCS p688.
Patella tendinopathy (jumper's knee)	Suggested by: pain on forceful movement of knee in sport.
	Confirmed by: tenderness over patellar tendon.
	Mangement: OHCS p688.
Ileotibial tract syndrome	*Suggested by:* pain when running.
	Confirmed by: tenderness over lateral femoral condyle.
	Mangement: OHCS p688.
Medial shelf syndrome	*Suggested by:* brief locking of knee.
	Confirmed by: inflamed synovial fold above medial meniscus on arthroscopy.
	Mangement: OHCS p688.
Hoffa's fat pad syndrome	*Suggested by:* brief locking of knee and pain under patella.
	Confirmed by: hypertrophic pad between articular surfaces on MRI or arthroscopy.
	Mangement: OHCS p688.

Acute arthritis due to sepsis, gout or rheumatoid arthritis	*Suggested by:* onset over hours or days of pain and swelling.
	Confirmed by: aspiration, microscopy and culture. Urate ↑ in gout. Rheumatoid factor +ve in RA.
	Mangement: OHCS p690.
Meniscal cyst	*Suggested by:* variable swelling, worse when knee flexed to 60°, less when flexed further. Knee clicking and giving way.
	Confirmed by: cyst present on MRI scan.
	Mangement: OHCS p690.
Ligament tears	*Suggested by:* sudden pain and swelling after forceful abduction or adduction at knee.
	Confirmed by: above history and tenderness on examination.
	Mangement: OHCS p752.
Anterior cruciate tears	*Suggested by:* history of posterior blow or rotational force when foot fixed to ground.
	Confirmed by: tibia moves forward when pulled (after effective analgesia or anaesthesia).
	Mangement: OHCS p752.
Meniscal tear	*Suggested by:* history of forceful twisting to a flexed knee. Knee locks when extension attempted.
	Confirmed by: tear visible on MRI scan.
	Mangement: OHCS p752.
Osteochondritis dessicans	*Suggested by:* pain and after exercise, intermittent knee swelling and locking.
	Confirmed by: defect on articular surface on X-ray.
	Mangement: OHCS p690.
Loose bodies due to osteochondritis dessicans, osteoarthritis, chip fractures, synovial chondromatosis	*Suggested by:* locking of knee during extension and flexion. Swelling and effusion.
	Confirmed by: seeing loose bodies on arthoscopy.
	Mangement: OHCS p690.
Bursitis (without or with infection) due to prepatellar bursitis (house-maid's knee) etc	*Suggested by:* localised pain and swelling over site of bursa (e.g. below patella).
	Confirmed by: localised pain and swelling over site of bursa. Improvement with rest, analgesia and physiotherapy.
	Mangement: OHCS p690.

Pain or limitation of movement of the foot

Watch gait, examine wear on shoe sole, and print on floor of damp foot. Ask to extend or dorsiflex (normal > 25°), flex (normal 30°) evert and invert. Ask to extend toes (normal > 60°) and stand on tiptoe. See also *OHCS* p640.

Some differential diagnoses and typical outline evidence

Hallux valgus Associated with bunion and osteoarthritis	*Suggested by:* big toe deviated laterally.
	Confirmed by: above clinical appearance (big toe deviated laterally).
	Mangement: OHCS p692.
Pes planus	*Suggested by:* loss of medial foot arch, (appearance of damp surface in contact with floor, normal in early childhood). Pain if foot and heel everted in some.
	Confirmed by: above clinical appearance and response to exercises and medial heel shoe wedges in some cases.
	Mangement: OHCS p692.
Pes cavus idiopathic, due to spina bifida, past polio	*Suggested by:* accentuated foot arches and other neurological disorders e.g spina bifida.
	Confirmed by: above clinical appearance.
	Mangement: OHCS p692.
Hammer toes	*Suggested by:* tip of toe points downwards.
	Confirmed by: toe extended at the M-P joint, flexed at the proximal I-P joint but extended at the distal I-P joint.
	Mangement: OHCS p692.
Claw toes	*Suggested by:* tip of toe points down and back.
	Confirmed by: toe extended at the M-P joint, flexed at the proximal I-P and distal I-P joint.
	Mangement: OHCS p692.
Hallux rigidus	*Suggested by:* pain localised proximal to big toe.
	Confirmed by: tenderness and swelling of 1st M-P joint. X-ray may show a distal ring of osteophytes.
	Mangement: OHCS p692.

Metatarsalgia due to shoe pressure, previous trauma, rheumatoid arthritis, sesamoid fracture, synovitis	*Suggested by:* pain in fore-foot.
	Confirmed by: tenderness of heads of metatarsals.
	Mangement: OHCS p694.
Morton's metatarsalgia due to inter-digital neuroma	*Suggested by:* localised sharp pain on dorsum of foot with radiation between 2 metatarsals down to toes.
	Confirmed by: tenderness on compression of site of neuroma between metatarsals.
	Mangement: OHCS p694.
March fracture	*Suggested by:* localised foot pain after excessive walking.
	Confirmed by: tenderness of 2nd or 3rd metatarsal. X-ray showing fracture.
	Mangement: OHCS p694.
Calcaneum disease; arthritis of subtalar joint; tear of calcaneal tendon; post calaneal bursitis; plantar fasciitis; etc.	*Suggested by:* localised heel pain.
	Confirmed by: **MRI scan** appearance.

General examination physical signs

General principles

The findings are discussed in a sequence of the general examination. You will have been looking at the patient's face during the history. If you are asked to look at the hands, look at the patient's face and note any recognisable features of significance as you introduce yourself and greet the patient. Then begin with finger nail and joints, backs and fronts of hands, arms, elbows, moving up to the neck and scalp, then down to the face, mouth, the throat, the breasts, axillae, trunk and groin. Note any skin abnormalities.

Fingernail abnormality

Classify fingernail changes by 'naming' them first (see *OHCM* p37). Some have very few causes.

Classification

Clubbing due to many causes (see pp234–5)	*Suggested by:* angle lost between nail and finger (no gap when nails of same finger on both hand apposed, bogginess of nail bed, increased nail curvature both longitudinally and transversely and drum-stick finger appearance—see *OHCM* p55).
	Confirmed by: see p223.
Terry's lines due to many causes (see p236)	*Suggested by:* nail tips having dark pink or brown bands.
	Confirmed by: see following page.
Nail fold infarcts due to vasculitis due to many causes (see following page)	*Suggested by:* dark blue-black areas in nail fold.
	Confirmed by: see following page.
Koilonychia due to iron deficiency anaemia (occasionally ischaemic heart disease or syphilis)	*Suggested by:* spoon shaped nails.
	Confirmed by: ↓*Hb*, ↓*ferritin* from iron deficiency (basal or exercise *ECG* for *IHD*; **serology** for syphilis).
Onycholysis due to psoriasis, hyperthyroidism	*Suggested by:* nail thickened, dystrophic and separated from the nail bed.
	Confirmed by: clinical appearance and evidence of cause e.g. skin changes of psoriasis or ↑*FT4*, ± ↑*FT3* and ↓*TSH*.
Beau's lines due to any period of severe illness	*Suggested by:* transverse furrows.
	Confirmed by: history of associated condition.
Longitudinal lines due to Lichen planus, alopecia areata, Darier's disease	*Suggested by:* transverse furrows (ending in triangular nicks and nail dystrophy in Darier's disease).

Onychomedesis due to any period of severe illness	*Suggested by:* shedding of nail.
	Confirmed by: history of associated condition.
Muehrcke's lines due to hypoalbuminaemia	*Suggested by:* paired white parallel transverse bands.
	Confirmed by: serum albumin <20g/L.
Nail pitting due to psoriais and alopecia areata	*Suggested by:* small holes in nail.
	Confirmed by: rash on extensor surfaces with silvery scales (psoriasis) or circumscribed areas of hair loss (alopecia areata).
Splinter haemorrhages due to infective endocarditis (sometimes due to manual labour)	*Suggested by:* fine longitudinal haemorrhagic streaks under the nail.
	Confirmed by: history of manual labour (or fever, changing heart murmurs and bacterial growth on several **blood cultures**).
Chronic paronychia due to chronic infection of nail bed	*Suggested by:* red, swollen and thickened skin in nail fold.
	Confirmed by: response to anitibiotics (erythromycin for bacterial infection or nystatin for fungal infection).
Mee's lines due to arsenic poisoning or renal failure, Hodgin's disease, heart failure	*Suggested by:* single, white transverse bands.
	Confirmed by: presence of associated conditions.
'Yellow' nails due to lymphoedema, bronchiectasis, hypoalbuminaemia	*Suggested by:* colour!
	Confirmed by: presence of associated condition.

Clubbing

Present when the angle is lost between nail and finger (no gap when nails of same finger on both hand apposed—see *OHCM* p55).

Some differential diagnoses and typical outline evidence

Subacute bacterial endocarditis	*Suggested by:* general malaise, weight loss, fever, PMH of heart valve disease or congenital heart disease, heart murmurs.
	Confirmed by: growth on **blood cultures** of organism e.g. *Strep. viridans*, etc. Endocardial vegetations on (but not always) on **echocardiography**.
	Management: OHCM p152.
Cyanotic congenital heart disease	*Suggested by:* long past history, central cyanosis.
	Confirmed by: **echocardiogram** appearances.
	Management: OHCM p160.
Bronchial carcinoma	*Suggested by:* malaise, increased cough, weight loss, haemoptysis. Smoking history. Opacity (suggestive of mass, ± pneumonia ± effusion) on **CXR** and **CT scan**.
	Confirmed by: **Bronchoscopy** appearances and histology.
	Management: OHCM p182.
Bronchiectasis	*Suggested by:* chronic cough, productive of copious purulent often rusty coloured sputum.
	Confirmed by: **CXR** and **CT scan** appearances (thickened 'tram line' (dilated) bronchi). **Bronchoscopy** appearances.
	Management: OHCM pp178, 179.
Lung abscess	*Suggested by:* cough, very ill, spiking fever, PMH of lung disease.
	Confirmed by: **CXR:** mass containing fluid level (air above pus).
	Management: OHCM p176.
Empyema	*Suggested by:* cough, very ill, fever, stony dull over one lung.
	Confirmed by: high neutrophil WBC. **CXR:** long opacity on one view. Aspiration of pus, culture and sensitivity.
	Management: OHCM p176.

Fibrosing alveolitis	*Suggested by:* cough, fine crackles, especially bases.
	Confirmed by: **CXR**: bilateral diffuse nodular shadows or honeycombing (late finding).
	Management: OHCM p200.
Cirrhosis	*Suggested by:* long history of alcohol intake, ascites, prominent abdominal veins. In males: spider naevi, gynaecomastia.
	Confirmed by: ↓**serum albumin**, abnormal **liver function tests** and ↑bilirubin (sometimes). **Liver biopsy** findings.
	Management: OHCM p232.
Crohn's disease	*Suggested by:* history of chronic diarrhoea and abdominal pain, low weight.
	Confirmed by: **colonoscopy** and biopsy, **barium** enema and **barium meal** and follow through.
	Management: OHCM p246.
Ulcerative colitis	*Suggested by:* history of intermittent diarrhoea with blood and mucus, low weight.
	Confirmed by: **colonoscopy** and biopsy.
	Management: OHCM p246.

Terry's lines: dark pink or brown bands on nails

Some differential diagnoses and typical outline evidence

Cirrhosis	*Suggested by:* long history of alcohol intake, ascites, prominent abdominal veins. In males: spider naevi, gynaecomastia.
	Confirmed by: ↓serum albumin, abnormal **liver function tests** and ↑bilirubin (sometimes). **Liver biopsy** findings.
	Management: OHCM p232.
Congestive cardiac failure	*Suggested by:* dyspnoea, orthopnoea, PND, ↑JVP, gallop rhythm, basal inspiratory crackles, ankle oedema.
	Confirmed by: **CXR** and echocardiography.
	Management: OHCM pp136–9.
Diabetes mellitus	*Suggested by:* thirst, polydipsia, polyuria, fatigue, FH.
	Confirmed by: **fasting blood glucose** ≥ 7.0mmol/L on two occasions OR fasting, random or **GTT** glucose ≥ 11.1mmol/L once only with symptoms.
	Management: OHCM pp292–9.
Cancer somewhere	*Suggested by:* weight loss and anorexia with symptoms developing over months, bone pain.
	Confirmed by: careful history, examination, **CXR, FBC, ESR** and follow up.
Old age	*Suggested by:* age >75 years.
	Confirmed by: normal follow up.

Vasculitic nodules on fingers

Nodules and dark lines in nail folds which are focal areas infarction, which suggest local vasculitis.

Some differential diagnoses and typical outline evidence

Systemic lupus erythematosis	*Suggested by:* swelling of distal inter-phalyngeal joints, any other large joints, malar rash, pleural effusion especially in Afro-Caribbean female. Multisystem dysfunction.
	Confirmed by: FBC: ↓Hb, ↓WBC. *ESR:*↑ or ↑*CRP*. ***Anti-nuclear antibody*** +ve, esp. if directed at **double stranded DNA**.
	Management: OHCM p422.
Subacute bacterial endocarditis ('Osler nodes')	*Suggested by:* general malaise, pallor, low grade fever, changing heart murmurs.
	Confirmed by: FBC: ↓Hb, ↑WBC. *ESR:*↑↑, ↑↑*CRP*. Growth of streptococci, e.g. viridians after **serial blood cultures**.
	Management: OHCM p152.

Hand arthropathy

Look at the finger joints (the inter-phalyngeal or I-P joints) the knuckles (the metacarpo-phalyngeal or M-P joints) and compare. Finally look at the wrist.

Some differential diagnoses and typical outline evidence

Primary (post menopausal) osteoarthrosis	*Suggested by:* Heberden's nodes (paired bony nodes on terminal I-P joints).
	Confirmed by: **X-ray** appearances of affected joints.
	Management: OHCM p416.
Rheumatoid arthritis	*Suggested by:* swelling and deformity phalyngeal joints (with ulnar deviation), wrist, and 'rheumatoid nodules'.
	Confirmed by: +ve **rheumatoid factor**. **X-ray** appearances of affected joints.
	Management: OHCM pp414–15.
Psoriatic arthropathy	*Suggested by:* swelling and deformity of distal (or all) I-P joints.
	Confirmed by: dry rash with silvery scales (especially near elbow extensor surface). **X-ray** appearances of affected joints.
Systemic lupus erythematosis	*Suggested by:* swelling and deformity of all (or distal) I-P joints, butterfly facial rash, signs of pleural/pericardial effusion, renal impairment.
	Confirmed by: +ve **anti-nuclear factor, ds DNA antibodies**.
	Management: OHCM p422.

Hand and upper limb rashes

Look at the back of the hands and forearm, the palms and forearm elbow flexures, the extensor surface of the elbows, then the upper arm.

Some differential diagnoses and typical outline evidence

Atopic eczema	*Suggested by:* vesicles, erythema, scaling, lichenification, fissures on flexor surfaces, wrists, palms. FH.
	Confirmed by: no evidence of contact precipitant.
	Management: OHCS p596.
Contact dermatitis and irritant	*Suggested by:* vesicles, erythema, scaling, lichenification, fissures related to contact with chemical or object. e.g. oil, nickel alloy.
	Confirmed by: response by improvement on removal of precipitant (and recurrence with re-exposure).
	Management: OHCS p596.
Psoriasis	*Suggested by:* dry rash with silvery scales (especially near elbow extensor surface).
	Confirmed by: clinical appearance if obvious, otherwise, **histology**.
	Management: OHCS p594.

Lumps around the elbow

Inspect and, with care not to hurt, palpate.

Some differential diagnoses and typical outline evidence

Osteoarthritis	*Suggested by:* joint deformity, intermittent pain and swelling, paired Heberden's nodes over distal I-P joints in primary osteoarthritis.
	Confirmed by: clinical appearance usually. If doubts, −ve **rheumatoid factor** and **X-ray** shows loss of joint space (due to atrophy of cartilage).
	Management: OHCM p416, OHCS p666.
Rheumatoid nodules	*Suggested by:* mobile subcutaneous nodule.
	Confirmed by: history or joint changes of rheumatoid arthritis and +ve **rheumatoid factor**.
	Management: OHCM pp414–15.
Xanthomatosis	*Suggested by:* pale subcutaneous plaques attached to underlying tendon.
	Confirmed by: **hyperlipidaemia** on blood testing.
	Management: OHCM pp706–7.
Gouty tophi	*Suggested by:* irregular hard nodules, risk factors or PMH of gout.
	Confirmed by: ↑**plasma urate**. **Biopsy:** urate crystals present.
	Management: OHCM p416.

Neck stiffness

Distinguish between limited range of neck movement and neck stiffness throughout range of movement.

- **Limited neck range of movement.**

Some differential diagnoses and typical outline evidence

Chronic cervical spondylosis with osteophytes	*Suggested by:* no fever or associated symptoms.
	Confirmed by: Limitation in range of neck movement but no stiffness within free range of movement. Normal **WBC**, no fever, no neurological signs, X-ray appearance of neck.
	Management: OHCM pp396, 397.

- **Neck stiffness throughout range of movement.**

Bacterial meningitis	*Suggested by:* gradual headache over days, photophobia, vomiting. Fever, high neutrophil count. Petechial rash in meningococcal meningitis.
	Confirmed by: **lumbar puncture:** turbid CSF. ↑CSF neutrophil count with ↓glucose. Bacteria on microscopy. Growth of bacteria on culture of CSF.
	Management: OHCM pp368–71.
Viral meningitis	*Suggested by:* gradual headache over days. Fever, high lymphocyte count, normal neutrophil count.
	Confirmed by: **lumbar puncture:** clear CSF. ↑ CSF lymphocyte count with normal glucose. No bacteria on microscopy. No growth of bacteria on CSF culture.
	Management: OHCM p368.
Meningism due to viral infection	*Suggested by:* gradual headache over days. Fever, high lymphocyte count, normal neutrophil count.
	Confirmed by: **lumbar puncture:** clear CSF. Normal CSF white cell count. No bacteria on microscopy. No growth of bacteria on CSF culture.
Subarachnoid haemorrhage	*Suggested by:* sudden onset of headache over seconds. Variable degree of consciousness. No fever. Normal white cell count.
	Confirmed by: **CT** or **MRI brain scan. Lumbar puncture:** blood stained CSF that does not clear in successive bottle collection, or presence of xanthochromia in CSF (12 hrs to 2 weeks after the haemorrhage).
	Management: OHCM pp362, 363, 752.

Acute cervical spondylitis	*Suggested by:* gradual neck pain (occasionally a headache) over hours or days. Immobile neck. Usually past history of similar episodes. No fever.
	Confirmed by: above history.
	Management: OHCM pp396, 397.
Posterior fossa tumour	*Suggested by:* headache, papilloedema.
	Confirmed by: CT or *MRI scan* appearances.
	Management: OHCM pp386, 387.
Anxiety with semi-voluntary resistance	*Suggested by:* improvement with reassurance or temporary distraction.
	Confirmed by: resolution after rest and observation.

Hair loss in a specific area

Examine overall and then gently part hair to examine scalp. Use magnifying glass if hair is abnormal.

Some differential diagnoses and typical outline evidence

Alopecia areata	*Suggested by:* well circumscribed loss with exclamation mark hairs.
	Confirmed by: above clinical appearance.
	Management: OHCS p602.
Alopecia totalis	*Suggested by:* total hair loss on head and body.
	Confirmed by: above clinical appearance.
	Management: OHCS p602.
Polycystic ovary syndrome	*Suggested by:* bitemporal recession and occipital thinning. Hirsutism on trunk. Onset near puberty. Obesity.
	Confirmed by: ↑testosterone and ↓SHBG. ↑LH, ovarian ultrasound scan.
	Management: OHCM p316; *OHCS* p252.
Testosterone secreting ovarian tumour	*Suggested by:* bitemporal recession and occipital thinning. Rapid onset over months.
	Confirmed by: ↑↑testosterone and ↓LH, ovarian ultrasound scan ± laparoscopy.
	Management: OHCS pp280–3.

Diffuse hair loss

Examine trunk, pubic and limb hair too.

Some differential diagnoses and typical outline evidence

Cytotoxic drugs	*Suggested by:* mainly head hair loss. History of recent cytotoxic drugs.
	Confirmed by: improvement after stopping cytotoxic drug.
Iron deficiency	*Suggested by:* mainly head hair loss. Koilonychia, pallor of conjunctivae.
	Confirmed by: ↓Hb, ↓MCV, ↓MCHC ↓ ferritin.
	Management: OHCM p624, 626.
Severe illness	*Suggested by:* mainly head hair loss. History of recent severe illness.
	Confirmed by: improvement with restoration of health.
Hypogonadism	*Suggested by:* loss of hair from axilla, pubic area.
	Confirmed by: testosterone ↓ or oestrogen ↓ with FSH ↑ and ↑ LH in primary gonadal failure; ↓LH or normal, ↓FSH or normal in secondary hypogonadism.
	Management: OHCM p318.
Recent pregnancy	*Suggested by:* mainly head hair loss. Recent pregnancy.
	Confirmed by: improvement after delivery.

External ear abnormalities

Inspect the pinna for scars and other abnormalities. Examine the auditory meatus by first pulling the pinna up and back to straighten the cartilaginous bend. (In infants, pinna is pulled back and down.) Swab any discharge, and remove any wax.

Some differential diagnoses and typical outline evidence

Congenital anomalies	*Suggested by:* accessory tags, auricles and pre-auricular pit, sinus, or fistula and atresia.
	Confirmed by: above clinical appearances.
	Management: OHCS p538.
Infected preauricular sinus	*Suggested by:* looking like infected sebaceous cyst.
	Confirmed by: deep tract that lies close to the facial nerve.
	Management: OHCS p538.
Chondrodermatitis nodularis chronica helicis	*Suggested by:* painful nodular lesions on the upper margin of the pinna in men.
	Confirmed by: excision of skin and underlying cartilage.
	Management: OHCS p538.
Pinna haematoma resulting in a 'cauliflower' ear	*Suggested by:* history of blunt trauma.
	Confirmed by: appearance of bleeding in the subperi-chondrial plane that elevates the perichondrium to form a haematoma.
	Management: OHCS p538.
Exostosis (localised bony hypertrophy) may cause build up of wax or debris or conductive deafness	*Confirmed by:* smooth, often multiple (bilateral) swellings of the bony ear canals.
	Management: OHCS p538.
Wax (cerumen)—may cause conductive deafness if it impacts	*Suggested by:* dark brown shiny soft mass.
	Confirmed by: improvement in hearing after removal.
	Management: OHCS p538.
Foreign bodies in the ear	*Suggested by:* visible foreign body and inflammation (in child or learning disabled patient).
	Confirmed by: retrieval of foreign body.
	Management: OHCS p538.

Painful ear

Consider referred pain from neck, (C3, C4 and C5), throat, and teeth and examine these too. Insert the largest comfortable aural speculum gently.

Some differential diagnoses and typical outline evidence

Otitis externa (Swimmer's ear) due to eczema, psoriasis, trauma, *Pseudomonas*, fungal infection	*Suggested by:* pain, discharge, and tragal tenderness.
	Confirmed by: acute inflammation of the skin of the meatus, *culture* of swab.
	Management: OHCS p542.
Malignant necrotising otitis externa	*Suggested by:* pain, discharge, and tragal tenderness in a diabetic, elderly or immunosuppressed person, facial palsy.
	Confirmed by: **X-ray** showing local bone erosion, isotope bone scan and white cell scan.
	Management: OHCS p542.
Furunculosis (staphylococcal abscess in hair follicle) often diabetic	*Suggested by:* acutely painful throbbing ear.
	Confirmed by: appearance of a boil in the meatus.
	Management: OHCS p542.
Bullous myringitis (associated with influenza infection or *Mycoplasma pneumoniae*)	*Suggested by:* extremely painful haemorrhagic blisters on the drum and deep meatal skin, and fluid behind the drum.
	Confirmed by: above clinical appearance.
	Management: OHCS p542.
Barotrauma (aerotitis)	*Suggested by:* history of ear pain during descent in an aircraft or diving.
	Confirmed by: relief by decompression (e.g. holding nose and swallowing).
	Management: OHCS p542.
Temporo-mandibular joint dysfunction	*Suggested by:* earache, facial pain, and joint clicking/popping related to malocclusion, teeth-grinding or joint derangement, and stress.
	Confirmed by: tenderness exacerbated by lateral movement of the open jaw, or trigger points in the pterygoids.
	Management: OHCS p542.

Discharging ear

Examine the eardrum quadrants in turn. Note colour, translucency, and any bulging or retraction of the membrane. Note size, position and site (marginal or central) of any perforations. Drum movement during a Valsalva manoeuvre also depends on a patient's eustachian tube.

Some differential diagnoses and typical outline evidence

Acute otitis media (due to pneumococcus, haemophilus, streptococcus and staphylococcus, occasionally complicated by mastoiditis)	*Suggested by:* rapid onset over hours of pain and fever, irritability, anorexia, or vomiting after viral upper respiratory tract infection. *Confirmed by:* bulging red drum or profuse purulent discharge for 48 hours after drum perforates. *Management:* OHCS p544.
Otitis media with effusion (serous, secretory, or glue ear) usually in young children	*Suggested by:* gradual onset over weeks or months of deafness and intermittent ear pain. *Confirmed by:* loss of drum's light reflex or retraction relieved by grommets. *Management:* OHCS p544.
Chronic suppurative otitis media (may be associated with cholesteatoma, petrositis, labyrinthitis; facial palsy; meningitis; intracranial abscess)	*Suggested by:* purulent discharge, hearing loss, but no pain. *Confirmed by:* central drum perforation. *Management:* OHCS p544.
Cholesteatoma (locally destructive stratified squamous epithelium)	*Suggested by:* foul discharge, deafness, headache, ear pain, facial paralysis, and vertigo. *Confirmed by:* continuing mucopurulent discharge, pearly white soft matter (keratin) in attic or posterior marginal perforation. *Management:* OHCS p544.

Chronic otitis externa	*Suggested by:* watery discharge, itching.
	Confirmed by: erythema and weeping of meatus.
	Management: OHCS p542.
Auditory canal trauma	*Suggested by:* bloody discharge.
	Confirmed by: history of trauma, laceration and erythema.
	Management: OHCS p544.
CSF otorrhoea	*Suggested by:* history of head or facial trauma or surgery.
	Confirmed by: halo sign on filter paper.
	Management: OHCS p544.

Striking facial appearance

Best recognised when meeting patient for the first time, but there is a wide normal variation.

Some differential diagnoses and typical outline evidence

Parkinson's disease	*Suggested by:* mask-like (akinetic) face ± hand or head tremor.
	Confirmed by: response to dopaminergic drugs.
	Management: OHCM p382.
Huntington's chorea (or drug effect)	*Suggested by:* choreiform—jerky, purposeless facial movement or athetosis (writhing facial movement).
	Confirmed by: family history, or response to withdrawal of drug or dose reduction (if due to drug effect).
	Management: OHCM p726.
Bilateral upper motor neurone lesion (due to motor neurone disease, cerebrovascular disease, myasthenia gravis)	*Suggested by:* paucity of movement of face.
	Confirmed by: other features of cause and *MRI* or *CT scan*.
Thyrotoxicosis	*Suggested by:* anxious looking with lid retraction and lag.
	Confirmed by: ↓TSH and ↑T3 or ↑T4 or both.
	Management: OHCM p304.
Hypothyroidism	*Suggested by:* puffy face, obesity, cold intolerance, tiredness, constipation, bradycardia.
	Confirmed by: ↑TSH, ↓FT4.
	Management: OHCM p306.
Acromegaly	*Suggested by:* large wide face, embossed forehead, jutting jaw (prognathism) widely spaced teeth and large tongue.
	Confirmed by: *IGF* ↑. Failure to suppress GH to <2mU/L with *oral GTT*. *Skull X-ray* confirm bony abnormalities. *Hand X-ray* shows typical tufts on terminal phalanges. *MRI* or *CT scan* showing enlarged pituitary fossa.
	Management: OHCM p324.

Cushing's syndrome pituitary-driven Cushing's disease, or autonomous adrenal Cushing's, or glucocorticoid therapy	*Suggested by:* round, florid face (and trunk with purple striae) with thin arms and legs, hirsutism in ♀. Inability to rise from squatting position (due to proximal myopathy). *Confirmed by:* midnight cortisol ↑ and/or failure to suppress on dexamethasone 0.5mg 6 hourly or drug history of glucocorticoids. *Management: OHCM* pp310, 311.

Proptosis of eye(s) or exophthalmos

Prominent eye suggested by sclera showing between the cornea and upper lid margin (may also be due to lid retraction due to sympathetic over-activity or lung disease). If in doubt look down on eyes from above. (In myopia there is a large eyeball but the sclera is not visible.)

Some differential diagnoses and typical outline evidence

Ophthalmic Graves disease (± thyrotoxicosis)	*Suggested by:* bilateral (usually) exophthalmos, goitre, pretibial myxoedema and lid retraction.
	Confirmed by: titre of thyroid antibodies ↑↑ (with ↓TSH or normal, and T3 or T4 ↑or normal). *CT* scan appearance.
	Management: OHCM p305.
Orbital cellulitis (medical emergency)	*Suggested by:* pain, fever, unilateral lid swelling, decreased vision and double vision. Neurological signs in advanced disease.
	Confirmed by: **CT or MRI scan** appearance and response to antibiotics.
	Management: OHCS p420.
Cortico-cavernous fistula	*Suggested by:* unilateral engorgement of eye surface vessels, lid and conjunctiva, pulsatile with bruit over eye.
	Confirmed by: **CT or MRI scan** appearance.
	Management: OHCS p420.
Orbital tumours—rarely primary, often secondary, especially reticulosis	*Suggested by:* unilateral proptosis and displacement of the eyeball. Lymph node, liver or spleen enlargement.
	Confirmed by: **CT or MRI scan** appearance.
	Management: OHCS p420.

Red eye

Gritty pain suggests external cause. Aching pain suggests internal cause. Light sensitivity always accompanies inflammation in the eye. Fluoresceine (Fl) yellow dye glows green with a blue examination light and stains all epithelial breaks.

Some differential diagnoses and typical outline evidence

Spontaneous sub-conjunctival haemorrhage	*Suggested by:* painless bright red area on conjunctiva (oxygenated blood) and no light sensitivity.
	Confirmed by: clinical appearance and resolution over days. No Fl staining of cornea (not done often).
	Management: OHCS p432.
Conjunctivitis due to bacterial infection	*Suggested by:* red eyes, dilated blood vessels on the eyeball and the tarsal (lid) conjunctiva with a purulent discharge ± bilateral ± gritty pain.
	Confirmed by: above clinical appearance. Not light sensitive and no Fl stain of cornea.
	Management: OHCS p432.
Conjunctivitis due to viral infection	*Suggested by:* red eyes with dilated vessels on the eyeball only, sometimes in one quadrant around the cornea with a watery 'tap running' discharge. Gritty pain ± impaired vision.
	Confirmed by: Fl stain showing dendritic (branching) pattern and resolution with topical antiviral.
	Management: OHCS p432.
Conjunctivitis due to allergy	*Suggested by:* red eyes with pink swollen conjunctiva and white stringy mucoid discharge.
	Confirmed by: no Fl stain and no visual loss and resolution with chromoglycate (over six weeks) or steroid eye drops.
	Management: OHCS p432.
Corneal ulcer (ulcerative keratitis) due to abrasion or Herpes simplex, *Pseudomonas*, *Candida*, *Aspergillus*, protozoa	*Suggested by:* painful, light-sensitive, deeply red eye with yellowish abscess in the cornea. Purulent discharge.
	Confirmed by: slit lamp examination after **fluorescein instillation showing** hypopyon (pus in the eye).
	Management: OHCS p432.

Episcleritis	*Suggested by:* localised red eye with superficial vessel dilatation. Mild pain. No visual loss or light sensitivity.
	Confirmed by: Instillation of one drop of phenylephrine 2.5% causing a blanching of the lesion.
	Management: OHCS p432.
Scleritis	*Suggested by:* localised area of dark red dilated superficial and deep vessel on the sclera with aching pain and tenderness.
	Confirmed by: failure to blanche with one drop of 2.5% phenylephrine.
	Management: OHCS p432.
Acute closed-angle glaucoma (emergency)	*Suggested by:* severely painful red eyeball with marked visual loss, accompanied by nausea and vomiting ± history of haloes around lights and severe headache with blurred vision.
	Confirmed by: dull grey cornea, non reacting and irregular pupil with raised ocular pressures.
	Management: OHCS p430.
Iritis or uveitis (see page 264)	*Suggested by:* redness around cornea and haze in front of iris and severe light sensitivity (photophobia).
	Confirmed by: small non-reacting and irregular pupil. Slit lamp examination showing flare, cells and hypopyon (pus in eye).
	Management: OHCS p430.

Iritis (anterior uveitis)

Redness in cornea next to iris (circumcorneal injection), with muddy appearance of fluid in front of iris. OHCS p430.

Some differential diagnoses and typical outline evidence

Trauma (usually surgical)	*Suggested by:* impact accident, recent surgery.
	Confirmed by: slit lamp examination showing blood in the front of the eye and 'D' shaped distortion of the pupil if torn from its base or perforation if the pupil is pointing.
Infection:	*Suggested by:* general malaise, fever, leucocytosis.
Herpes simplex, zoster, TB, syphilis, leprosy, protozoa, fungi	*Confirmed by:* **bacteriological culture** of eye swab or **viral immunology**.
Autoimmune diseases:	*Suggested by:* arthritis, anaemia, no obvious fever, raised ESR.
ankylosing spondylitis, Reiter's disease, juvenile chronic arthritis, immune ocular disease	*Confirmed by:* **immunology** (seronegative for Rheumatoid factor). **Protein electrophoresis**.
Sarcoidosis	*Suggested by:* history of dry cough, breathlessness, malaise, fatigue, weight loss, enlarged lacrimal glands, erythema nodosum. Raised serum ACE.
	Confirmed by: **CXR** appearances (e.g. bilateral lymphadenopathy), **tissue biopsy** showing non-caseating granuloma. Slit lamp shows large keratic precipitates.
	Management: OHCM p198.
Ulcerative colitis	*Suggested by:* history of diarrhoea with mucus and blood.
	Confirmed by: **colonoscopy** and **histology of biopsy**.
	Management: OHCM p244.
Crohn's disease	*Suggested by:* history of abdominal pain, diarrhoea, weight loss.
	Confirmed by: **colonoscopy, barium enema** and **meal** and follow through.
	Management: OHCM p246.

Clinical anaemia

Subconjunctival pallor (± face, nail and hand pallor).

Some differential diagnoses and typical outline evidence

Microcytic due to iron deficiency, thalassaemia, etc (see p624)	*Suggested by:* history of blood loss or FH of haemoglobinopathy (esp. in Mediterranean origin) and sideroblastic anaemia.
	Confirmed by: FBC: ↓Hb and ↓MCV, in thalassaemia ↓↓MCV.
Macrocytic (see p626)	*Suggested by:* FH of pernicious anaemia, antifolate and cytotoxic drugs or alcohol.
	Confirmed by: FBC: ↓Hb and ↑MCV. *Film:* hypersegmented polymorphs in B_{12} deficiency.
Normocytic (see p628)	*Suggested by:* history of chronic intercurrent illness e.g. chronic renal failure, anaemia of chronic disease etc.
	Confirmed by: FBC: ↓Hb and MCV normal.
Hypoplastic or aplastic	*Suggested by:* gradual onset without blood loss and potentially causal medication.
	Confirmed by: FBC: ↓Hb and MCV normal and **bone marrow** atrophic.
	Management: OHCM p662.
Leukaemia	*Suggested by:* gradual onset and large spleen or LN (can fall ill suddenly with rapid deterioration in acute leukaemia).
	Confirmed by: ↓Hb and MCV normal, ↑↑WBC and bone marrow replaced by leukaemic cells.
	Management: OHCM p652–6.

Fever

Temperature >37°C. Fever is not a 'good lead'. The causes suggested here are broad.

Some differential diagnoses and typical outline evidence

Infection	*Suggested by:* low grade or high fever with raised white cell count and usually symptoms and signs pointing to a focus.
	Confirmed by: **serology ± cultures** of blood and other body fluids.
Thrombus, tissue necrosis, neoplasm, autoimmune diseases, drugs	*Suggested by:* low grade fever, history of severe illness or trauma.
	Confirmed by: specific tests, e.g. **chest X-ray, Doppler ultrasound scan of leg veins**.

Possible hypothermia

Temperature <35°C—but confirm with low reading thermometer—it could be lower. Also confirm with rectal temperature.

Some differential diagnoses and typical outline evidence

True hypothermia due to prolonged exposure to cold or hypothyroidism	*Suggested by:* history of immersion or cold weather exposure. Temperature <35°C with low reading rectal thermometer.
	Confirmed by: temperature chart using low reading rectal thermometer.
	Management: OHCM p836.

Mouth lesions

Examine lips, buccal mucosa, teeth, tongue, tonsils and pharynx.

Some differential diagnoses and typical outline evidence

Local aphthous ulcers	*Suggested by:* red, painful ulcer with associated lymph node enlargement.
	Confirmed by: spontaneous resolution within days.
Local infection and gingivitis	*Suggested by:* vesicles in herpes simplex, creamy white plaques in oral candidiasis.
	Confirmed by: spontaneous resolution or after antibiotic or antifungal treatment within days.
Carious teeth	*Suggested by:* intermittent toothache, broken and or severely discoloured teeth.
	Confirmed by: formal dental examination.
Traumatic ulceration	*Suggested by:* jagged ulcers or lacerations.
	Confirmed by: history of trauma, injury, ill-fitting dentures, shallow, painful ulcers.
Vitamin deficiency e.g. B_{12}, riboflavine, nicotinic acid	*Suggested by:* atrophic glossitis, fissured tongue; 'raw beef' in B_{12} deficiency, magenta in riboflavin deficiency.
	Confirmed by: response to vitamin supplements.
	Management: OHCM pp250, 738.
Hereditary haemorrhagic telangiectasia	*Suggested by:* telangiectasia on the face, around the mouth, on the lips and tongue, epistaxis, anaemia.
	Confirmed by: family history and examination of relatives.
Peutz–Jegher's syndrome (associated with intestinal polyps)	*Suggested by:* peri-oral pigmentation (not the tongue).
	Confirmed by: finding polyps on **colonoscopy**.
	Management: OHCM p732.

Red pharynx and tonsils

Some differential diagnoses and typical outline evidence

Viral pharyngitis	*Suggested by:* sore throat, pain on swallowing, fever, cervical lymphadenopathy and injected fauces. ↑ lymphocytes, leucocytes normal in WBC.
	Confirmed by: negative **throat swab** for bacterial culture, self-limiting: resolution within days.
Acute follicular tonsillitis (streptococcal)	*Suggested by:* severe sore throat, pain on swallowing, fever, enlarged tonsils with white patches (like strawberries and cream). Cervical lymphadenopathy especially in angle of jaw. Fever, ↑ leucocytes in WBC.
	Confirmed by: **throat swab** for culture and sensitivities of organisms.
	Management: OHCS p564.
Infectious mononucleosis (glandular fever) due to Epstein–Barr virus	*Suggested by:* very severe throat pain with enlarged tonsils covered with creamy membrane. Petechiae on palate. Profound malaise. Generalised lymphadenopathy, splenomegaly.
	Confirmed by: ↑ atypical lymphocytes in **WBC**. **Paul–Bunnel** test positive. **Viral titres**.
	Management: OHCM p570.
Candidiasis of buccal or oesophageal mucosa	*Suggested by:* painful dysphagia, white plaque, history of immunosuppression/diabetes/recent antibiotics.
	Confirmed by: **oesophagoscopy** showing erythema and plaques, **brush cytology ± biopsy** shows spores and hyphae.
	Management: OHCM p210.
Agranulocytosis	*Suggested by:* sore throat, background history of taking a drug or contact with noxious substance.
	Confirmed by: low or absent neutrophil count.
	Management: OHCM p662.
Meningococcal meningitis	*Suggested by:* headache, photophobia, vomiting, sore throat, red fauces without purulent patches, neck stiffness. High blood neutrophil count.
	Confirmed by: lumbar puncture showing pus or neutrophil count and organisms on microscopy or culture.
	Management: OHCM p370.

'Parotid' swelling

Swelling from anterior border of masseter muscle (teeth clenched), to lower half of ear and from zygoma to angle of jaw.

Some differential diagnoses and typical outline evidence

Parotid duct obstruction (usually due to stone)	*Suggested by:* intermittent infection or no discharge from duct.
	Confirmed by: **plain X-ray** showing radio-opaque stone or **sialography** to show filling defect.
Parotid tumour	*Suggested by:* no obvious features of alterative non-malignant or infective condition.
	Confirmed by: urgent surgical referral for **biopsy** or exploration.
Mumps parotitis	*Suggested by:* acute painful swelling of whole gland(s), contact with others cases.
	Confirmed by: bilateral swelling or associated pancreatitis or orchitis. (Rising mumps **viral titre** if doubt.)
Suppurative parotid infection	*Suggested by:* hot tender fluctuant swelling with high fever. No discharge from duct orifice.
	Confirmed by: ↑WBC, response to **drainage** ± antibiotics.
Non-suppurative parotitis from ascending infection along parotid duct	*Suggested by:* unilateral swelling, oral sepsis or poor general condition.
	Confirmed by: fever, ↑WBC discharge from duct orifice. Resolution with antibiotics.
Parotid Sjögren's syndrome	*Suggested by:* dry mouth and eyes with no tears.
	Confirmed by: rheumatoid factor +ve ± anti Ro(SSA) and anti-La(SSB) +ve.
Parotid sarcoidosis	*Suggested by:* history of dry cough, enlarged lacrimal glands erythema nodosum raised serum ACE.
	Confirmed by: **CXR** appearances (e.g. bilateral lymphadenopathy) and tissue biopsy showing non-caseating granuloma.

Lump in the face (non-parotid lesion)

Swelling anterior to border of masseter muscle (teeth clenched).

Some differential diagnoses and typical outline evidence

Preauricular lymph node inflammation	*Suggested by:* tender nodular swelling in front of ear.
	Confirmed by: above clinical features.
Preauricular lymphoma	*Suggested by:* non-tender nodular swelling in front of ear.
	Confirmed by: **biopsy** with or without or excision.
Basal cell carcinoma	*Suggested by:* painless ulcer with rolled edge.
	Confirmed by: **biopsy**.
	Management: OHCM p430.
Sebaceous cyst	*Suggested by:* fluctuant swelling with central punctum.
	Confirmed by: **incision**.
	Management: OHCM p510.
Subcutaneous abscess	*Suggested by:* tender fluctuant swelling.
	Confirmed by: **incision** when pointing.
	Management: OHCM p510.
Dental abscess	*Suggested by:* tenderness of underlying tooth (tap gently).
	Confirmed by: **dental exploration**.
Skin melanoma	*Suggested by:* painless swelling with pigment and red edge.
	Confirmed by: **wide excision biopsy**.
	Management: OHCM p430.

Submandibular lump—not moving with tongue nor on swallowing

Below the mandible and above the digastric muscle.

Some differential diagnoses and typical outline evidence

Mumps sialitis	*Suggested by:* acute painful swelling of whole gland(s), contact with others cases.
	Confirmed by: bilateral swelling or associated pancreatitis or orchitis. (Rising *mumps titre* if doubt.)
Non-suppurative sialitis from ascending infection along duct	*Suggested by:* unilateral swelling, oral sepsis or poor general condition.
	Confirmed by: discharge from duct orifice. Resolution with antibiotics.
	Management: OHCM p515.
Suppurative salivary infection	*Suggested by:* hot tender fluctuant swelling with high fever. No discharge from duct orifice.
	Confirmed by: **ultrasound scan**, response to drainage ± antibiotics.
Salivary duct obstruction (usually due to stone)	*Suggested by:* intermittent infection or no discharge from duct.
	Confirmed by: **ultrasound scan** response to stomaplasty.
	Management: OHCM p515.
Salivary Sjögren's syndrome	*Suggested by:* dry mouth and eyes with no tears.
	Confirmed by: rheumatoid factor +ve, anti-Ro(SSA) and anti-La(SSB) +ve.
Salivary sarcoidosis	*Suggested by:* dry cough, enlarged lacrimal glands and erythema nodosum.
	Confirmed by: **CXR** appearances (e.g. bilateral lymphadenopathy) and tissue biopsy showing non-caseating granuloma.
Salivary tumour due to adeno-carcinoma, squamous cell tumour, etc.	*Suggested by:* no obvious features of alternative non-malignant or infective condition.
	Confirmed by: urgent surgical referral for **biopsy** or **exploration**.
	Management: OHCM p515.

Submandibular lymph node inflammation	*Suggested by:* tender solid nodular swelling between rami of mandible, especially <20 years of age.
	Confirmed by: above clinical features or ***ultrasound scan***.
Submandibular lymph node malignancy	*Suggested by:* non-tender solid nodular swelling between rami of mandible, especially age >20 years.
	Confirmed by: ***ultrasound scan, biopsy*** ± excision.
Ranula	*Suggested by:* transilluminable cyst lateral to midline, with domed bluish discolouration in floor of mouth lateral to frenulum.
	Confirmed by: clinical appearance, ***ultrasound scan,*** and ***histology*** after excision.
Submental dermoid	*Suggested by:* midline cyst and age <20 years.
	Confirmed by: ***histology*** after excison.

Anterior neck lump—moving with tongue and swallowing

Suggest extrathyroid tissue.

Some differential diagnoses and typical outline evidence

Thyroglossal cyst	*Suggested by:* fluctuant cystic lump in midline or just to the left.
	Confirmed by: *ultrasound scan, radioisotope scan* (cyst is cold), CT scan, *histology* of excised tissue.
Ectopic thyroid tissue	*Suggested by:* solid lump in midline or just laterally.
	Confirmed by: *ultrasound scan, radioisotope scan* (nodule may take up iodine), CT scan, *histology* of excised tissue.

Neck lump—moving with swallowing but not with tongue

Suggests a goitre (or attached to thyroid gland). The following are preliminary diagnoses (see also pp284 and 286):

Some differential diagnoses and typical outline evidence

Thyrotoxic goitre	*Suggested by:* sweating, fine tremor, tachycardia, weight loss, lid lag.
	Confirmed by: ↑*FT4*, ± ↑*FT3* and ↓↓*TSH*. US scan, Isotope scan.
	Management: OHCM p304.
Hypothyroid goitre	*Suggested by:* cold intolerance, tiredness, constipation, bradycardia.
	Confirmed by: ↑*TSH*, ↓*FT4*. US scan ± Thyroid antibodies +ve.
	Management: OHCM p304.
Euthyroid goitre	*Suggested by:* no sweating, no fine tremor, no weight change, no cold intolerance, no tiredness, no lid lag, normal bowel habit, normal pulse rate.
	Confirmed by: normal *FT4*, and normal *TSH*.
	Management: OHCM p304.

Bilateral neck mass—moving with swallowing but not with tongue

(Central mass crossing the midline)

Some differential diagnoses and typical outline evidence

Graves disease	*Suggested by:* clinical thyrotoxicosis, exophthalmos, pretibial myxoedema. No nodules.
	Confirmed by: ↑FT4 or ↑FT3 and ↓↓TSH and TSH receptor antibody +ve. Diffuse increased uptake on **thyroid isotope** scan.
	Management: OHCM pp302, 304.
Hashimoto's thyroiditis	*Suggested by:* clinically euthyroid or hypothyroid (or rarely transient thyrotoxicosis). Multiple nodules in large gland.
	Confirmed by: FT4↑ transiently then ↓FT4 and ↑TSH, **thyroid antibodies** titre ↑↑. Diffuse poor uptake on **thyroid isotope scan**.
	Management: OHCM p306.
'Simple' goitre	*Suggested by:* clinically euthyroid. Not nodular.
	Confirmed by: normal FT4 or FT3 and normal TSH and −ve **thyroid antibodies**.
	Management: OHCM p304.
Toxic multinodular goitre	*Suggested by:* multiple nodules and clinically thyrotoxic.
	Confirmed by: ↑FT4 or ↑FT3, and ↓TSH and nodules on **ultrasound scan** or **thyroid isotope scan**.
	Management: OHCM pp304, 516.
Non-toxic multinodular goitre	*Suggested by:* multiple nodules and clinically euthyroid
	Confirmed by: normal FT4 or FT3 and normal TSH. Nodules on **ultra-sound scan** or **thyroid isotope scan.**
	Management: OHCM p516.
Thyroid enzyme deficiency (rare)	*Suggested by:* presentation in childhood, clinically hypothyroid or euthyroid. Not nodular.
	Confirmed by: ↓FT4 or ↓FT3 and ↑TSH but with abnormal (high or low) **radio-iodine uptake**.

Solitary thyroid nodule

(see *OHCM* p516).

Some differential diagnoses and typical outline evidence

Autonomous toxic thyroid nodule	*Suggested by:* single nodule and clinically thyrotoxic (weight loss, frequent bowel movement, ↑ pulse rate, sweats, tremor).
	Confirmed by: ↑ FT4 or FT3, ↓ TSH and single hot nodule thyroid isotope (iodine or technetium) scan.
Thyroid carcinoma: papillary 60% follicular 25% medullary 5% lymphoma 5% anaplastic <1%	*Suggested by:* single nodule and clinically euthyoid.
	Confirmed by: normal FT4 or FT3, normal TSH and single cold nodule thyroid isotope (iodine or technetium) scan. Solid on ultrasound scan. Malignant cells on needle aspiration or removal.
Thyroid adenoma	*Suggested by:* single nodule and clinically euthyoid.
	Confirmed by: normal FT4 or FT3, normal TSH and single cold nodule thyroid isotope (iodine or technetium) scan. Solid on ultrasound scan. No malignant cells on needle aspiration or removal.
Thyroid cyst	*Suggested by:* single nodule and clinically euthyoid.
	Confirmed by: normal FT4 or FT3, normal TSH and single cold nodule thyroid isotope (iodine or technetium) scan. Cystic on ultrasound scan. Disappears on needle aspiration and no malignant cells then or if removed.

Lump in anterior triangle

Below digastric and in front of sternomastoid muscles.

Some differential diagnoses and typical outline evidence

Lymph node inflammation	*Suggested by:* tender, solid nodular swelling especially <20 years of age.
	Confirmed by: above clinical features, CT scan.
Acute abscess	*Suggested by:* hot, tender fluctuant swelling with high fever.
	Confirmed by: clinical features and discharge of pus after incision, US scan, CT scan.
TB ('cold') abscess	*Suggested by:* fluctuant swelling with low grade or no fever.
	Confirmed by: **AFB,** culture and sensitivity of aspirate.
Branchial cyst	*Suggested by:* fluctuant swelling at anterior border of sternomastoid muscle, <20 years of age.
	Confirmed by: US scan, CT scan, surgical anatomy, appearance and **histology** on excision.
Cystic hygroma	*Suggested by:* fluctuant swelling that transilluminates well, <20 years of age.
	Confirmed by: US scan, CT scan, surgical anatomy, appearance and histology on excision or regression with sclerosant.
Pharyngeal pouch	*Suggested by:* intermittent fluctuant swelling (usually on left) and dysphagia.
	Confirmed by: **barium swallow** fills pouch.
Carotid body tumour (chemo-dectoma)	*Suggested by:* mobile arising from carotid bifurcation soft (upper third of sternomastoid) and gently pulsatile.
	Confirmed by: US scan, CT scan, surgical anatomy, appearance and **histology** on excision.

Hodgkin's or non-Hodgkin's lymphoma	*Suggested by:* non-tender solid nodular swelling between rami of mandible, especially >20 years of age, ± fever, weight loss. Chest pain with alcohol in Hodgkin's.
	Confirmed by: US scan, CT scan, ***biopsy*** with or without or excision.
	Management: OHCM pp658, 660.

Lump in posterior triangle of neck

Behind sternomastoid and in front of trapezius.

Some differential diagnoses and typical outline evidence

Acute abscess	*Suggested by:* hot, tender fluctuant swelling with high fever.
	Confirmed by: clinical features and discharge of pus after incision, US scan, CT scan.
Cystic hygroma	*Suggested by:* fluctuant swelling that transilluminates well, <20 years of age.
	Confirmed by: US scan, CT scan, surgical anatomy, appearance and *histology* on excision or regression with sclerosant.
Lymph node inflammation	*Suggested by:* tender, solid nodular swelling especially <20 years of age.
	Confirmed by: clinical features, US scan, CT scan.
Hodgkin's or non-Hodgkin's lymphoma	*Suggested by:* non-tender, solid nodular swelling. Chest pain with alcohol in Hodgkin's.
	Confirmed by: US scan, CT scan, *biopsy* with or without or excision.
	Management: OHCM p658, 660.
Metastasis in lymph node	*Suggested by:* non-tender, solid nodular swelling.
	Confirmed by: US scan, CT scan, *biopsy* ± excision.
Tuberculous ('cold') abscess	*Suggested by:* non-tender, cystic swelling >50 years of age.
	Confirmed by: US scan, CT scan, *aspiration biopsy* or excision, culture of *AFB*.
	Management: OHCM pp564, 566.

Supra clavicular lump(s)

Some differential diagnoses and typical outline evidence

Lymph node inflammation	*Suggested by:* tender, solid nodular swelling especially <20 years of age.
	Confirmed by: clinical features.
Lymphoma	*Suggested by:* rubbery, matted nodes.
	Confirmed by: lymph node **biopsy**.
	Management: OHCM p660.
Lymph node secondary to gastric or lung carcinoma	*Suggested by:* rock-hard, fixed nodes, Virchow's node in left supraclavicular fossa (Troisier's sign).
	Confirmed by: lymph node **biopsy, gastroscopy, bronchoscopy**.
Aneurysm of subclavian artery	*Suggested by:* pulsatile cyst.
	Confirmed by: **ultrasound scan** and **MRI scan** or **angiography**.

Galactorrhoea

Spontaneous or expressible milky fluid.

Some differential diagnoses and typical outline evidence

Primary hyper-prolactinaemia	*Suggested by:* infertility, oligomenorrhoea or amenorrhoea.
	Confirmed by: ↑*prolactin* and normal *TSH* and *T4*. **Pituitary CT or MRI scan:** normal or microadenoma.
	Management: OHCM p322.
Prolactinoma	*Suggested by:* infertility, oligomenorrhoea or amenorrhoea. In large tumours, field defects and loss of secondary sexual characteristics.
	Confirmed by: ↑*prolactin* and normal *TSH* and *T4*. Micro or macro adenoma on **CT or MRI scan pituitary**.
	Management: OHCM p322.
Pregnancy	*Suggested by:* amenorrhoea, frequency of urine etc. in woman of childbearing age.
	Confirmed by: pregnancy test +ve.
Primary hypothyroidism	*Suggested by:* cold intolerance, tiredness, constipation, bradycardia.
	Confirmed by: ↑*TSH*, ↓*FT4*.
	Management: OHCM p306.
Drugs	*Suggested by:* taking chlorpromazine and other major tranquilisers, metoclopramide, domperidone.
	Confirmed by: ↑*prolactin* and ↑*TSH* and ↓*T4*, resolution and lowering of *prolactin* after stopping suspected drug.
	Management: OHCM p322.
'Idiopathic galactorrhoea'	*Suggested by:* galactorrhoea alone, no other findings.
	Confirmed by: normal *prolactin* and *TSH* and *T4*.
	Management: OHCM p322.

Nipple abnormality

Some differential diagnoses and typical outline evidence

Paget's disease of nipple with underlying carcinoma	*Suggested by:* breast nipple 'eczema'.
	Confirmed by: in-situ malignant change on **histological examination** of skin scrapings.
	Management: OHCM p732.
Duct ectasia and chronic infection	*Suggested by:* green or brown nipple discharge.
	Confirmed by: chronic inflammation on **histology** of excised ducts.
	Management: OHCM p504.
Duct papilloma	*Suggested by:* bleeding from nipple.
	Confirmed by: excision of affected ducts. Benign **histology** of excised ducts.
Mamillary fistula	*Suggested by:* discharge from para-areolar region aged 30–40.
	Confirmed by: excision of affected ducts. Benign **histology** of excised ducts.

Breast lump(s)

(see *OHCM* pp504–5)

Some differential diagnoses and typical outline evidence

Benign fibrous mammary dysplasia	*Suggested by:* generally painful breast lumpiness, greatest near axilla. Cyclically related to periods.
	Confirmed by: relief on **aspiration** of cysts, diuretics or oestrogen suppression.
Fibroadenoma	*Suggested by:* smooth and mobile lump ('breast mouse') usually in ages 15–30 years.
	Confirmed by: appearance on mammogram confirmed by benign **histology** after excision.
Cyst(s)	*Suggested by:* spherical, fluctuant lump, single or multiple, painful before periods.
	Confirmed by: cysts on **mammography**, benign tissue after excision.
Acute or chronic abscess	*Suggested by:* fluctuant lump, hot and tender, acute presentation often in puerperium. Chronic after antibiotics.
	Confirmed by: response to drainage, Chronic abscess excision and **histology** to exclude carcinoma.
Fat necrosis or sclerosing adenosis	*Suggested by:* firm, solitary localised lump.
	Confirmed by: appearance on mammogram confirmed by benign **histology** after excision.
Carcinoma infiltrating ductal cancer or invasive lobar cancers	*Suggested by:* some of the following: fixed, irregular, hard, painless lump, nipple retraction, fixed to skin (peau d'orange) or muscle and local, hard or firm, fixed nodes in axilla. Metastases to lymph nodes, or via blood to bones, brain liver, lung and abdominal cavity.
	Confirmed by: ill-defined speculate borders, faint linear or irregular calcification and abnormal adjacent structures on mammography. Malignant **histology after aspiration** or excision.

Gynaecomastia

These findings should have been discovered during the general examination. Breast swelling in male with disc of firm tissue. If there is no disc, it is fatty tissue only.

Some differential diagnoses and typical outline evidence

Immature testis	*Suggested by:* adolescence and no testicular lump.
	Confirmed by: normal testosterone, estrogen and LH levels normal ultrasound scan of testis.
Digoxin, Spironolactone	*Suggested by:* taking of drug and no testicular lump.
	Confirmed by: improvement when drug stopped.
High alcohol intake	*Suggested by:* high alcohol intake and no testicular lump.
	Confirmed by: improvement when alcohol stopped.
Hepatic cirrhosis	*Suggested by:* long history of high alcohol intake (usually), spider naevi, abnormal liver size (large or small) and consistency (fatty or hard).
	Confirmed by: very abnormal biochemical liver function tests, ↓*LH*, ↑*oestrogens*, ↓*testosterone*.
	Management: OHCM p232.
Testicular tumours	*Suggested by:* scrotal mass ± pain, tenderness if haemorrhage occurs. (Sometimes arising in undescended testis).
	Confirmed by: testicular ultrasound, inguinal exploration, ↑*α-fetoprotein*, ↑*β-hCG*.
	Management: OHCM 512.
Hypogonadism (primary to testicular disease, or secondary to low LH from pituitary defect or tumour)	*Suggested by:* sparse pubic hair, no drug or alcohol history, poor libido.
	Confirmed by: **Testosterone↓**, LH↑ (in primary testicular disease), LH↓ or normal (when secondary to pituitary diseases).
	Management: OHCM pp316, 318.
Bronchial carcinoma	*Suggested by:* smoking history, haemoptysis, weight loss, clubbing.
	Confirmed by: **CXR, bronchoscopy** with biopsy.
	Management: OHCM p182.

Klinefelter's syndrome	*Suggested by:* poor sexual development, infertility, eunuchoid.
	Confirmed by: 47, XXY **karyotype**.
Obesity	*Suggested by:* no breast tissue, only mammary fat.
	Confirmed by: improvement with weight loss.
	Management: OHCM p208.

Axillary lymphadenopathy

Axillary lymphadenopathy ± tenderness.

Some differential diagnoses and typical outline evidence

Reaction to infection e.g. viral prodrome, HIV infection, etc.	*Suggested by:* tender solid nodular swelling(s) especially <20 years of age. *Confirmed by:* clinical features.
Infiltration by secondary tumour e.g. breast	*Suggested by:* non-tender solid nodular swelling(s). *Confirmed by:* **excision biopsy**.
Reticulosis or primary tumour	*Suggested by:* non-tender solid nodular swelling(s). *Confirmed by:* **excision biopsy**.
Drug effect	*Suggested by:* DH e.g. phenytoin, retroviral drug. *Confirmed by:* improvement when drug withdrawn.

Hirsuitism in female

Upward extension of pubic hair in female. Hirsute upper lip, sideburns, chin.

Some differential diagnoses and typical outline evidence

Racial skin sensitivity	*Suggested by:* family history, normal menstrual periods (and fertility if applicable).
	Confirmed by: **LH** normal, **testosterone** normal.
Polycystic ovary syndrome	*Suggested by:* gradual increase in hirsutism since puberty, thin head hair, irregular periods, infertility.
	Confirmed by: **testosterone** ↑, **SHBG**↓, **LH**↑ (tests done in follicular phase of menstrual cycle). US scan showing cystic ovaries.
	Management: OHCS p252.
Ovarian or adrenal carcinoma	*Suggested by:* change in hair pattern over months, voice deeper, breast atrophy, no periods cliteromegally.
	Confirmed by: ↓**LH** and ↑↑**testosterone**. US scan and laparoscopy findings.
	Management: OHCS p283.
Cushing's syndrome pituitary-driven Cushing's disease, or autonomous adrenal Cushing's, or glucocorticoid therapy	*Suggested by:* round, florid face (and trunk with purple striae) with thin arms and legs hirsuitism in ♀. Inability to rise from squatting position (due to proximal myopathy).
	Confirmed by: ↑ 24 hour urinary free cortisol, midnight cortisol ↑, and/or failure to suppress cortisol after 48 hours on dexamethazone 0.5mg 6 hourly or drug history of glucocorticoids.
	Management: OHCM pp310–11.

Abdominal striae

White striae are healed pink or purple striae.

- Pink striae

Some differential diagnoses and typical outline evidence

Pregnancy	*Suggested by:* no periods and obvious pregnant uterus.
	Confirmed by: **pregnancy test** +ve and US scan abdomen/pelvis.
Simple obesity	*Suggested by:* large abdomen and usually rapid weight increase.
	Confirmed by: above clinical findings.
	Management: OHCM p208.

- Purple striae

Some differential diagnoses and typical outline evidence

Glucocorticoid steroid therapy	*Suggested by:* truncal obesity, purple striae, bruising moon face and buffalo hump.
	Confirmed by: drug history: taking high dose of glucocorticoid.
Cushing's disease (ACTH driven)	*Suggested by:* truncal obesity, purple striae, bruising, moon face and buffalo hump. Pigmented creases indicate high ACTH especially in ectopic ACTH (from a carcinoma or carcinoid tumour).
	Confirmed by: ↑ 24 hour urinary free cortisol, midnight cortisols ↑ and/or failure to suppress cortisol after dexamethazone 0.5mg 6 hourly for 48 hours and ↑ACTH and bilaterally large adrenals on *CT MRI scan*.
Cushing's syndrome due to adrenal adenoma	*Suggested by:* truncal obesity, purple striae and bruising. No pigmentation in skin creases.
	Confirmed by: ↑ 24 hour urinary free cortisol, midnight cortisols ↑ and/or failure to suppress cortisol after dexamethazone 0.5mg 6 hourly for 48 hours and ↓ACTH and unilateral large adrenal on *CT MRI scan*.
	Management: OHCM pp310, 311.

Obesity

Definition: BMI >30 kgm^{-2}.

Some differential diagnoses and typical outline evidence

Simple obesity	*Suggested by:* limb and truncal obesity.
	Confirmed by: TSH and FT4 normal. 24 hour urinary cortisol normal.
	Management: OHCM p208.
Hypothyroidism	*Suggested by:* cold intolerance, tiredness, constipation, bradycardia.
	Confirmed by: ↑TSH, ↓FT4
	Management: OHCM p306.
Cushing's syndrome	*Suggested by:* 'moon face', truncal obesity, hirsutism, 'Buffalo hump', abdominal striae, proximal weakness.
	Confirmed by: ↑ 24 hour urinary free cortisol, midnight cortisol ↑ and/or failure to suppress cortisol after dexamethazone 0.5mg 6 hourly for 48 hours.

Pigmented creases and flexures (and buccal mucosa)

Suggests excess ACTH secretion.

Some differential diagnoses and typical outline evidence

Addison's disease = primary adrenal failure due to autoimmune destruction or tuberculosis	*Suggested by:* fatigue, low BP and postural drop.
	Confirmed by: low 9am cortisol with poor response to Synacthen stimulation test and ACTH↑.
	Management: OHCM p312.
(Pituitary) 'Cushing's disease'	*Suggested by:* facial and truncal obesity with striae, limb wasting and proximal myopathy.
	Confirmed by: ↑ 24 hour urinary free cortisol and/or failure to suppress cortisol after dexamethazone 0.5mg 6 hourly for 48 hours. Midnight cortisol ↑ and ACTH ↑.
	Management: OHCM p310.
Ectopic ACTH secretion	*Suggested by:* general weakness, proximal myopathy, usually evidence of lung cancer or other malignancy.
	Confirmed by: ↓ serum potassium and ↑↑ midnight cortisols and ↑ACTH.
	Management: OHCM p310.

Spider naevi

Red pin-head sized spots with radiating blood vessels that empty when centre pressed by pin-head sized object.

Some differential diagnoses and typical outline evidence

Normal	*Suggested by:* small numbers on chest (≤3), usually in a young woman on chest and upper back.
	Confirmed by: no increase with time.
Taking oestrogens	*Suggested by:* small numbers on chest in a young woman on pill.
	Confirmed by: decrease when pill stopped in due course (no urgency).
Pregnancy	*Suggested by:* moderate numbers in a pregnant woman.
	Confirmed by: decrease when pregnancy over.
Liver failure	*Suggested by:* large numbers on chest, also on neck and face, jaundice, features of liver failure.
	Confirmed by: ↓*albumin*, ↑*prothrombin time*.
	Management: OHCM p231.

Thin, wasted, cachectic

Some differential diagnoses and typical outline evidence

Low calorie intake e.g. anorexia nervosa alcholism, drug abuse, any prolonged systemic illness e.g. severe COPD	*Suggested by:* dietary history.
	Confirmed by: dietician's assessment, as in-patient if necessary.
Thyrotoxicosis	*Suggested by:* normal appetite and adequate intake, frequent loose bowel movement, lid retraction and lag, sweats, tachycardia.
	Confirmed by: ↓↓TSH, ↑FT4.
	Management: OHCM p304.
AIDS	Suggested by: signs of opportunistic infection e.g. oral candidiasis, oral hairy leukoplakia, Kaposi's sarcoma, lymphadenopathy.
	Confirmed by: detection of *HIV antibodies* in serum, *HIV RNA in plasma*.
	Management: OHCM p578–84.
Malignancy	*Suggested by:* progressive weight loss and malaise, poor appetite.
	Confirmed by: metastases in liver on *ultrasound scan*, bone secondaries on *plain X-rays*, *endoscopy* for gut tumours, *bronchoscopy*, etc.
Tuberculosis	*Suggested by:* cough, night sweats, haemoptysis, CXR: abnormal shadowing.
	Confirmed by: AFB in sputum on microscopy, mycobacteria on culture, response to antibiotics.
	Management : OHCM pp564, 566.

Purpura

Covers a spectrum from small pin-point petechiae to large areas of 'bruising' in skin do not blanch when compressed.

Some differential diagnoses and typical outline evidence

Thrombocytopenia due to autoimmune process or idiopathic (ITP), SLE	*Suggested by:* petechiae and history of associated condition. *Confirmed by:* ↓*platelet count* but *RBC* and *WBC* normal. *Management:* OHCM p644.
Pancytopenia due to aplastic anaemia, hypersplenism, myelodysplasia, disseminated vascular anticoagulation	*Suggested by:* petechiae and history of associated condition. *Confirmed by:* ↓*platelet count* ↓*WBC* and ↑*Hb*. *Management:* OHCM p662.
Platelet dysfunction due to aspirin, NSAIDs, renal failure	*Suggested by:* bruising and drug history. *Confirmed by:* less bruising when aspirin stopped or other cause removed.
Congenital vasculopathy due to Osler–Weber–Rendu syndrome etc.	*Suggested by:* bruising from punctiform malformations on mucous membranes. Nose bleeds, GI bleeding. *Confirmed by:* clinical findings and normal **platelet count** and clotting.
Acquired vasculopathy due to senile changes, autoimmune vasculitis (Henoch–Schönlein), steroids, scurvy	*Suggested by:* bruising into associated thin skin with atrophied subcutaneous tissue. *Confirmed by:* normal **platelet count** and **clotting**.
Acquired coagulopathy due to liver disease, vitamin K deficiency, DIC	*Suggested by:* bruising and history of associated condition. *Confirmed by:* prolonged **prothrombin time**.

Congenital coagulopathy e.g. Von Willebrand's disease	*Suggested by:* lifelong bruising and bleeding (after tooth extraction, heavy periods).
	Confirmed by: abnormal platelets function (count normal) and long activated partial thromboplastin time.
Drug effect	*Suggested by:* drug history e.g. warfarin, steroids.
	Confirmed by: improvement or drug withdrawal.

Generalised lymphadenopathy

Some differential diagnoses and typical outline evidence

Infectious mononucleosis (glandular fever) due to Epstein–Barr virus	*Suggested by:* very severe throat pain with enlarged tonsils covered with creamy membrane. Petechiae on palate. Profound malaise. Generalised lymphadenopathy, splenomegally. *Confirmed by:* **Paul–Bunnel** test +ve. **Viral titres**. *Management:* OHCM p570.
Hodgkin's lymphoma	*Suggested by:* anaemia, splenomegaly, multiple lymph node enlargement. *Confirmed by:* histology showing Reed–Sternberg cells. *Management:* OHCM p658.
Non-Hodgkin's lymphoma	*Suggested by:* anaemia, multiple lymph node enlargement. *Confirmed by:* histology with no Reed–Sternberg cells. *Management:* OHCM p660.
Chronic myeloid leukaemia (CML)	*Suggested by:* splenomegaly, variable hepatomegaly, bruising, anaemia. *Confirmed by:* presence of Philadelphia chromosome, ↑↑WBC e.g. >100 × 10^9/L. *Management:* OHCM p656.
Chronic lymphocytic leukaemia (CLL)	*Suggested by:* anorexia, weight loss, enlarged rubbery non-tender lymph nodes. Hepatomegaly, late splenomegaly. Bruising, anaemia. *Confirmed by:* marked lymphocytosis. Bone marrow infiltration. *Management:* OHCM p656.
Acute myeloid leukaemia (AML)	*Suggested by:* variable hepatomegaly, bruising, anaemia. *Confirmed by:* Blast cells in bone marrow biopsy. *Management:* OHCM p654.
Acute lymphoblastic leukaemia (ALL)	*Suggested by:* variable hepatomegaly, bruising, anaemia. *Confirmed by:* presence of immunological marker of Common (CD10), T-cell, β-cell, null-cell. *Management:* OHCM p652.

Sarcoidosis	*Suggested by:* dry cough, breathlessness, malaise, fatigue, weight loss, enlarged lacrimal glands, erethyma nodosum.
	Confirmed by: **CXR** appearances (e.g. bilateral lymphandenopathy), and **tissue biopsy** showing non-caseating granuloma.
	Management: OHCM p198.
Drug effect	*Suggested by:* DH e.g. phenytoin, retroviral drug.
	Confirmed by: improvement when drug withdrawn.

Localised groin lymphadenopathy

Non-specific finding.

Some differential diagnoses and typical outline evidence

Infection somewhere in lower limb or pelvis (usually in past and node remained large)	*Suggested by:* enlarged nodes confined to groins.
	Confirmed by: local infection in foot or leg, or no symptoms or signs of generalised condition.

Pressure sores

Blisters or ulcers on heel or sacrum. (OHCM p486).

Some differential diagnoses and typical outline evidence

Prolonged contact	*Suggested by:* history ± sensory loss e.g. spinal cord injury, CVA.
	Confirmed by: response to frequent turning and dressings/wound care.
Poor nutrition	*Suggested by:* ↓Hb. Low total serum protein and low potassium.
	Confirmed by: formal dietary assessment, response to improved nutrition, nurses 'turning' patient frequently and dressings/wound care.

Chapter 8

Cardiovascular signs

Thoughts on interpreting cardiovascular signs

The findings are discussed in a sequence of the CV examination, thinking of cardiac output, beginning with hand warmth, checking the radial pulse, measuring the BP. Continuing to think of cardiac output, examine the carotids. Next think of venous return by inspecting the JVP. Finally, inspect, palpate, percuss and auscultate the heart. Examine the legs and again think of cardiac output (e.g. temperature of skin and peripheral pulses) venous return (e.g. pitting oedema, leg veins and liver enlargement).

Peripheral cyanosis

Cyanosis of hands but not tongue.

Main differential diagnoses and typical outline evidence

Raynaud's phenomenon due to exposure of hands to cold or vibration	*Suggested by:* normal pulse and BP, history of blue hands after exposure to cold, vibrating tools, etc.
	Confirmed by: hands and feet assume normal colour in warm room.
	Management: OHCM p732, 733.
Arterial obstruction due to atheroma or small vessel disease in diabetics	*Suggested by:* absent or poor pulsation of radial or dorsalis pedis. Absent hair and skin atrophy in chronic cases.
	Confirmed by: **Doppler ultrasound** measure of blood flow low and **angiography**.
Haemorrhage due to external or internal bleeding	*Suggested by:* pallor, sweating, low BP high pulse rate, observable external bleeding or malaena or massive trauma expected to cause internal bleeding.
	Confirmed by: low **Hb** (although initial Hb is often normal) and **response to blood transfusion** or plasma expander and control of bleeding.
Low cardiac output due to large myocardial infarction or major loss of myocardial mass or severe valve stenosis or incompetence	*Suggested by:* pallor, sweating, low BP, orthopnoea, raised JVP and large liver, basal fine lung crepitations, displaced apex beat.
	Confirmed by: cardiomegaly and pulmonary oedema on **CXR** and poor LV function on **echocardiogram**. Abnormal **ECG**.
Septicaemia due to gram negative organisms commonly	*Suggested by:* warm, well-perfused peripheries, bounding pulse, low BP, tachycardia.
	Confirmed by: +ve blood cultures and response to plasma expanders and control of infection.

Central cyanosis

Cyanosis of tongue and hands.

Main differential diagnoses and typical outline evidence

Right to left cardiac shunt due to congenital heart disease e.g. Tetralogy of Fallot, Eisenmenger's syndrome, tricuspid atresia, Ebstein's anomaly, pulmonary AV fistula, transposition of the great vessels	*Suggested by:* breathlessness, clubbing, systolic or continuous murmur, right ventricular heave. *Confirmed by:* **echocardiogram** and **cardiac catheterisation**.
Right to left pulmonary shunt due to no perfusion of lung tissue from extensive collapse or consolidation due to alveolar infection or bronchial obstruction	*Suggested by:* breathlessness, poor chest movement, dullness to percussion and absent breath sounds over a large area of the chest. *Confirmed by:* **chest X-ray** and **bronchoscopy**.
Haemoglobin abnormalities due to congenital NADH diaphorase, Hb M disease or acquired methaemo-globinaemia or sulfhaemo-globinaemia	*Suggested by:* no clubbing, no murmurs normal chest movement, no chest signs. History from childhood or exposure to toxic drugs e.g. aniline dyes, phenacatin etc. *Confirmed by:* **Hb electrophoresis**. *Management:* OHCM pp640–3.

Pulse rate >120bpm

Main differential diagnoses and typical outline evidence

Fever	*Suggested by:* warm skin, erythema, sweats, temperature >38°C.
	Confirmed by: temperature chart, fever pattern and pulse rate↑.
Haemorrhage	*Suggested by:* signs of blood loss, pallor, sweats, low BP, poor peripheral perfusion.
	Confirmed by: low **Hb** (can be normal in initial stages), low central venous pressure.
Hypoxia	*Suggested by:* cyanosis, respiratory distress.
	Confirmed by: ↓P_aO_2.
Thyrotoxicosis	*Suggested by:* sweating, fine tremor, weight loss, lid lag, frequent bowel movements, sweats.
	Confirmed by: ↑*FT4*, ± ↑*FT3* and ↓*TSH*.
	Management: OHCM p304.
Severe anaemia	*Suggested by:* subconjunctival and nail-bed pallor.
	Confirmed by: ↓**Hb** (and indices).
Heart failure (LVF, RHF, CCF) associated with ischaemic heart disease, myocarditis etc.	*Suggested by:* 3rd heart sound, fine crackles at bases, raised JVP.
	Confirmed by: **CXR** showing large heart, pulmonary shadowing, upper lobe vein dilatation.
Pulmonary embolism	*Suggested by:* history of sudden breathlessness, cyanosis, raised JVP, loud P2. **ECG**: right axis deviation and RBBB.
	Confirmed by: **V/Q scan** showing mismatched defects, **pulmonary angiography** of spinal CT showing filling defect in pulmonary artery.
	Management: OHCM pp96, 194, 802, 803.
Drugs e.g. amphetamines, β-agonists	*Suggested by:* drug history.
	Confirmed by: normal pulse rate if drug stopped.

Bradycardia (<60bpm)

Main differential diagnoses and typical outline evidence

Athletic heart	*Suggested by:* young/fit, asymptomatic.
	Confirmed by: above clinical findings.
Drugs	*Suggested by:* history e.g. beta blockers.
	Confirmed by: improvement when drug withdrawn.
Sinoatrial disease	*Suggested by:* elderly, ischaemic heart disease.
	Confirmed by: **ECG**: abnormal P wave or P-R interval.
	Management: OHCM p127.
Ventricular or supraventricular begemini	*Suggested by:* known ischaemic heart disease.
	Confirmed by: **ECG**: premature ectopics with compensatory pause.
	Management: OHCM p126.
Myocardial infarction	*Suggested by:* central, crushing chest pain (can be atypical pain).
	Confirmed by: **ECG**: Q waves, raised ST segments, and inverted T waves. ↑CPK and **troponin**.
	Management: OHCM pp120–124.
Hypothyroid	*Suggested by:* constipation, weight gain, dry skin, dry hair, slow relaxing reflexes.
	Confirmed by: ↑TSH, ↓T4.
	Management: OHCM p306.
Hypothermia	*Suggested by:* history of exposure to cold temperature and immobility.
	Confirmed by: Core temperature <35°C.
	Management: OHCM p836.

Pulse irregular

Main differential diagnoses and typical outline evidence

Atrial fibrillation caused by ischaemic heart disease, thyrotoxicosis, etc.	*Suggested by:* irregularly irregular pulse.
	Confirmed by: **ECG** showing no P waves, and irregularly irregular normal QRS complexes.
	Management: OHCM p130.
Atrial flutter with variable heart block caused by ischaemic heart disease, etc.	*Suggested by:* irregularly irregular pulse.
	Confirmed by: **ECG** showing 'saw tooth' F waves, and irregularly irregular normal QRS complexes.
	Management: OHCM p130.
Atrial or ventricular ectopics caused by ischaemic heart disease, etc.	*Suggested by:* regular rate with irregular dropped beat.
	Confirmed by: **ECG** showing normal sinus rhythm with irregular QRS complexes not preceded by P wave, and then compensatory absence of subsequent QRS.
	Management: OHCM p132.
Wenkenbach heart block caused by ischaemic heart disease, etc.	*Suggested by:* regular rate with regular dropped beat.
	Confirmed by: **ECG** showing progressive prolongation of P-R interval with normal QRS complex followed by an absent QRS complex.
	Management: OHCM p126–7.

Pulse volume high

This is an indication of the width of the pulse pressure. It can be confirmed by a large difference between the systolic and diastolic blood pressure.

Main differential diagnoses and typical outline evidence

Aortic incompetence	*Suggested by:* striking 'water hammer' quality. Systolic BP high (say >160mmHg) and diastolic BP very low (say <50mmHg) early diastolic murmur, forceful, displaced apex impulse.
	Confirmed by: **echocardiogram** and **cardiac catheterisation** showing loss of valvular function.
	Management: OHCM p148.
Arteriosclerosis	*Suggested by:* thickened arterial wall. Systolic BP high (say >160mmHg) and diastolic BP not low (say >80mmHg).
	Confirmed by: **echocardiogram** to exclude aortic incompetence.
	Management: OHCM pp114, 148.
Severe anaemia	*Suggested by:* pallor. systolic BP high (say >160mmHg) and diastolic BP normal (say <85mmHg).
	Confirmed by: **Hb↓** (say <10grm/dL).
Bradycardia of any cause with normal myocardium	*Suggested by:* slow heart rate (e.g <50bpm).
	Confirmed by: **ECG** showing slow rate and type of rhythm.
Hyperkinetic circulation e.g. due to hypercapnia, thyrotoxicosis, fever, Paget's disease, AV fistula	*Suggested by:* warm peripheries and features of cause e.g. cyanosis, tremor, lid lag, fever, skull deformity, etc.
	Confirmed by: high **pCO_2** (if hypercapnia) or **↑FT4**, ± **↑FT3** and **↓TSH** (if thyrotoxic) or fever or ↑ hydroxyproline (if Paget's).

Pulse volume low

This is an indication of the width of the pulse pressure. It can be confirmed by a small difference between the systolic and diastolic blood pressure.

Main differential diagnoses and typical outline evidence

Poor cardiac contractility due to ischaemic heart disease, cardiomyopathy, cardiac tamponade, constrictive pericarditis	*Suggested by:* quiet heart sounds, ↑JVP, peripheral oedema, basal lung crackles. *Confirmed by:* **ECG**, **echocardiogram** to show evidence of cardiac muscle disease.
Hypovolaemia due to blood loss, dehydration	*Suggested by:* cold peripheries, thirst, dry skin, low urine output. *Confirmed by:* **urea**↑, **Hb**↓ (in loss) or ↑ (if haemo-concentrated).
Poor vascular tone due to septicaemic shock	*Suggested by:* warm peripheries, thirst, dry skin, ↓ eye tension, ↓ urine output. *Confirmed by:* **urea** ↑.
Aortic stenosis	*Suggested by:* slow rising pulse, systolic murmur. *Confirmed by:* **echocardiogram** and **cardiac catheterisation**. *Management:* OHCM p148.

Blood pressure high—hypertension

(systolic >150mmHg and diastolic >90mmHg)
The level treated depends on presence of risk factors. Generally any sustained systolic BP over 150 is treated, but in diabetics >140 systolic or >85 diastolic.

Main differential diagnoses and typical outline evidence

Temporary hypertension with no risk factors	*Suggested by:* normal blood pressure <150mmHg systolic and <90mmHg diastolic when repeated. *Confirmed by:* **24 hour ambulatory blood pressure monitoring**.
Essential hypertension 95% cases	*Suggested by:* sustained hypertension. If well established, then AV nipping present. *Confirmed by:* **24 hour ambulatory blood pressure monitoring**. No symptoms or signs of 2° cause, normal urea and electrolytes, and prompt control on treatment. *Management:* OHCM pp140–3.
Hypertension of pregnancy (pre-eclampsia sometimes progressing to eclampsia)	*Suggested by:* only occurring during pregnancy. Very high BP and fits in eclampsia. *Confirmed by:* resolution or improvement when pregnancy over or brought to an early end.
Renal hypertension due to renovascular stenosis or primary renal disease	*Suggested by:* established renal impairment too soon to be caused by hypertension. *Confirmed by:* **urea** and **creatinine** raised, **Hb↓** (in established renal failure). **Ultrasound** or **isotope scan** of kidneys and ureters. *Management:* OHCM pp260, 282.
Endocrine hypertension due to primary hyperaldosteronism (Conn's syndrome if tumour too), Cushing's syndrome, phaeochromocytoma	*Suggested by:* proximal muscle weakness in Cushing's syndrome or severe aldosteronism. Paroxysms of vascular symptoms in 'phaeo'. *Confirmed by:* ↑ **aldosterone** and ↓ **renin**, ↑ 24 hour urinary free cortisol etc in Cushing's syndrome. **↑VMA** and **metanephrins** ↑ in 'phaeo'. *Management:* OHCM pp310, 314.

Vascular hypertension due to coarctation of the aorta, subclavian artery stenosis	*Suggested by:* upper body hypertension (right arm) normal in legs (and left arm in subclavian artery stenosis). *Confirmed by:* **MRA/angiography**.
Drug induced due to NSAIDs, oestrogen pill, steroids, erythropoetin	*Suggested by:* drug history. *Confirmed by:* resolution or improvement when drug stopped.

Blood pressure very low

Main differential diagnoses and typical outline evidence

Cardiogenic—low output due to poor myocardium stenosis or regurgitation, etc.	*Suggested by:* very low BP, fast or slow heart rate, peripheral and central cyanosis, quiet heart sound ± abnormal murmur. JVP high, crepitations at lung bases.
	Confirmed by: high CVP, ECG abnormal ± rhythm abnormalities, large heart ± 'pulmonary oedema' on CXR. Abnormal myocardium ± valvular lesions on echocardiogram.
Low circulating blood volume due to haemorrhage (GI etc.) dehydration etc.	*Suggested by:* very low BP, fast heart rate, peripheral cyanosis, JVP low. Background evidence of cause.
	Confirmed by: low CVP, ECG normal heart on CXR. Improvement with blood, plasma expander, IV fluids with CVP monitoring.
Loss of vascular tone due to septicaemia, adrenal failure etc.	*Suggested by:* very low BP, fast heart rate, peripheral cyanosis, JVP low. Background evidence of cause.
	Confirmed by: low CVP, ECG normal heart on CXR. Improvement with IV blood, plasma expander, IV fluids with CVP monitoring, glucocorticoids and antibiotics.

Postural fall in blood pressure

To be significant the blood pressure must fall >30mmHg and stay down for at least 1 minute and be accompanied by dizziness.

Main differential diagnoses and typical outline evidence

Drug induced due to excessive dose of hypotensive agent, L-dopa, carbidopa, phenothiazines, antidepressants	*Suggested by:* drug history.
	Confirmed by: by resolution or improvement after stopping or reducing drug.
Autonomic neuropathy due to diabetes mellitus or tabes dorsalis (rarely)	*Suggested by:* history of long standing diabetes (common) or tabes dorsalis (rare). Also, diarrhoea, abdominal distension and vomiting (gastroparesis), impotence, urine frequency.
	Confirmed by: **ECG monitor of beat to beat variation:** <10 beats per minute change in heart rate on deep breathing at 6 breaths per minute or getting up from lying.
	Management: OHCM p298.
Idiopathic orthostatic hypotension	*Suggested by:* no other features except elderly.
	Confirmed by: isolated phenomenon.

BP/pulse difference between arms

R > L by 15mmHg.

Main differential diagnoses and typical outline evidence

Old or acute thrombosis in atheromatous artery or aneurysm or dissection of ascending aorta	*Suggested by:* associated peripheral vascular disease. *Confirmed by:* **MRA/angiography**.
Supravalvular aortic stenosis (congenital)	*Suggested by:* 'elfin-like' facies, ejection systolic murmur, angina and syncope. *Confirmed by:* **angiography**.
Subclavian steal syndrome	*Suggested by:* associated neurological symptoms. Exercising right arm induces cerebral ischaemia. *Confirmed by:* **angiography** showing abnormal subclavian artery. *Management:* OHCM p333.
Thoracic inlet syndrome	*Suggested by:* bracing shoulder aggravating BP difference. *Confirmed by:* **MRA/angiography** showing abnormal subclavian artery.
Aortic arch syndrome, Takayasu's syndrome	*Suggested by:* in young Asian female with cerebral and peripheral ischaemic symptoms. *Confirmed by:* **angiography** showing abnormal subclavian artery. *Management:* OHCM p736.

BP/pulse difference between arm and legs

R > L by 15mmHg. Need wide cuff for thigh. NB patient arms and leg must be level.

Main differential diagnoses and typical outline evidence

Old or acute thrombosis in atheromatous artery or aneurysm or dissection of descending thoracic or abdominal aorta or iliac arteries especially in diabetics	*Suggested by:* associated peripheral vascular disease. Atrophic skin and hair loss on lower legs. *Confirmed by:* Doppler ultrasound of legs to try to find remediable flow reduction. **Angiography** to try to identify surgically remediable arterial stenosis.
Coarctation of aorta	*Suggested by:* ejection systolic murmur presenting in childhood or early adult life. *Confirmed by:* rib notching on chest X-ray and stenosis on angiography.

Prominent leg veins ± unilateral leg swelling

Main differential diagnoses and typical outline evidence

Varicose veins ± competent communicating valves	*Suggested by:* veins distended and tortuous made worse when standing. Cough impulse felt and Trendelenberg test shows filling down along extent of communicating valve leaks.
	Confirmed by: clinical findings usually but if doubt **Doppler ultrasound** probe to confirm if incompetence is present or not in the sapheno-femoral junction or the short saphenous vein behind the knee.
	Management: OHCM p528.
Thrombophlebitis	*Suggested by:* tender hot veins with redness of surrounding skin.
	Confirmed by: resolution on antibiotics.
Deep vein thrombosis	*Suggested by:* immobility, prominent dilated veins, warm tender swollen calf.
	Confirmed by: reduced flow on compression **Doppler**, blockage seen on **venography**.
	Management: OHCM p456.

Unilateral leg and ankle swelling

Main differential diagnoses and typical outline evidence

Deep vein thrombosis	*Suggested by:* immobility, prominent dilated veins, warm tender swollen calf and positive Homan's sign.
	Confirmed by: reduced flow on compression *Doppler*, blockage seen on **venography**.
	Management: OHCM p456.
Ruptured Baker's cyst	*Suggested by:* sudden onset while straightening knee, warm tender swollen calf.
	Confirmed by: **D-dimer** titres not raised, normal flow on compression *Doppler*, no blockage seen on **venography**. Leaking from joint capsule on arthrography.
	Management: OHCM p718.
Cellulitis from infection secondary or primarily due to insect bites	*Suggested by:* tender hot red leg and fever.
	Confirmed by: resolution on antibiotics.
Unilateral varicose veins	*Suggested by:* distended and tortuous veins made worse when standing.
	Confirmed by: **Doppler ultrasound probe** to confirm where incompetence is present.
	Management: OHCM p528.
Chronic venous insufficiency from old deep vein thromboses	*Suggested by:* past history, veins distended and made worse on standing.
	Confirmed by: **Doppler ultrasound** probe to where incompetence is present.
Venous insufficiency from obstruction by tumour or lymph node	*Suggested by:* onset over weeks, veins distended.
	Confirmed by: **Doppler ultrasound** and **venography** to explore where obstruction is present.
Immobility	*Suggested by:* history of immobility and cause (e.g. disabling CVA, hemiplegic site).
	Confirmed by: response to elevation legs, **elastic stockings** etc.

Lymphoedema due to lymphatic obstruction due to primary lymphatic hypoplasia	*Suggested by:* unilateral swelling worse pre-menstrually, in warm weather and immobility. No venous dilatation.
	Confirmed by: **Doppler ultrasound** to show normal venous flow. **Lymphography** to show hypoplastic lymphatics.
	Management: OHCM p456.
Subacute lymphatic obstruction secondary to neoplastic obstruction	*Suggested by:* unilateral swelling developing over months. No venous dilatation.
	Confirmed by: **Doppler ultrasound** to show normal venous flow. **Lymphography** to show site of obstruction.
	Management: OHCM p456.
Acute lymphatic obstruction due to streptococcal lymphangitis	*Suggested by:* sudden unilateral swelling developing over hours. No venous dilatation but lymphangitic streaks.
	Confirmed by: clinical features and response to penicillin. **Doppler ultrasound** to show normal venous flow.
	Management: OHCM p456.

Bilateral leg and ankle swelling

Main differential diagnoses and typical outline evidence

Bilateral varicose veins or old deep vein thromboses	*Suggested by:* veins distended and tortuous made worse when standing.
	Confirmed by: **Doppler ultrasound** probe to confirm where incompetence is present.
	Management: OHCM p528.
Low albumin due to poor nutrition, malabsorption, liver failure, nephrotic syndrome, protein losing enteropathy	*Suggested by:* history of facial puffiness in morning and evidence of possible cause of low albumin.
	Confirmed by: low **serum albumin** (<30g/L to be significant).
Congestive cardiac failure due to ischaemic heart disease, mitral stenosis, cardiomyopathy etc.	*Suggested by:* raised JVP, liver large, fine crackles at bases, 3rd heart sound.
	Confirmed by: **CXR**: large heart, linear upper lobe shadows and fluffy lung shadows. **Echocardiogram**: ventricular dysfunction.
	Management: OHCM pp136–9.
Cor pulmonale (right heart failure, due to pulmonary hypertension due to long standing lung disease, old pulmonary emboli etc.)	*Suggested by:* raised JVP, liver large, 3rd heart sound, loud pulmonary second sound and RV heave.
	Confirmed by: **chest X-ray** showing pulmonary disease, **ECG** showing right axis deviation. **Echocardiogram**: ventricular dysfunction.
	Management: OHCM p204.
Lymphoedema due to primary lymphatic hypoplasia	*Suggested by:* bilateral swelling worse pre-menstrually, in warm weather and immobility. No venous dilatation.
	Confirmed by: **Doppler ultrasound** to show normal venous flow. Occasional **lymphangiography** to show hypoplastic lymphatics.
	Management: OHCM p456.
Immobility	*Suggested by:* history of immobility and cause (e.g. disabling CVA).
	Confirmed by: response to elevation legs, **elastic stockings** etc.

Raised jugular venous pressure

Measured with patient lying at 45°. Undetectably low if external jugular empties when compressing finger released.

Main differential diagnoses and typical outline evidence

Fluid volume overload	*Suggested by:* pulsatile JVP with 'a' waves. History of high input of IV fluids.
	Confirmed by: response to less fluid and spontaneous diuresis (or diuretics).
	Management: OHCM p680.
Congestive cardiac failure	*Suggested by:* pulsatile JVP with 'a' and 'v' waves.
	Confirmed by: **echocardiogram** showing ventricular dysfunction.
	Management: OHCM pp136–9.
Cor pulmonale due to high right atrial pressure	*Suggested by:* large 'a' waves present.
	Confirmed by: **ECG** showing tall P wave.
	Management: OHCM p204
Atrial fibrillation	*Suggested by:* 'a' waves absent, irregularly irregular pulse.
	Confirmed by: **ECG** showing no P waves and normal QRS complexes.
	Management: OHCM p130.
Complete heart block	*Suggested by:* intermittent giant 'v' waves. Bradycardia.
	Confirmed by: **ECG** showing no association between P wave, and QRS complex.
	Management: OHCM p134.
Tricuspid regurgitation	*Suggested by:* large 'v' waves. Pan-systolic murmur present.
	Confirmed by: **echocardiogram** showing large right atrium and tricuspid incompetence.
	Management: OHCM p150.
Pericardial effusion	*Suggested by:* pulsatile JVP with 'a' and rapid descent. Very breathless. Quiet heart sounds.
	Confirmed by: globular heart shadow on **CXR**. Low voltage QRS complexes on **ECG**.
	Management: OHCM pp42, 110, 158.

Constrictive pericarditis	*Suggested by:* JVP rising with inspiration (Kussmaul sign), 'a' waves have rapid descent. Quiet heart sounds. Large liver and ascites.
	Confirmed by: small heart shadow on **CXR**. **Echocardiogram** shows small cavity and little contraction.
	Management: OHCM p158.
Jugular vein obstruction	*Suggested by:* no JVP pulsation, external jugular vein also distended.
	Confirmed by: **ultrasound** scan to explore site of obstruction.

Abnormal apex impulse

Look for displacement from normal site in mid-clavicular line, heave and character of impulse (tapping, double).

Main differential diagnoses and typical outline evidence

Obesity, emphysema, pleural effusion, pericardial effusion or dextrocardia	*Suggested by:* impalpable apex.
	Confirmed by: evidence of intervening factors or apex palpable on right.
Large left ventricle due to mitral incompetence, aortic incompetence, right to left VSD shunt	*Suggested by:* apex displaced and heaving.
	Confirmed by: large left ventricle on **echocardiogram** with corresponding valve lesion.
Hypertrophied left ventricle due to hypertension aortic stenosis	*Suggested by:* apex not displaced but heaving.
	Confirmed by: hypertrophied left ventricular wall on **echocardiogram**.
Hypertrophic cardiomyopathy (HOCM)	*Suggested by:* double apex beat, angina, breathless, syncope on exercise, jerky pulse, high JVP with 'a' wave, thrill and murmur best at left sternal edge.
	Confirmed by: **echocardiogram** showing hypertrophied septum and ventricular walls with small ventricular cavities esp. on left.
	Management: OHCM p156.
Ventricular aneurysm	*Suggested by:* double impulse.
	Confirmed by: paradoxical movement of ventricular wall on **echocardiogram**. Persistently raised ST segments on **ECG**.
	Management: OHCM p124.

Mitral stenosis	*Suggested by:* tapping left ventricular impulse (palpable 1st heart sound) and rumbling diastolic murmur.
	Confirmed by: **ECG** findings and **echocardiogram** and **cardiac catheterisation**.
	Management: OHCM p146.
Right ventricular hypertrophy due to pulmonary stenosis or hypertension	*Suggested by:* left parasternal heave.
	Confirmed by: **ECG** findings and **echocardiogram**.
Major valve or septal defects	*Suggested by:* palpable thrill (i.e. palpably loud murmur).
	Confirmed by: **ECG** findings and **echocardiogram** and **cardiac catheterisation**.

Extra heart sounds

Main differential diagnoses and typical outline evidence

Normal young heart	*Suggested by:* 4th heart sound.
	Confirmed by: normal *CXR*, and *echocardiogram*.
Heart failure, cardiomyopathy, constrictive pericarditis	*Suggested by:* 3rd heart sound.
	Confirmed by: clinical findings, *ECG* and *echocardiogram*.
Severe heart failure	*Suggested by:* 3rd and 4th heart sound giving 'gallop'.
	Confirmed by: raised JVP, crackles at lung bases, pulmonary oedema on *CXR* and slow contraction of large ventricles on *echocardiogram*.

Diastolic murmur

Find where it is heard best (e.g. apex or left sternal edge).

Main differential diagnoses and typical outline evidence

Mitral stenosis	*Suggested by:* mitral facies, tapping apex beat, loud 1st heart sound, rumbling mid-diastolic murmur best at apex with patient lying on left side.
	Confirmed by: **echocardiogram** and cardiac catheter displaying valve lesion.
	Management: OHCM p146.
Mitral stenosis with pliable valve	*Suggested by:* opening snap.
Aortic incompetence	*Suggested by:* high BP, collapsing pulse, displaced apex beat, early diastolic murmur best at left sternal edge.
	Confirmed by: **echocardiogram** and **cardiac catheter** displaying valve lesion.
	Management: OHCM p148.

Mid-systolic murmur

Main differential diagnoses and typical outline evidence

Aortic stenosis	*Suggested by:* cool extremities, slow rising pulse, low BP and pulse pressure, heaving apex and soft or absent aortic component of the second heart sound (A_2).
	Confirmed by: **ECG** (tall R waves and left axis deviation). **Echocardiogram** and **cardiac catheter** stenosed valve.
	Management: OHCM p148.
Hypertrophic cardiomyopathy (HOCM)	*Suggested by:* angina, breathless, syncope on exercise, jerky pulse, high JVP with 'a' wave, double apex beat, thrill normal aortic component of second heart sound (A_2) and systolic murmur best at left sternal edge.
	Confirmed by: **echocardiogram** showing hypertrophied septum and ventricular walls with small ventricular cavities esp. on left.
	Management: OHCM p156.
Aortic sclerosis	*Suggested by:* normal pulse and BP ± no heaving apex.
	Confirmed by: normal **ECG** and **echocardiogram**.
Pulmonary high flow	*Suggested by:* normal pulse, and BP, normal JVP and no left para-sternal heave.
	Confirmed by: normal **ECG** and **echocardiogram**.
Atrial septal defect (rare) causing high pulmonary flow	*Suggested by:* normal pulse and BP, normal JVP and left para-sternal heave present.
	Confirmed by: **ECG**: peaked P waves, right axis deviation in secundum defect, left axis deviation in primum defect. **Echocardiogram** and **cardiac catheter** findings.
	Management: OHCM p160.
Pulmonary stenosis	*Suggested by:* low pulse, high JVP and left parasternal heave.
	Confirmed by: RBB block and right axis deviation on **ECG**. **Echocardiogram** and **cardiac catheter**.
	Management: OHCM p150.

Pan-systolic murmur

Main differential diagnoses and typical outline evidence

Mitral incompetence due to rheumatic heart disease, valve dysfunction after myocardial infarction	*Suggested by:* pan-systolic murmur at apex with radiation to axilla. No large JVP 'V' waves. Displaced heaving apex beat. *Confirmed by:* **CXR**: large round opacity 'behind heart' (big left atrium). **ECG**: 'M' shaped P wave. ***Echocardiogram*** and **cardiac catheter**. *Management:* OHCM p146.
Tricuspid incompetence (rare alone) sometimes alone in severe cor pulmonale or after pulmonary embolus	*Suggested by:* pan-systolic murmur at left sternal edge (louder on inspiration), no radiation to axilla. Large JVP 'V' waves. Left parasternal heave. *Confirmed by:* **ECG**: tall peaked 'P' waves, right axis deviation and RBBB. ***Echocardiogram*** and **cardiac catheter** show incompetence. *Management:* OHCM p150.
Mitral and tricuspid incompetence due to rheumatic heart disease or dilated ventricles in severe heart failure	*Suggested by:* pan-systolic murmur with radiation to axilla. Large JVP 'V' waves. Displaced heaving apex beat. *Confirmed by:* normal **ECG** and **echocardiogram** show incompetence. *Management:* OHCM pp146, 150.
Ventricular septal defect usually congenital, sometimes rupture of septum after infarction	*Suggested by:* pan-systolic murmur loud and rough. Raised JVP. Central cyanosis if right to left shunt. Displaced heaving apex beat. *Confirmed by:* RBB block and right axis deviation on **ECG**. ***Echocardiogram*** and **cardiac catheter** shows defect. *Management:* OHCM p160.

Murmurs not entirely in systole or diastole

Main differential diagnoses and typical outline evidence

Patent ductus arteriosus	*Suggested by:* new born infant, high pulse volume, diastolic and systolic murmur to give continuous murmur: 'shee-shoo, shee-shoo'.
	Confirmed by: **echocardiogram** and **cardiac catheter**.
Pericarditis with pericardial friction rub	*Suggested by:* 'scratching murmur' heard in systole ± diastole. Chest pain worse when lying back and relieved by lying forward.
	Confirmed by: raised ST segments on **ECG** but no inversion of T waves.
	Management: OHCM p159.

Respiratory physical signs

Examination of respiratory system

The findings are discussed in a sequence of those found on inspection, palpation, percussion and then auscultation. While inspecting, think of blood gas status and when palpating think of the mechanisms of ventilation. When percussing think of the pleural surfaces, contents of the pleural cavity and lung tissue. When auscultating think of the state of the lung tissue and the airways.

Appearance suggestive of blood gas disturbance

Look at hands for cyanosis, feel for warmth, ask patient to hold arms out and extended at the wrists to see if there is a coarse tremor and muscle twitching in the arms. Look at the tongue and lips for central cyanosis.

Some differential diagnoses and typical outline evidence

Hypoxic	*Suggested by:* blue hands and tongue (central cyanosis), restless, confused, drowsy or unconscious.
	Confirmed by: ↓P_aO_2 <8kPa on **blood gas analysis** (or **pulse oximetry** of <90% (mild) or <80% (severe)).
	Management: OHCM p192.
Carbon dioxide retention	*Suggested by:* warm hands, bounding pulse, dilated veins on hands and face, twitching of facial muscles, drowsy.
	Confirmed by: ↑P_aCO_2 >6.5kPa on **blood gas analysis**.
	Management: OHCM p192.
Hypocapnia	*Suggested by:* hyperventilation, dizzy, paraesthesiae around lips.
	Confirmed by: ↓P_aCO_2 <4.5kPa on **blood gas analysis**.
	Management: OHCM p192.

Respiratory rate low (<10/minute)

Count the number of respirations for a minute if rate appears low.

Some differential diagnoses and typical outline evidence

Carbon dioxide narcosis (very high blood carbon dioxide)	*Suggested by:* warm hands, bounding pulse, dilated veins on hands and face, twitching of facial muscles, drowsy.
	Confirmed by: $\downarrow P_aCO_2$ >6.5kPa on **blood gas analysis**.
	Management: OHCM p192.
Drugs e.g. opiates alcohol, benzodiazepines	*Suggested by:* Pin-point pupils (in opiates—track marks). History of ingestion, empty medication bottle.
	Confirmed by: **response to drug withdrawal** or antidotes e.g. naloxone, flumazenil. Drug levels on **toxicology screen**.
Raised intra-cranial pressure	*Suggested by:* papilloedema, focal neurology, severe headaches and vomiting.
	Confirmed by: **CT brain** (loss of normal sulci, oedema).

Chest wall abnormalities

Inspect the chest shape and then its change on movement for asymmetry, looking up over the abdomen.

Some differential diagnoses and typical outline evidence

Pectus carinatum developmental or associated with emphysema	*Suggested by:* prominent sternum, often associated with indrawing of the ribs causing Harrison's sulci above the costal margins. *Confirmed by:* **CXR**.
Pectus excavatum developmental defect	*Suggested by:* depression of the lower end or whole sternum. *Confirmed by:* **CXR**.
Kyphosis congenital or due to anterior collapse of spinal vertebrae e.g. spinal TB	*Suggested by:* spine curved forward and laterally. *Confirmed by:* **CXR, spinal X-ray**.
Scoliosis congenital, neuromuscular disease, previous surgery, TB	*Suggested by:* spine curved laterally. *Confirmed by:* **CXR, spinal X-ray**.
Absence of part of chest wall bone structure congenital (Poland's syndrome) or post surgery	*Suggested by:* absence of ribs, pectoralis muscle, clavicle etc. *Confirmed by:* **CXR, spinal X-ray**.

Bilateral poor chest expansion

Some differential diagnoses and typical outline evidence

Obesity	*Suggested by:* insidious onset of breathlessness.
	Confirmed by: examination (*BMI* >30kg/m^2).
	Management: OHCM p208.
Emphysema	*Suggested by:* hyperinflation, poor air entry, hyper-resonance, pursed lip breathing. Hyperinflation and paucity of lung markings on *CXR*.
	Confirmed by: **CT thorax,** obstructive deficit with reduced transfer factor and no reversibility on **lung function**.
	Management: OHCM p188.
Pulmonary fibrosis	*Suggested by:* clubbed (60–70%), fine late inspiratory bibasal crepitations. Loss of lung volume on *CXR* (not corresponding to a single lobe).
	Confirmed by: **HR-CT thorax.** Restrictive deficit with reduced transfer factor **on lung function**.
	Management: OHCM p202.
Muscular dystrophy (other rarer myopathies)	*Suggested by:* early age onset, FH, calf hypertrophy, LMN signs. Restrictive deficit **on lung function** (especially when lying flat). Sparing of corrected transfer factor.
	Confirmed by: **muscle biopsy.**
	Management: OHCM p398.
Motor neurone disease	*Suggested by:* late onset mixed UMN/LMN signs, tongue fasciculation, bulbar palsy. Restrictive deficit on lung function (especially when lying flat). Sparing of corrected transfer factor.
	Confirmed by: **EMG.**
	Management: OHCM p394.
Multiple sclerosis	*Suggested by:* onset in early adulthood onwards, hyper-reflexia, hypertonia, optic atrophy. Restrictive deficit on lung function (especially when lying flat). Sparing of corrected transfer factor.
	Confirmed by: **MRI brain, visual evoked responses.**
	Management: OHCM p384–5.

Guillain–Barré syndrome	*Suggested by:* ascending weakness, autonomic disturbances and recent infection. Restrictive deficit on lung function (especially when lying flat). Rapid deterioration on **lung function** (FVC or PEFR). Sparing of corrected transfer factor.
	Confirmed by: history, **response to steroids and plasmapheresis/globulin infusions.**
	Management: OHCM p727.

Unilateral poor chest expansion

Some differential diagnoses and typical outline evidence

Pleural effusion	*Suggested by:* reduced breath sounds, reduced tactile vocal fremitus, stony dull percussion note.
	Confirmed by: hazy opacification on **CXR** and fluid on **USS chest**.
	Management: OHCM p196.
Pneumothorax	*Suggested by:* reduced breath sounds, reduced tactile vocal fremitus, resonant percussion note.
	Confirmed by: **CXR** showing no lung markings next to chest wall, and line of demarcation with lung tissue. Best seen at lung apex.
	Management: OHCM pp750, 798.
Extensive consolidation	*Suggested by:* reduced breath sounds, bronchial breathing, increased tactile vocal fremitus, reduced percussion note.
	Confirmed by: **CXR**.
Fractured ribs	*Suggested by:* antecedent trauma, focal tenderness.
	Confirmed by: **CXR**.
Flail segment following trauma	*Suggested by:* paradoxical movement of part of chest wall.
	Confirmed by: **CXR, spinal X-ray**.
Musculoskeletal e.g. previous thoracoplasty	*Suggested by:* history, scar.
	Confirmed by: **CXR**.

Trachea displaced

Palpate with middle finger with index and ring finger either side of trachea. Localize apex beat to see if lower mediastinum also displaced.

Some differential diagnoses and typical outline evidence

Scoliosis	*Suggested by:* chest wall deformity and curved spine.
	Confirmed by: **spinal X-ray, CXR**.
Pulled by ipsilateral pneumothorax	*Suggested by:* reduced breath sounds, reduced tactile vocal fremitus, resonant percussion note.
	Confirmed by: **CXR** showing space with absent lung markings 'pulling' on mediastinum.
	Management: OHCM pp750, 798.
Pulled by ipsilateral upper lobe fibrosis, collapse or removal	*Suggested by:* tuberculosis (chronic), radiation fibrosis (skin changes, tattoo marks), surgery (scar), ankylosing spondylitis, sarcoidosis. Reduced upper chest wall expansion.
	Confirmed by: **chest X-ray** showing diminished abnormal chest anatomy 'pulling' on mediastinum.
	Management: OHCM pp750, 798.
Pushed by contralateral tension pneumothorax	*Suggested by:* in extremis with high pulse rate and hypotension, reduced breath sounds, reduced tactile vocal fremitus, resonant percussion note.
	Confirmed by: **insertion of a venflon into 2nd intercostal space**.
	Management: OHCM pp750, 798.
Pushed by contralateral pleural effusion	*Suggested by:* reduced breath sounds, reduced tactile vocal fremitus, stony dull percussion note.
	Confirmed by: **CXR** showing large homogenous white opacification 'pushing' on mediastinum.
	Management: OHCM p196.

Reduced tactile vocal fremitus

Some differential diagnoses and typical outline evidence

Pleural effusion	*Suggested by:* reduced breath sounds, reduced expansion, stony dull percussion note.
	Confirmed by: **CXR** and **USS chest**.
	Management: OHCM p196.
Pneumothorax	*Suggested by:* reduced breath sounds, reduced expansion, resonant percussion note. Trachea and apex displaced.
	Confirmed by: **CXR** showing no lung markings next to chest wall, and line of demarcation with lung tissue. Best seen at lung apex.
	Management: OHCM pp750, 798.
Collapsed lobe with no consolidation	*Suggested by:* reduced breath sounds, reduced expansion, normal percussion note.
	Confirmed by: **CXR** (see p634: collapse of different lobes will have different patterns radiologically e.g. showing fan-shaped shadow arising from mediastinum, mediastinal shift, raised hemidiaphragm, displaced horizontal fissure or 'sail sign'). **CT thorax** confirms lobar collapse.

Stony dull percussion

Implies pleural effusion.

Some differential diagnoses and typical outline evidence

Transudates	*Suggested by:* bilateral effusions, underlying clinical cause.
	Confirmed by: **protein in effusion** <30g/L or <0.5 ratio to serum protein (except in treated heart failure).
Left heart failure, SVC obstruction, pericarditis, peritoneal dialysis	*Suggested by:* peripheral oedema, raised JVP, basal crackles, 3rd heart sound.
	Confirmed by: **CXR, echocardiogram, CT thorax**.
Low albumin states e.g. liver cirrhosis, nephrotic syndrome	*Suggested by:* malnutrition, generalised oedema.
	Confirmed by: low **serum albumin**.
Miscellaneous causes: myxoedema, 1° pulmonary hypertension	

Exudates	*Suggested by:* unilateral effusion (but may be bilateral).
	Confirmed by: (**protein in effusion** >30g/dL or >0.5 ratio to serum protein)
Infective: bacterial/ empyema, TB, viral, etc.	*Suggested by:* history, fever pH↓, glucose in pleural fluid↓. Many lymphocytes in exudates often seen in TB, caseating granuloma on pleural biopsy.
	Confirmed by: gram stain/**ZN stain and cultures of pleural fluid and blood or cultures from pleural biopsy**.
Neoplastic: lung primary or secondaries, breast, ovarian, reticuloses, Kaposi's, local chest wall tumours, mesothelioma	*Suggested by:* history, especially weight loss. Signs of local or distal spread.
	Confirmed by: **pleural aspiration, biopsy or other tissue histology**.
Rheumatoid, SLE, etc.	*Suggested by:* history, other organ specific involvement, +ve rheumatoid factor in fluid, very low fluid glucose.
	Confirmed by: **auto-antibodies, response to immunosuppression**.
Pulmonary infarction	*Suggested by:* history. Sudden onset of pleuritic chest pain, and breathlessness. Associated risk factors. Usually hypoxic. **CXR** may show other evidence e.g. Fleischner lines, Hampton's hump, wedge-shaped shadowing.
	Confirmed by: **CT-PA**.
	Management: OHCM pp194, 802.

Dull to percussion but not stony dull

Some differential diagnoses and typical outline evidence

Consolidation	*Suggested by:* reduced breath sounds, bronchial breathing, increased tactile vocal fremitus. Fever, cough (may be productive).
	Confirmed by: air bronchogram on **CXR and CT**.
Pulmonary oedema usually due to left ventricular failure	*Suggested by:* displaced apex beat, S3, basal crepitations.
	Confirmed by: **CXR, echocardiogram**.
	Management: OHCM pp136–8, 786.
Elevated hemi-diaphragm	*Suggested by:* absent breath sounds (asymptomatic).
	Confirmed by: **CXR**.
Severe fibrosis/ collapse	*Suggested by:* reduced breath sounds, crepitations, poor expansion, tracheal deviation.
	Confirmed by: **CXR, CT thorax**.
Mesothelioma/ severe pleural thickening	*Suggested by:* chest pain, weight loss, asbestos exposure, clubbing, reduced breath sounds.
	Confirmed by: **CT thorax and pleural biopsy**.

Hyper-resonant percussion

Some differential diagnoses and typical outline evidence

Emphysema	*Suggested by:* >10 pack year smoking history, chronic, progressive breathlessness, cough with sputum, reduced breath sounds, hyper-resonance, pursed lip breathing, tracheal tug. Hyperinflation and paucity of lung markings on **CXR**.
	Confirmed by: **CT thorax**, obstructive deficit with reduced transfer factor and no reversibility on **lung function**.
	Management: OHCM p188.
Large bullae	*Suggested by:* other signs of emphysema.
	Confirmed by: **CT thorax**.
Pneumothorax	*Suggested by:* acute breathlessness, chest pain, **unilateral signs** such as reduced breath sounds, reduced tactile vocal fremitus, poor expansion.
	Confirmed by: **CXR** showing no lung markings next to chest wall and line of demarcation with lung tissue.
	Management: OHCM pp750, 798.

Diminished breath sounds

Ensure patient breathes with mouth open, regularly and deeply and does not vocalize (e.g. groaning).

Some differential diagnoses and typical outline evidence

Poor respiratory effort	*Suggested by:* reduced consciousness/cooperation, any cause of poor chest wall expansion (see p376). *Confirmed by:* **ABGs** (type 2 failure).
Pleural effusion	*Suggested by:* reduced expansion, stony dull percussion, reduced tactile vocal fremitus. *Confirmed by:* **CXR, USS chest**. *Management:* OHCM p196.
Endobronchial obstruction e.g. tumour, retained secretions, inhaled foreign body	*Suggested by:* cough, stridor, unilateral dullness to percussion, crackles and reduced breath sounds. *Confirmed by:* **CT thorax, bronchoscopy**.
Severe asthma (broncho-constriction)	*Suggested by:* history, sudden onset, often precipitating factor. Patient *in extremis*, reduced consciousness. *Confirmed by:* **peak flow rate** undetectable. **ABGs** show type 2 respiratory failure. *Management:* OHCM pp184–6.
Emphysema	*Suggested by:* >10 pack year smoking history, chronic, progressive breathlessness, cough with sputum, hyper-inflation, hyper-resonance, and pursed lip breathing, tracheal tug. Hyperinflation and paucity of lung markings on **CXR**. *Confirmed by:* **CT thorax**, obstructive deficit with reduced transfer factor and no reversibility on **lung function**. *Management:* OHCM p188.
Mesothelioma/ severe pleural thickening	*Suggested by:* chest pain, weight loss, asbestos exposure, clubbing, reduced breath sounds. *Confirmed by:* **CT thorax and pleural biopsy**. *Management:* OHCM p202.
Bullae	*Suggested by:* localised bronchial breathing (if large). *Confirmed by:* **CXR, CT thorax**.

Consolidation	*Suggested by:* reduced percussion, increased tactile vocal fremitus, bronchial breathing.
	Confirmed by: **CXR**.
Pneumothorax	*Suggested by:* acute breathlessness, chest pain, reduced expansion, hyper-resonance.
	Confirmed by: **CXR**.
	Management: OHCM pp750, 798.
Elevated hemidiaphragm ?phrenic nerve paresis	*Suggested by:* being asymptomatic. Scar from phrenic nerve surgery/injury.
	Confirmed by: **CXR**.

Bronchial breathing

Prolonged expiration phase with definite silence between inspiration and expiration (same as sound heard with stethoscope bell over trachea).

Some differential diagnoses and typical outline evidence

Consolidation	*Suggested by:* fever, reduced breath sounds, reduced percussion, crepitations, increased tactile vocal fremitus.
	Confirmed by: **CXR**.
Lung cavity	*Suggested by:* localised bronchial breathing, otherwise normal examination.
	Confirmed by: **CXR, CT thorax**.
Pulmonary fibrosis	*Suggested by:* reduced expansion, normal or reduced percussion, late inspiratory fine crepitations, clubbing.
	Confirmed by: **HR-CT thorax**.
	Management: OHCM p202.

Fine inspiratory crackles or crepitations

Very fine crackles are like the sound made when hair next to the ear is rolled between finger and thumb or velcro pad!

Some differential diagnoses and typical outline evidence

Incidental	*Suggested by:* late in inspiration, disappears on coughing.
	Confirmed by: **CXR** showing normal lung fields.
Pulmonary oedema	*Suggested by:* late in inspiration, dullness to percussion at lung bases (in associated effusion) 3rd heart sound.
	Confirmed by: **CXR** showing fluffy shadows, large heart and linear opacities in upper lobes. *Echocardiogram* shows reduced contraction.
	Management: OHCM pp136–8, 786.
Pulmonary fibrosis	*Suggested by:* very fine crackles late in inspiration, reduced chest expansion, finger clubbing.
	Confirmed by: **CXR** and **HR-CT thorax**.
	Management: OHCM p202.
Chronic bronchitis	*Suggested by:* fine to coarse crackles early in inspiration, productive cough for 3 months over 2 consecutive years.
	Confirmed by: above history.
	Management: OHCM p188.
Emphysema	*Suggested by:* hyperinflation, poor air entry, hyper-resonance, and pursed lip breathing. Hyperinflation and paucity of lung markings on **CXR**.
	Confirmed by: **CT thorax**, obstructive deficit with reduced transfer factor and no reversibility on lung function.
	Management: OHCM p188.
Consolidation	*Suggested by:* early inspiratory crackles, fever, reduced breath sounds, reduced percussion, increased tactile vocal fremitus.
	Confirmed by: **CXR**.

Coarse crackles

Bubbly crackles.

Some differential diagnoses and typical outline evidence

Bronchiectasis	*Suggested by:* copious amounts of mucopurulent sputum, chest pain, wheeze. Previous chest infections, asthma, surgery or cystic fibrosis. Crepitations not disappearing after coughing, clubbed.
	Confirmed by: **HR-CT thorax.**
	Management: OHCM pp178, 179.

Pleural rub

Sounds like two wet leather surfaces rubbing together (or crunching through snow). Caused by inflammation of the pleura.

Some differential diagnoses and typical outline evidence

Pleuritic infection with adjacent pneumonia	*Suggested by:* fever, reduced breath sounds, reduced percussion, crepitations, increased tactile vocal fremitus.
	Confirmed by: **CXR, sputum and blood cultures.**
Pulmonary embolus	*Suggested by:* signs of DVT, loud P2, tachycardia, dyspnoea, hypoxic, $\downarrow P_aCO_2$, $\uparrow$FDPs.
	Confirmed by: **V/Q, CT(PA), pulmonary angiogram.**
	Management: OHCM pp194, 802.
Pleural tumours e.g. secondaries or mesothelioma	*Suggested by:* history e.g. asbestos exposure.
	Confirmed by: **CT thorax, pleural biopsy.**
	Management: OHCM p202.

Stridor ± inspiratory wheeze

Suggests obstruction in or near larynx.

Some differential diagnoses and typical outline evidence

Epiglottitis	*Suggested by:* fever, URTI coryzal symptoms, drooling.
	Confirmed by: **indirect laryngoscopy** under controlled (anaesthetic) conditions.
Croup	*Suggested by:* high-pitched cough in infants.
	Confirmed by: above presentation and findings.
Inhaled foreign body	*Suggested by:* history of inhaling peanut, bead, etc.
	Confirmed by: **CXR, CT thorax, bronchoscopy.**
Rapidly progressive laryngomalacia	*Suggested by:* change in voice over months to years.
	Confirmed by: **indirect laryngoscopy, CT thorax.**
Laryngeal papillomas	*Suggested by:* change in voice over weeks to months.
	Confirmed by: **indirect laryngoscopy.**
Laryngeal oedema due to anaphylaxis	*Suggested by:* flushing of face and trunk, uritcarial rash, lip and facial swelling, tachycardia, BP↓
	Confirmed by: improvement with adrenaline IM and removal of precipitating allergen.

Inspiratory monophonic wheeze

Suggests large airway obstruction. Lesion above the carina can be immediately lifethreatening as neither lung can be ventilated.

Some differential diagnoses and typical outline evidence

Acute bilateral vocal cord paralysis	*Suggested by:* change in voice which becomes weaker over minutes to hours.
	Confirmed by: **laryngoscopy**.
Inhalation of foreign body	*Suggested by:* history of inhaling peanut, bead or other foreign body.
	Confirmed by: **CXR, CT thoracic inlet, bronchoscopy**.
Tracheal tumours or stenosis after ventilation	*Suggested by:* Stridor, over weeks to months, bilateral reduced breath sounds.
	Confirmed by: **bronchoscopy**.
Extrinsic compression by mediastinal masses	*Suggested by:* neck/chest discomfort ± swelling over weeks to months.
	Confirmed by: **CT thoracic inlet**.
Extrinsic compression by oesophageal tumours	*Suggested by:* dysphagia, weight loss over weeks to months.
	Confirmed by: **CT thoracic inlet**.
Tracheal blunt trauma	*Suggested by:* history, pain and swelling, change in voice over minutes or hours after trauma.
	Confirmed by: **laryngoscopy, bronchoscopy**.
Laryngeal oedema due to anaphylaxis	*Suggested by:* flushing of face and trunk, uritcarial rash, lip and facial swelling, tachycardia, BP↓
	Confirmed by: improvement with adrenaline IM and removal of precipitating allergen.

Expiratory monophonic wheeze

Large airway obstruction.

Some differential diagnoses and typical outline evidence

Endobronchial carcinoma (benign lesions very rare)	*Suggested by:* smoker, weight loss, cough, chest pain, haemoptysis, clubbed. Unilateral wheeze and reduced breath sounds. Signs of consolidation. *Confirmed by:* **bronchoscopy and biopsy**. *Management:* OHCM p182.
Acute bilateral vocal cord paralysis	*Suggested by:* change in voice, bilateral reduced breath sounds and wheeze. *Confirmed by:* **laryngoscopy**.
Inhalation of foreign body	*Suggested by:* history of sudden cough and stridor, when eating. *Confirmed by:* **CXR, CT thoracic inlet, bronchoscopy**.
Tracheal tumours	*Suggested by:* cough, haemoptysis. *Confirmed by:* **bronchoscopy**.
Extrinsic compression by mediastinal masses	*Suggested by:* neck/chest discomfort ± swelling *Confirmed by:* **CT thoracic inlet**.
Extrinsic compression by oesophageal tumours	*Suggested by:* dysphagia, weight loss over weeks to months. *Confirmed by:* **CT thoracic inlet**.
Tracheal blunt trauma	*Suggested by:* history, pain and swelling, change in voice over minutes or hours after trauma. *Confirmed by:* **laryngoscopy**.

Expiratory polyphonic, high pitched wheeze

Suggest small airways obstruction.

Some differential diagnoses and typical outline evidence

Bronchial asthma	*Suggested by:* non-productive cough or white sputum, worse in morning. Some episodes not related to infection.
	Confirmed by: FEV_1 response to bronchodilators.
	Management: OHCM pp184–7.
'Wheezy bronchitis'	*Suggested by:* association with infective episodes of bronchitis alone.
	Confirmed by: FEV_1 response to bronchodilators and antibiotics.
	Management: OHCM pp184–7.
Anaphylaxis	*Suggested by:* history of allergen exposure, feeling of dread, hypotension, facial/generalised oedema, flushed, urticaria.
	Confirmed by: above history, **response to adrenaline and removal of precipitating cause**.
	Management: OHCM p780.
Left ventricular failure and pulmonary oedema	*Suggested by:* 'cardiac asthma': pink frothy sputum, 3rd heart sound, displaced apex beat.
	Confirmed by: **echocardiogram, CXR**.
	Management: OHCM p136–8, 786.

GI and GU signs

General examination checklist

Preliminary findings should have been discovered during the general examination. These include jaundice, anaemia, clubbing, xanthelasma, gynaecomastia, lips, buccal mucosa, fauces, tongue, supraclavicular lump(s).

Distended abdomen

Inspect the abdomen from a sitting position next to the bed or couch. Consider the general shape then look at the skin. Next, consider movement of the abdomen. The causes are the traditional 6 'F's: Fat, Fluid, Flatus, Faeces, Fibroids, Fetus.

Some differential diagnoses and typical outline evidence

Fat (obese)	*Suggested by:* usually sunken umbilicus, dullness to percussion throughout.
	Confirmed by: **CT abdomen**.
	Management: OHCM p208.
Fluid (ascites)	*Suggested by:* bilateral bulging flanks, shifting dullness, fluid thrill
	Confirmed by: **ultrasound liver and abdomen**.
	Management: OHCM p232.
Flatus (gas) due to normal dietary variation	*Suggested by:* tympanic sound throughout. Often associated constipation.
	Confirmed by: **AXR** shows normal gas shadow.
Small bowel obstruction ('flatus' again)	*Suggested by:* mild distension, early vomiting, central, high abdominal pain, resonant percussion, increased bowel sounds. Supine **AXR** showing central gas but no peripheral abdominal large bowel shadow (i.e. without haustra partly crossing) but valvulae conniventes of small intestine entirely crossing the lumen. Fluid levels on erect film.
	Confirmed by: **abdominal ultrasound and laparotomy findings**.
	Management: OHCM p492.
Large bowel obstruction	*Suggested by:* severe distension, late vomiting, visible peristalsis, resonant percussion, increased bowel sounds. Supine **AXR** showing peripheral abdominal large bowel shadow (with haustra partly crossing the lumen). Fluid levels on erect film.
	Confirmed by: **abdominal ultrasound and laparotomy findings**.
	Management: OHCM p492.

Faecal impaction	*Suggested by:* paucity of bowel movement and constipation. **AXR** shows stippled pattern of 'faecal loading'.
	Confirmed by: resolution of swelling with evacuation or partly with flatus tube.
Fibroids, large ovarian cyst	*Suggested by:* mass in pelvis in middle-aged female.
	Confirmed by: **abdominal ultrasound**.
Fetus	*Suggested by:* amenorrhoea and mass in pelvis (cannot get below it).
	Confirmed by: +ve **urine pregnancy test** or ↑*plasma* *β-hCG*. Also **abdominal ultrasound**.

Distended abdominal veins

Some differential diagnoses and typical outline evidence

Portal hypertension	*Suggested by:* veins radiating out from umbilicus (caput Medusa), ± ascites, ± splenomegaly, other stigmata of chronic liver disease, venous hum over collaterals.
	Confirmed by: **ultrasound scan** appearance of liver which is small cirrhotic with dilated portal veins.
	Management: OHCM p226.
Inferior vena cava obstruction	*Suggested by:* distended veins with blood flow up from groin towards chest when compressed and one end released.
	Confirmed by: **CT abdomen**.
Superior vena cava obstruction	*Suggested by:* distended veins with blood flow from chest towards groin when compressed and one end released.
	Confirmed by: **CT thorax**.
	Management: OHCM p436.

Abdominal bruising

Also consider the general causes of bruising as indicated in the general examination findings.

Some differential diagnoses and typical outline evidence

Retroperitoneal haemorrhage e.g. in acute pancreatitis	*Suggested by:* abdominal tenderness and rigidity, bruises in and around the umbilicus (Cullen's sign), on one or both flanks (Grey Turner's sign).
	Confirmed by: ↑**serum amylase, CT abdomen**.
Ruptured or dissecting abdominal aortic aneurysm	*Suggested by:* hypotension and abdominal pain, tenderness and rigidity, bruises in and around the umbilicus (Cullen's sign), on one or both flanks (Grey Turner's sign). Expansile pulsatile mass >3cm diameter, bruit over the mass.
	Confirmed by: **abdominal ultrasound** or **CT abdomen**.
	Management: OHCM p480.

Poor abdominal movement

From the sitting position watch and ask about any areas of tenderness and begin furthest away palpating gently looking at the patient's face to see if there is any reaction. 'Rigidity' is when there is no initial lack of resistance but reflex rigidity from the outset.

Some differential diagnoses and typical outline evidence

Small bowel obstruction ('flatus' again)	*Suggested by:* mild distension, early vomiting, central, high abdominal pain, resonant percussion, increased bowel sounds. Supine **AXR** shows central gas but no peripheral abdominal large bowel shadow (i.e. without haustra partly crossing) but valvulae conniventes of small intestine crossing the entire lumen. Fluid levels on erect film.
	Confirmed by: **abdominal ultrasound and laparotomy findings.**
	Management: OHCM p492.
Large bowel obstruction ('flatus' again)	*Suggested by:* severe distension, late vomiting, visible peristalsis, resonant percussion, increased bowel sounds. Supine **AXR** shows peripheral abdominal large bowel shadow (with haustra partly crossing the lumen). Fluid levels on erect film.
	Confirmed by: **abdominal ultrasound and laparotomy findings.**
	Management: OHCM p492.
Peritonitis from perforated stomach, duodenum, diverticulum; intraperitoneal haemorrhage or bowel infarction	*Suggested by:* decreased or absent abdominal movement, generalised tenderness and rigidity, absent bowel sounds and board-like rigidity.
	Confirmed by: **erect AXR or CXR** show gas under diaphragm and laparotomy.
	Management: OHCM p474.

Localised tenderness in the hypogastrium (suprapubic area)

Some differential diagnoses and typical outline evidence

Acute bladder distension (due to prostatic hypertrophy in males)	*Suggested by:* suprapubic mass (cannot get below), dull to percussion.
	Confirmed by: **bladder US scan, urethral catheterisation** and drainage of high volume of urine (e.g. >1 litre).
	Management: OHCM p496.
Cystitis	*Suggested by:* frequency of urine, dysuria, turbid urine, haematuria on 'dipstick'.
	Confirmed by: excess **WBC** and organisms on microscopy and growth of 'significant' bacterial colonies on **MSU culture**.
	Management: OHCM p262.

Localised tenderness in the right upper quadrant

Guarding is when there is reflex rigidity on palpation.

Some differential diagnoses and typical outline evidence

Acute cholecystitis	*Suggested by:* fever, guarding and positive Murphy's sign (abrupt stopping of inspiration when the palpating hand meets the inflamed gallbladder descending with the liver from behind the sub-costal margin on the right side—but not on the left side).
	Confirmed by: **ultrasound gallbladder and biliary ducts.**
	Management: OHCM p484.
Acute alcoholic hepatitis	*Suggested by:* history of recent drinking binge, tender hepatomegaly, jaundice.
	Confirmed by: rise and fall in liver function tests to coincide with binge, –ve **hepatitis serology.**
	Management: OHCM p255.
Acute viral hepatitis A (or serum B, C, D or E)	*Suggested by:* –ve history of recent binge drinking, fever, tender hepatomegaly, jaundice.
	Confirmed by: +ve **hepatitis serology A, B C, D or E.**
	Management: OHCM p576.
Acute liver congestion	*Suggested by:* tender hepatomegaly, ↑JVP, leg oedema.
	Confirmed by: **CXR showing large heart, liver ultrasound showing distension.**
	Management: OHCM p136.

Localised tenderness in the left upper quadrant

Some differential diagnoses and typical outline evidence

Pyelonephritis	*Suggested by:* fever, rigor, ↑vomiting, loin pain, tenderness at renal angle, ↑**WBC** proteinuria, haematuria, leucocytes on **urine testing**.
	Confirmed by: above clinical picture and 'significant' growth of organisms on **urine culture**. US scan for possible anatomical abnormality.
	Management: OHCM p242.
Splenic rupture	*Suggested by:* history of trauma, plain **AXR** showing loss of left psoas shadow, **peritoneal tap** demonstrates free blood.
	Confirmed by: **CT scan** and laparotomy.
	Management: OHCM p474.
Splenic infarct	*Suggested by:* presence of predisposing cause especially sickle cell disease and crisis.
	Confirmed by: **CT** abdomen.
	Management: OHCM p440.

Localised tenderness in the epigastrium or central abdomen

Some differential diagnoses and typical outline evidence

Gastritis	*Suggested by:* epigastric pain, dull or burning discomfort, nocturnal pain.
	Confirmed by: **oesophagogastroscopy, barium meal and pH study**.
	Management: OHCM p214.
Duodenal ulcer	*Suggested by:* epigastric pain, dull or burning discomfort, typically relieved by food, nocturnal pain.
	Confirmed by: oesophagogastroscopy, barium meal and pH study. **Helicobacter pylori** present in mucosa or **serology**.
	Management: OHCM p214.
Gastric ulcer	*Suggested by:* epigastric pain, dull or burning discomfort, typically exacerbated by food.
	Confirmed by: **oesophagogastroscopy, barium meal and pH study**.
	Management: OHCM p214.
Pancreatitis	*Suggested by:* rigidity or guarding ± bruises e.g. Cullen or Grey Turner's signs.
	Confirmed by: ↑**serum amylase, CT pancreas** showing enlargement cyst/pseudocyst.
	Management: OHCM p478, 479.
Small bowel infarction	*Suggested by:* abdominal distension, absent bowel sounds. Predisposing cause e.g. atrial fibrillation, extensive atheroma in diabetes.
	Confirmed by: **AXR** showing dilated loop of small bowel with valvulae conniventes but no large bowel (with haustra etc.).
	Management: OHCM p488.
Ruptured or dissecting abdominal aortic aneurysm	*Suggested by:* hypotension and abdominal pain, tenderness and rigidity, bruises in and around the umbilicus (Cullen's sign), on one or both flanks (Grey Turner's sign). Expansile pulsatile mass >3cm diameter, bruit over the mass.
	Confirmed by: **abdominal ultrasound** or **CT abdomen**.
	Management: OHCM p480.

Localised tenderness in the left or right loin

Some differential diagnoses and typical outline evidence

Pyelonephritis	*Suggested by:* fever, rigor, vomiting, loin pain, tenderness at renal angle, ↑*WBC* proteinuria, haematuria, leucocytes on **urine testing**. *Confirmed by:* clinical picture and 'significant' growth of organisms on **urine culture**. US scan for possible anatomical abnormality. *Management: OHCM* p262.
Renal calculus	*Suggested by:* colicky pain beginning in loin and radiating down to lower abdomen. Tenderness at renal angle. *Confirmed by:* haematuria, dilated ureter on **renal ultrasound**, filling defect on **IVU**. *Management: OHCM* p264.
Ruptured or dissecting abdominal aortic aneurysm	*Suggested by:* hypotension and abdominal pain, tenderness and rigidity, bruises in and around the umbilicus (Cullen's sign), on one or both flanks (Grey Turner's sign). Expansile pulsatile mass >3cm diameter, bruit over the mass. *Confirmed by:* **abdominal ultrasound** or CT **abdomen**. *Management: OHCM* p480.

Localised tenderness in left or right lower quadrant

Some differential diagnoses and typical outline evidence

Appendicitis	*Suggested by:* abdominal pain, then localised to right (rarely left in situs inversus) lower quadrant, fever, guarding, +ve Rovsing's sign (tenderness on contralateral side), psoas sign (pain from passive extension of right hip), adductor pain (pain on passive internal rotation of flexed thigh); anterior tenderness on rectal examination.
	Confirmed by: macroscopic and microscopic appearances at **laparotomy**.
	Management: OHCM p476.
Diverticulitis	*Suggested by:* left iliac fossa tenderness ± tender mass.
	Confirmed by: flexible sigmoidoscopy, barium enema.
	Management: OHCM p482.
Ureteric calculus	*Suggested by:* colicky pain with radiation to lower abdomen, microscopic or frank haematuria.
	Confirmed by: ureteric dilation on **renal ultrasound**, filling defect on **IVU**.
	Management: OHCM p264.
Mesenteric adenitis	*Suggested by:* symptoms and signs similar to early appendicitis but without guarding or rectal tenderness.
	Confirmed by: clinical findings or made at laparotomy or laparoscopy
	Management: OHCM p476.
Salpingitis	*Suggested by:* severe adnexal tenderness, cervical motion tenderness, cervical discharge.
	Confirmed by: **cervical swab culture, laparoscopy**.
	Management: OHCM p488.

Ectopic pregnancy	*Suggested by:* enlarged uterus (but often small for dates), vaginal bleeding, faintness/shock in acute rupture.
	Confirmed by: pregnancy test +ve, mass on bimanual examination. **Pelvic ultrasound** shows empty uterus with thickened decidua.

Hepatomegaly—smooth and tender

Some differential diagnoses and typical outline evidence

Right heart failure due to pulmonary hypertension acutely due to pulmonary embolism	*Suggested by:* ↑JVP, leg oedema.
	Confirmed by: large heart on **CXR** and associated large pulmonary arteries or pulmonary oedema if CCF.
	Management: OHCM pp255, 136.
Alcoholic hepatitis	*Suggested by:* history of drinking binge, ↑MCV, jaundice.
	Confirmed by: abnormal *liver function tests:* ↑↑ AST: ↑ALP, *liver biopsy* later.
Infectious hepatitis	*Suggested by:* sharp edge, no or slight splenomegaly, jaundice.
	Confirmed by: abnormal liver function tests, hepatitis A serology positive.
	Management: OHCM p576.
Glandular fever (infectious mononucleosis)	*Suggested by:* cervical lymphadenopathy, sharp edge, ± Splenomegaly, ± jaundice.
	Confirmed by: **Paul–Bunnell**, +ve **heterophil antibody** test.
	Management: OHCM p570.
Right heart failure due to tricuspid regurgitation	*Suggested by:* pulsatile liver, ± jaundice ↑JVP with prominent v waves, systolic murmur louder on inspiration.
	Confirmed by: **echocardiography**.
	Management: OHCM p150.

Hepatomegaly—smooth but *not* tender

Some differential diagnoses and typical outline evidence

Cirrhosis of the liver (early + fatty change)	*Suggested by:* firm, round edge, ± splenomegaly, other stigmata of chronic liver disease (e.g. spider naevi).
	Confirmed by: small liver with abnormal parenchyma on **liver ultrasound and biopsy** appearance.
	Management: OHCM pp254–5.
Lymphoma	*Suggested by:* generalised lymphadenopathy, splenomegaly.
	Confirmed by: **lymph node biopsy, bone marrow biopsy, CT thorax/abdomen.**
	Management: OHCM p660.
Leukaemia	*Suggested by:* anaemia, lymphadenopathy, splenomegaly.
	Confirmed by: abnormal **WBC** on blood film, **bone marrow examination.**
	Management: OHCM pp652–6.
Haemochromatosis	*Suggested by:* bronze skin pigmentation, evidence of diabetes mellitus, cardiac failure, arthropathy.
	Confirmed by: elevated **serum ferritin** (>500µg/L), **liver biopsy with hepatic iron measurement.**
	Management: OHCM p234.
Primary biliary cirrhosis	*Suggested by:* xanthelasmata and xanthomas, scratch marks, arthralgia, ± splenomegaly.
	Confirmed by: +ve **anti-mitochondrial antibody, ↑↑serum IgM, liver biopsy.**
	Management: OHCM p238.
Amyloidosis 1° or 2° to chronic inflammation	*Suggested by:* evidence of underlying chronic infective disease if 2°.
	Confirmed by: **biopsy of rectal mucosa**, stained with Congo red dye.
	Management: OHCM p668.

Hepatomegaly—irregular, not tender

Some differential diagnoses and typical outline evidence

Metastatic carcinoma	*Suggested by:* hard, ± nodular, cachexia.
	Confirmed by: **liver ultrasound ± biopsy**.
	Management: OHCM p242.
Hepatoma	*Suggested by:* firm, nodular edge, ± arterial bruit ↑serum AFP.
	Confirmed by: alpha-fetoprotein ↑, **liver ultrasound and biopsy**.
	Management: OHCM p242.
Hydatid cyst	*Suggested by:* sometimes hard, nodular.
	Confirmed by: **liver ultrasound** showing cyst and daughter cysts inside, eosinophilia, **serology** (Echinococcus granulosus), **Casoni intradermal test**.
	Management: OHCM p616.

Splenomegaly—slight (<3 fingers)

Spleen enlarges diagonally downwards towards the RLQ. Begin there so as not to miss edge of massive enlargement.

Some differential diagnoses and typical outline evidence

Glandular fever	*Suggested by:* cervical lymphadenopathy, hepatomegaly with sharp edge.
	Confirmed by: **Paul–Bunnell, +ve heterophil antibody test (monospot).**
	Management: OHCM p570.
Brucella	*Suggested by:* occupation e.g. farmer, hepatomegaly.
	Confirmed by: **brucella serology.**
	Management: OHCM p592.
Hepatitis A, B, C or D	*Suggested by:* jaundice, tender hepatomegaly, lymphadenopathy
	Confirmed by: abnormal **liver function tests, hepatitis A, B, C and D serology.**
	Management: OHCM p576.
Bacterial endocarditis	*Suggested by:* splinter haemorrhages, heart murmur, anaemia, microscopic haematuria.
	Confirmed by: **blood cultures, trans-oesophageal echocardiography.**
	Management: OHCM pp152–3.
Amyloidosis 1° or 2° to chronic inflammation	*Suggested by:* evidence of underlying chronic infective disease if 2°.
	Confirmed by: **biopsy of rectal mucosa**, stained with Congo red dye.
	Management: OHCM p668.
Haemolytic anaemia	*Suggested by:* anaemia, jaundice.
	Confirmed by: **FBC** showing reticulocytosis, anaemia, **liver function tests** showing ↑unconjugated bilirubin, ↓haptoglobin.
	Management: OHCM p638.

Splenomegaly—moderate (3–5 fingers)

Some differential diagnoses and typical outline evidence

Lymphoma	*Suggested by:* generalised lymphadenopathy, non-tender hepatomegaly.
	Confirmed by: **lymph node biopsy, bone marrow biopsy, CT thorax/abdomen**.
	Management: OHCM p660.
Chronic leukaemia	*Suggested by:* lymphadenopathy, non-tender hepatomegaly.
	Confirmed by: abnormal FBC and **blood film, bone marrow examination**.
	Management: OHCM p656.
Cirrhosis ± portal hypertension	*Suggested by:* hard, round edge, ± hepatomegaly, other stigmata of chronic liver disease.
	Confirmed by: small nodular **liver** on **ultrasound ± biopsy**.
	Management: OHCM p232.

Splenomegaly—massive (>5 fingers)

Spleen enlarges diagonally downwards towards the RLQ. Begin there so as not to miss edge of massive enlargement.

Some differential diagnoses and typical outline evidence

Chronic myeloid leukaemia	*Suggested by:* variable hepatomegaly, bruising, anaemia.
	Confirmed by: presence of **Philadelphia chromosome, ↑↑WBC**.
	Management: OHCM p656.
Myelofibrosis	*Suggested by:* anaemia, ± hepatomegaly, ± lymphadenopathy.
	Confirmed by: **bone marrow tap** is usually dry, **bone marrow biopsy** shows fibrosis.
	Management: OHCM p664.
Malaria	*Suggested by:* anaemia, jaundice, hepatomegaly, paroxysmal rigors.
	Confirmed by: **thick and thin blood films** showing Plasmodium.
	Management: OHCM p560.
Kala-azar (visceral leishmaniasis)	*Suggested by:* pancytopenia, hepatomegaly.
	Confirmed by: demonstration of *Leishmania donovani* in **Giemsa-stained smears**, specific **serological test**.
	Management: OHCM pp610–11.

Bilateral masses in upper abdomen

The lower half of normal right kidney is often palpable. Renal mass is bimanually ballotable, moves slightly downwards on inspiration.

Some differential diagnoses and typical outline evidence

Polycystic renal disease	*Suggested by:* masses are bimanually ballotable, hypertension.
	Confirmed by: **ultrasound/CT kidneys**.
	Management: OHCM p286.
Amyloidosis, 1° or 2° to chronic inflammation	*Suggested by:* evidence of underlying chronic infective disease.
	Confirmed by: **biopsy of kidney or rectal mucosa**, stained with Congo red dye.
	Management: OHCM p668.
Bilateral hydronephroses	*Suggested by:* masses bimanually ballotable, renal impairment.
	Confirmed by: dilated ureters ± renal calyces on **abdominal ultrasound**.
	Management: OHCM p266.

Unilateral mass in right or left upper quadrant

Some differential diagnoses and typical outline evidence

Renal carcinoma	*Suggested by:* haematuria, PUO, ± polycythaemia.
	Confirmed by: **renal ultrasound/CT with biopsy**.
	Management: OHCM p498.
Unilateral hydronephrosis	*Suggested by:* no other symptoms and signs except bimanually ballotable mass.
	Confirmed by: unilateral dilated ureter ± renal calyx on **abdominal ultrasound.**
	Management: OHCM p266.
Renal cyst	*Suggested by:* tense, fluctuant feel.
	Confirmed by: cyst on **abdominal ultrasound**.
	Management: OHCM p260.
Distended gall bladder (on right side)	*Suggested by:* right sided pear-shaped rounded mass that continues with the liver above (Courvoisier's sign—implies extra-hepatic biliary obstruction).
	Confirmed by: **ultrasound gallbladder and biliary ducts.**
	Management: OHCM p484.

Mass in epigastrium (± umbilical area)

Some differential diagnoses and typical outline evidence

Gastric carcinoma	*Suggested by:* anorexia, weight loss over weeks to months, hard, irregular mass, left supraclavicular node (Virchow's node giving Troisier's sign).
	Confirmed by: **gastroscopy with biopsy**.
	Management: OHCM p508.
Carcinoma of pancreas	*Suggested by:* progressive painless jaundice ± abdominal or back pain later.
	Confirmed by: **ERCP or MRCP**.
	Management: OHCM p248.
Aortic aneurysm	*Suggested by:* >3cm in diameter, pulsatile swelling with bruit.
	Confirmed by: **abdominal ultrasound** or **CT abdomen**.
	Management: OHCM p480.

Mass in right lower quadrant

Some differential diagnoses and typical outline evidence

Appendix mass	*Suggested by:* recent history of fever and RIF pain.
	Confirmed by: **ultrasound** or **CT abdomen and finding at laparotomy**.
	Management: OHCM p476.
Crohn's granuloma	*Suggested by:* aphthous ulcers, wasting, anaemia, tender mass, scars of previous surgery, anal fissures, fistulae.
	Confirmed by: **barium follow through** and **small bowel enema, colonoscopy with biopsy**.
	Management: OHCM p247.
Carcinoma of caecum	*Suggested by:* asymptomatic right iliac fossa mass, iron-deficiency anaemia.
	Confirmed by: **colonoscopy with biopsy**.
	Management: OHCM pp506, 507.
Transplanted kidney	*Suggested by:* obvious history of transplant and scar over mass, usually in iliac fossa.
	Confirmed by: **abdominal ultrasound**.
	Management: OHCM p279.
Other causes: intussusception, carcinoma of ascending colon, caecal volvulus	

Mass in hypogastrium (suprapubic region)

Some differential diagnoses and typical outline evidence

Distended bladder	*Suggested by:* suprapubic dullness, resonance in flank, tender mass and acute retention of urine.
	Confirmed by: mass disappears on **bladder ultrasound scan and catheterisation, abdominal/pelvic ultrasound**.
	Management: OHCM p496.
Pregnant uterus	*Suggested by:* suprapubic dullness, resonance in flank.
	Confirmed by: pregnancy test +ve, bimanual examination, **abdominal/pelvic ultrasound scan**.
Uterine fibroid	*Suggested by:* asymptomatic, hard rounded non-tender mass on bimanual palpation.
	Confirmed by: **pelvic examination and ultrasound**.
Uterine neoplasm	*Suggested by:* postmenopausal bleeding, blood-stained vaginal discharge, irregular bleeding.
	Confirmed by: pelvic examination and **pelvic ultrasound**.
Ovarian cyst	*Suggested by:* tense, fluctuant feel, fluid thrill if cyst is large.
	Confirmed by: pelvic examination and **ultrasound of ovary**.

Mass in left lower quadrant

Some differential diagnoses and typical outline evidence

Diverticular abscess	*Suggested by:* fever, tender mass.
	Confirmed by: ultrasound/**CT abdomen/pelvis**.
	Management: OHCM p482.
Carcinoma of descending or sigmoid colon	*Suggested by:* hard mass, not tender.
	Confirmed by: **barium enema, colonoscopy with biopsy.**
	Management: OHCM pp506, 507.
Faecal impaction	*Suggested by:* paucity of bowel movement and constipation. **AXR** shows stippled pattern of 'faecal loading'.
	Confirmed by: resolution of swelling with evacuation or partly with flatus tube.

Central dullness, resonance in flank

Some differential diagnoses and typical outline evidence

Distended bladder	*Suggested by:* suprapubic mass, tender in acute retention of urine.
	Confirmed by: mass disappears on **bladder ultrasound scan and catheterisation**.
	Management: OHCM p496.
Pregnant uterus	*Suggested by:* suprapubic mass.
	Confirmed by: serum or urine β-hCG↑, pelvic/**abdominal ultrasound.**
Massive ovarian cyst	*Suggested by:* tense, fluctuant feel, fluid thrill.
	Confirmed by: **pelvic/abdominal ultrasound.**

Shifting dullness

Implies ascites

Some differential diagnoses and typical outline evidence

Carcinomatosis with spread to peritoneum	*Suggested by:* cachexia.
	Confirmed by: **diagnostic paracentesis including cytology, liver ultrasound with biopsy.**
Cirrhosis	*Suggested by:* stigmata of chronic liver disease, ± splenomegaly.
	Confirmed by: **paracentesis, liver ultrasound with biopsy.**
	Management: OHCM p232.
Congestive cardiac failure	*Suggested by:* ↑JVP, leg oedema, ± tender hepatomegaly.
	Confirmed by: **liver function tests, FBC, diagnostic paracentesis, CXR.**
	Management: OHCM p136–9.
Nephrotic syndrome	*Suggested by:* generalised oedema including face on rising from bed.
	Confirmed by: **proteinuria, hypoalbuminaemia.**
	Management: OHCM p270.
TB peritonitis	*Suggested by:* fever, history of tuberculosis, generalised tenderness.
	Confirmed by: **diagnostic paracentesis including microscopy, bacterial and AFB cultures.**
	Management: OHCM p564.
Peritoneal dialysis	*Suggested by:* renal failure, CAPD.
	Confirmed by: elevated **serum creatinine.**
	Management: OHCM p278.

Silent abdomen with no bowel sounds

Some differential diagnoses and typical outline evidence

Peritonitis e.g. due to bowel perforation	*Suggested by:* decreased or absent abdominal movement, generalised tenderness with 'board-like' rigidity.
	Confirmed by: **AXR**, erect **CXR** shows gas under diaphragm.
	Management: OHCM p474.
Bowel infarction	*Suggested by:* decreased or absent abdominal movement, generalised tenderness with 'board-like' rigidity.
	Confirmed by: **AXR**, erect **CXR** shows *no* gas under diaphragm.
	Management: OHCM p488.

High-pitched bowel sounds

Some differential diagnoses and typical outline evidence

Small bowel obstruction	*Suggested by:* mild distension, early vomiting, central, high abdominal pain, resonant percussion, increased bowel sounds. Supine *AXR* showing central gas but no peripheral abdominal large bowel shadow (i.e. without haustra partly crossing) but valvulae conniventes of small intestine entirely crossing the lumen. Fluid levels on erect film.
	Confirmed by: **abdominal ultrasound and laparotomy findings.**
	Management: OHCM p492.
Large bowel obstruction	*Suggested by:* severe distension, late vomiting, resonant percussion, increased bowel sounds. Supine *AXR* showing peripheral abdominal large bowel shadow (with haustra partly crossing the lumen). Fluid levels on erect film.
	Confirmed by: **abdominal ultrasound and laparotomy findings.**
	Management: OHCM p492.
Adhesions of bowel	*Suggested by:* scars, **signs of bowel obstruction**.
	Confirmed by: **abdominal ultrasound and laparotomy findings.**
	Management: OHCM p492.
Tumour in bowel	*Suggested by:* palpable abdominal mass, **signs of bowel obstruction**.
	Confirmed by: **abdominal ultrasound and laparotomy findings.**
	Management: OHCM p492.
Hernial orifice strangulation	*Suggested by:* hernia visible, not reducible, very ill, peritonism, **signs of bowel obstruction**.
	Confirmed by: **laparotomy findings.**
	Management: OHCM p524.

Sigmoid volvulus	*Suggested by:* **signs of severe bowel obstruction.** Supine *AXR* showing U shaped gas shadow.
	Confirmed by: **sigmoidascopy and reduction with flatus tube or and laparotomy findings.**
	Management: OHCM p492.
Irritable bowel syndrome	*Suggested by:* slight distension, history of abdominal pain and small hard motions.
	Confirmed by: abdominal ultrasound and spontaneous resolution.
	Management: OHCM p248, 249.
Faecal impaction	*Suggested by:* paucity of bowel movement and constipation. Hard faeces on rectal examination. *AXR* shows stippled pattern of 'faecal loading'.
	Confirmed by: resolution of swelling with evacuation or partly with flatus tube.

Abdominal/loin bruit

Some differential diagnoses and typical outline evidence

Aortic aneurysm	*Suggested by:* systolic bruit in the epigastrium (over mass), expansile pulsatile swelling.
	Confirmed by: **ultrasound/CT abdomen**.
	Management: OHCM p480.
Renal artery stenosis	*Suggested by:* systolic bruit in the right upper quadrant, hypertension. Expansile swelling.
	Confirmed by: **renal arteriography—digital subtraction angiography**.
	Management: OHCM p282.
Dissecting aorta	*Suggested by:* tearing abdominal pain radiating to back and hypotension. Brachial—ankle gradient and pulse delay.
	Confirmed by: urgent **ultrasound/CT abdomen**.
	Management: OHCM p480.

Lump in the groin

Some differential diagnoses and typical outline evidence

Inguinal hernia	*Suggested by:* origin horizontally just above and medial to pubic tubercle, impulse on coughing or bearing down, reducible.
	Confirmed by: above clinical examination and surgery.
	Management: OHCM p526.
Femoral hernia	*Suggested by:* origin horizontally just below and lateral to pubic tubercle, cough impulse rarely detectable, usually irreducible (because of narrow femoral canal).
	Confirmed by: above clinical examination and surgery.
	Management: OHCM p524.
Strangulated hernia	*Suggested by:* irreducible, tense and tender, red, followed by symptoms and signs of bowel obstruction.
	Confirmed by: above clinical examination and surgery.
	Management: OHCM p524.
Lymph node inflammation	*Suggested by:* enlarged, tender, mobile, nodes, usually multiple.
	Confirmed by: above clinical examination.
Lymphoma or secondary tumour	*Suggested by:* fixed nodes when infiltrated by tumour.
	Confirmed by: **ultrasound, exploration of groin**.
Femoral artery aneurysm	*Suggested by:* lump lies below the midpoint of the inguinal ligament, expansile pulsation.
	Confirmed by: above clinical examination. **Duplex ultrasound scan**.

Saphena varix (dilatation of long saphenous vein in the groin)	*Suggested by:* soft and diffuse swelling that lies below inguinal ligament, empties with minimal pressure and refills on release, disappears on lying down, cough impulse.
	Confirmed by: above clinical examination.
	Management: OHCM p528.
Cold abscess of psoas sheath	*Suggested by:* fluctuant tender swelling arising below the inguinal ligament.
	Confirmed by: **ultrasound, exploration of groin.**

Scrotal mass

Some differential diagnoses and typical outline evidence

Inguinal hernia descended into scrotum	*Suggested by:* inability to get above it. Does not transilluminate.
	Confirmed by: above clinical examination.
Testicular torsion	*Suggested by:* exquisitely tender, unilateral mass in the scrotal sac, chord thickened, opposite testis lies horizontally (bell-clapper testis).
	Confirmed by: above clinical examination, **Doppler ultrasound** reveals a ↓ blood flow.
Haematocele	*Suggested by:* history of trauma or scrotal surgery. Tenderness.
	Confirmed by: above history and examination, Doppler ultrasound.
Acute epididymitis	*Suggested by:* diffuse tenderness in the epididymis, marked redness and oedema.
	Confirmed by: **urine microscopy and culture** (white cells and organisms).
Acute orchitis	*Suggested by:* large and tender testes fever.
	Confirmed by: above history and examination.
Chronic epididymitis	*Suggested by:* chronic, diffuse scrotal tenderness.
	Confirmed by: identification of infecting organism by **urine cultures or culture of urethral discharge** after prostatic massage.
Varicocele (90% on the left)	*Suggested by:* non-tender, unilateral fleshy mass that feels like a bag of worms, decreases in size with scrotal elevation.
	Confirmed by: above clinical examination (patient must be examined while standing).

Hydrocele	*Suggested by:* non-tender, unilateral mass in scrotal sac.
	Confirmed by: above clinical and demonstration of transillumination.
	Management: OHCM p512.
Spermatocele	*Suggested by:* non-tender, small nodules posterior to the head of the epididymis.
	Confirmed by: above clinical examination, may or may not transilluminate.
	Management: OHCM p512.
Epididymal cyst	*Suggested by:* non-tender nodule in the head of epididymis, adjacent to inferior pole of testis and transillumination.
	Confirmed by: above clinical examination and demonstration of transillumination.
	Management: OHCM p512.
Seminoma	*Suggested by:* firm, non-tender, non-transilluminable nodule or mass adjacent to a testis.
	Confirmed by: **ultrasound of scrotal contents** showing a solid testicular mass, **direct surgical examination**, normal **serum alpha-fetoprotein**.
	Management: OHCM p512.
Teratoma	*Suggested by:* firm, non-tender, non-transilluminable nodule or mass adjacent to a testis.
	Confirmed by: **ultrasound of scrotal contents** showing a solid testicular mass, **direct surgical examination**, ↑**serum alpha-fetoprotein**.
	Management: OHCM p512.

Anal appearance

The rectal examination (with a chaperone) begins with an examination of the anus by parting the buttocks with the patient lying in the left lateral position with knees flexed.

Some differential diagnoses and typical outline evidence

Prolapsed internal haemorrhoids	*Suggested by:* segmental, plum-coloured rectal protrusion.
	Confirmed by: proctoscopy.
	Management: OHCM p522.
Acute anal fissure	*Suggested by:* acute pain during defaecation, exquisite anal tenderness. Mucosal fissure with skin tag if chronic (sentinel pile).
	Confirmed by: above history and clinical **examination under anaesthesia**.
	Management: OHCM p520.
Spontaneous perianal haematoma	*Suggested by:* blue-black lump in the skin near the anal margin.
	Confirmed by: above history and examination.
	Management: OHCM p520.
Perianal abscess	*Suggested by:* tender, fluctuant, perianal mass.
	Confirmed by: above clinical examination.
	Management: OHCM p520.
Rectal prolapse	*Suggested by:* smooth, elongated rectal protrusion continuous with anal skin.
	Confirmed by: above clinical examination.
	Management: OHCM p520.

Enlargement of prostate

The rectal examination continues by feeling for a prostatic protrusion anteriorly and sweeping around for other masses including impacted faeces.

Some differential diagnoses and typical outline evidence

Prostatitis	*Suggested by:* smooth, enlarged and tender.
	Confirmed by: **+ve urine culture, culture of prostatic secretions.**
	Management: OHCM p262.
Benign prostatic hypertrophy	*Suggested by:* smooth, enlarged, firm, non-tender usually with a palpable median groove.
	Confirmed by: normal or slight ↑ in **serum prostatic-specific antigen (PSA), prostatic biopsy.**
	Management: OHCM p496.
Prostatic carcinoma	*Suggested by:* irregular, hard, sometimes obliteration of median groove, non-tender.
	Confirmed by: ↑↑ **serum prostatic-specific antigen (PSA), prostatic biopsy.**
	Management: OHCM p498.

Melaena on finger

The rectal examination ends by inspecting the faecal smear on the examining gloved finger for colour, especially bright red blood or tarry melaena.

Some differential diagnoses and typical outline evidence

Bleeding duodenal ulcer	*Suggested by:* epigastric pain and tenderness, nausea.
	Confirmed by: **oesophagogastroscopy**.
	Management: OHCM pp214, 224.
Gastric erosion	*Suggested by:* history of NSAIDs or alcohol ingestion, epigastric pain, dull or burning discomfort, nocturnal pain.
	Confirmed by: **oesophagogastroscopy, barium meal and pH study**.
	Management: OHCM p224.
Gastric ulcer	*Suggested by:* epigastric pain, dull or burning discomfort, nocturnal pain.
	Confirmed by: **oesophagogastroscopy, barium meal and pH study**.
	Management: OHCM pp214, 220.
Mallory–Weiss tear	*Suggested by:* preceding marked vomiting, later bright red blood.
	Confirmed by: **oesophagogastroscopy**.
Gastro-oesophageal reflux	*Suggested by:* heartburn, anorexia, nausea, ± regurgitation of gastric content.
	Confirmed by: **oesophagogastroscopy, barium meal and oesophageal pH study**.
	Management: OHCM p216.
Hiatus hernia	*Suggested by:* heartburn, worsens with stooping or lying, relieved by antacids.
	Confirmed by: **oesophagogastroscopy, barium meal**.
	Management: OHCM p216.
False haematemesis	*Suggested by:* swallowed nose bleed (epistaxis) or haemoptysis.
	Confirmed by: normal **oesophagogastroscopy and ENT endoscopy**.

Oesophageal carcinoma	*Suggested by:* progressive dysphagia with solids, which sticks, weight loss.
	Confirmed by: **barium swallow, fibreoptic gastroscopy with mucosal biopsy.**
	Management: OHCM pp214, 508.
Gastric carcinoma	*Suggested by:* marked anorexia, fullness, pain, Troissier's sign (enlarged left supraclavicular lymph (Virchow') node).
	Confirmed by: **oesophagogastroscopy with biopsy.**
	Management: OHCM pp214, 508.
Ingestion of corrosives	*Suggested by:* history of ingestion etc.
	Confirmed by: **oesophagogastroscopy later.**
Oesophageal varices	*Suggested by:* liver cirrhosis, splenomegaly, prominent upper abdominal veins.
	Confirmed by: **oesophagogastroscopy.**
	Management: OHCM p226.
Bleeding diathesis	*Suggested by:* symptoms or signs of bleeding elsewhere (or bruising), DH of warfarin etc.
	Confirmed by: abnormal clotting screen and/or low platelets and/or improvement on withdrawal of a potentially causal drug (but NB possibility of another cause).

Fresh blood on finger on rectal examination

Usually suggestive of lower GI bleeding but occasionally from massive upper GI bleeding passing through rapidly without alteration.

Some differential diagnoses and typical outline evidence

Haemorrhoids	*Suggested by:* rectal bleeding follows defecation, perianal protrusion with pain.
	Confirmed by: anal inspection and **proctoscopy** (haemorrhoids drop over edge of proctoscope as it is withdrawn).
	Management: OHCM p522.
Rectal carcinoma	*Suggested by:* rectal bleeding with defaecation, blood often limited to surface of stool.
	Confirmed by: **sigmoidoscopy with rectal biopsy**.
	Management: OHCM p506.
Colonic carcinoma	*Suggested by:* alternate diarrhoea and constipation with red blood.
	Confirmed by: **colonoscopy with biopsy, barium enema**.
	Management: OHCM p506.
Ulcerative colitis	*Suggested by:* loose blood-stained stools, anaemia, arthropathy, uveitis and iritis.
	Confirmed by: **colonoscopy with biopsy, barium studies**.
	Management: OHCM pp244–5.
Crohn's disease	*Suggested by:* aphthous ulcers, anaemia, tender mass, scars of previous surgery, anal fissures, fistulae.
	Confirmed by: **colonoscopy with biopsy, barium studies**.
	Management: OHCM pp246–8.
Angiodysplasia	*Suggested by:* chronic recurrent GI bleeding.
	Confirmed by: **endoscopy, mesenteric angiography**.
	Management: OHCM p482.

Diverticulitis	*Suggested by:* history of red 'splash' in the toilet pan, left iliac fossa tenderness ± tender mass.
	Confirmed by: **flexible sigmoidoscopy, barium enema**.
	Management: OHCM pp482–3.
Ischaemic colitis	*Suggested by:* left-sided abdominal pain, loose stools, dark clots.
	Confirmed by: **barium enema** (may show 'thumb printing' sign), **colonoscopy**.
	Management: OHCM p488.
Meckel's diverticulum	*Suggested by:* usually asymptomatic, anaemia, rectal bleeding.
	Confirmed by: **technetium-labelled red blood cell scan, laparotomy**.
Intussusception (in children or elderly)	*Suggested by:* child, usually between 6–18 months of life, acute onset of colicky intermittent abdominal pain, red currant 'jelly' PR bleed, ± a sausage-shaped mass in upper abdomen.
	Confirmed by: **barium or air enema**, may reduce the intussusceptions with appropriate hydrostatic pressure.
	Management: OHCM p494.
Mesenteric infarction (acute occlusion)	*Suggested by:* acute abdominal pain, generalised tenderness, shock, profuse diarrhoea (patient often in atrial fibrillation).
	Confirmed by: **mesenteric angiography, exploratory laparotomy**.
	Management: OHCM p488.
Massive upper GI bleed	*Suggested by:* hypotension or associated haematemesis.
	Confirmed by: **upper GI endoscopy**.
Trauma	*Suggested by:* pain, history or physical signs of trauma (e.g. sexual assault).
	Confirmed by: sigmoidoscopy.

Vulval skin abnormalities

Some differential diagnoses and typical outline evidence

Thrush, *Candida albicans* often in pregnancy, contraceptive and steroids, immunodeficiencies, antibiotics and diabetes mellitus	*Suggested by:* vulva and vagina red, fissured and sore. *Confirmed by:* mycelia or spores on **microscopy and culture.** *Management:* OHCS p266.
Allergy	*Suggested by:* being worse after nylon underwear, chemicals and soap. *Confirmed by:* response to avoidance of precipitants. *Management:* OHCS p266.
Lichen sclerosis	*Suggested by:* being intensely itchy. Bruised red purpuric appearance. Bullae, erosions, and ulcerations. Later white, flat and shiny with an hourglass shape around the vulva and anus. *Confirmed by:* above clinical appearance and **biopsy.** *Management:* OHCS p266.
Leukoplakia	*Suggested by:* itchiness and white vulval patches due to skin thickening and hypertrophy. *Confirmed by:* above clinical appearance and **biopsy.** *Management:* OHCS p266.
Carcinoma of the vulva	*Suggested by:* an indurated ulcer with an everted edge. *Confirmed by:* **biopsy.** *Management:* OHCS p266.
Obesity, incontinence, diabetes mellitus psoriasis, lichen planus, scabies, pubic lice, threadworms	

Ulcers and lumps of the vulva

Some differential diagnoses and typical outline evidence

Vulval warts (condylomata acuminata) due to human papilloma virus	*Suggested by:* warts on vulva, perineum, anus, vagina, or cervix. Florid in pregnancy or if immunosuppressed.
	Confirmed by: above clinical appearance. Managed initially by annual **cervical smears** and observation of the vulva and anus.
	Management: OHCS p268.
Urethral caruncle caused by meatal prolapse	*Suggested by:* small red swelling at the urethral orifice. Tender and pain on micturition.
	Confirmed by: above clinical appearance.
	Management: OHCS p268.
Bartholin's cyst and abscess caused by blocked duct	*Suggested by:* extreme pain (cannot sit) and a very swollen, hot red labium.
	Confirmed by: above clinical appearance.
	Management: OHCS p268.
Herpes simplex (herpes type II)	*Suggested by:* vulva ulcerated and exquisitely painful. Urinary retention may occur.
	Confirmed by: above clinical appearance.
	Management: OHCS p268.

Other causes of vulval lumps: local varicose veins; boils; sebaceous cysts; keratoacanthomata, condylomata, latent syphilis; primary chancre; molluscum contagiosum; abscess; uterine prolapse or polyp; inguinal hernia; varicocele; carcinoma. Also causes of vulval ulcers: syphilis, herpes simplex, chancroid; lymphogranuloma venereum; granuloma inguinale; TB, Behçet's syndrome; aphthous ulcers; Crohn's disease

Lumps in the vagina

Some differential diagnoses and typical outline evidence

Cystocele	*Suggested by:* frequency and dysuria. Bulging upper front wall of the vagina.
	Confirmed by: **cystogram** showing residual urine within the cystocele.
	Management: OHCS p290.
Urethrocele	*Suggested by:* stress incontinence (leaks when laughing). Bulging of the lower anterior vaginal wall.
	Confirmed by: **micturating cystogram** showing displaced urethra and impaired sphincter mechanisms.
	Management: OHCS p290.
Rectocele	*Suggested by:* patient may have to reduce herniation prior to defecation by putting a finger in the vagina. Bulging middle posterior wall.
	Confirmed by: **barium enema or MRI scan** showing rectum bulging through weak levator ani.
	Management: OHCS p290.
Enterocele	*Suggested by:* bulging of the upper posterior vaginal wall.
	Confirmed by: **barium enema or MRI scan** showing loops of intestine in the pouch of Douglas.
	Management: OHCS p290.
Uterine prolapse	*Suggested by:* 'dragging' or 'something coming down', is worse by day. Cystitis, frequency, stress incontinence, and difficulty in defecation.
	Confirmed by: seeing the cervix well down in the vagina (first degree prolapse) or cervix protruding from the introitus when standing or straining (second degree) or the uterus lying outside the vagina which is keratinised and the cervix ulcerated (third degree prolapse or procidentia).
	Management: OHCS p290.

Vaginal carcinoma	*Suggested by:* vaginal bleeding. Tumour in the upper third of the vagina.
	Confirmed by: squamous cell carcinoma on **biopsy**.
	Management: OHCS p275.

Ulcers and lumps in the cervix

Some differential diagnoses and typical outline evidence

Cervical ectropion ('erosion' innocuous)	*Suggested by:* red ring of soft glandular tissue around cervical opening often found with puberty, combined Pill, during pregnancy. May be bleeding, producing excess mucus or infected.
	Confirmed by: (in cases of doubt) **histology** showing columnar epithelium.
	Management: OHCS p270.
Nabothian cysts	*Suggested by:* smooth spherical (mucus retention).
	Confirmed by: above clinical appearance.
	Management: OHCS p270.
Cervical polyps	*Suggested by:* increased mucus discharge or post-coital bleeding. Pedunculated polyp arising from mouth of cervix.
	Confirmed by: **histology** showing pedunculated benign tumour arising from endocervical junction.
	Management: OHCS p270.
Cervicitis	*Suggested by:* increased mucus discharge or post-coital bleeding. Very red swollen cervix with overlying mucous and blood.
	Confirmed by: histology being follicular or mucopurulent. Vesicles in herpes. **Culture** may produce chlamydia, gonococci, etc.
	Management: OHCS p270.
Cervical intraepithelial neoplasia (CIN)	*Suggested by:* overlying cervicitis, older women, smokers, under-privileged background, prolonged pill use, high parity, many sexual partners or a partner having many other partners, early first coitus, sexually transmitted diseases.
	Confirmed by: **Papanicolaou smear** showing degree of dyskaryosis but no malignancy on **cervical biopsy**.
	Management: OHCS p270.

Cervical carcinoma	*Suggested by:* inter-menstrual or post-coital bleeding. Firm or friable mass which bleeds on contact.
	Confirmed by: **Papanicolaou smear** showing severe dyskaryosis and malignancy on **cervical biopsy**.
	Management: OHCS pp272–3.

Tender or bulky mass (uterus, fallopian tubes or ovary) on pelvic examination

Some differential diagnoses and typical outline evidence

Pregnancy	*Suggested by:* amenorrhoea in sexually active woman. Uterus at 6 weeks of pregnancy is like an egg, at 8 weeks like a peach, at 10 weeks it is like a grapefruit, and at 14 weeks it fills the pelvis.
	Confirmed by: pregnancy test +ve, pregnancy sac seen on abdominal or *transvaginal ultrasound*.
	Management: OHCS p8.
Ovarian tumour, benign functional cysts, theca-lutein cysts, epithelial cell tumours (serous and mucinous), cystadenomas, mature teratomas, fibromas malignant cystadenomas, germ cell or sex cord malignancies, secondaries from the uterus or stomach, Krukenberg tumours spreading via the peritoneum	*Suggested by:* painless pelvic mass often to one side. May or may not have amenorrhoea.
	Confirmed by: **abdominal or transvaginal ultrasound**.
	Management: OHCS p280–3.

Endometritis (uterine infection) after abortion and childbirth, IUCD insertion, or surgery. May involve Fallopian tubes and ovaries. Low-grade infection is often due to chlamydia	*Suggested by:* lower abdominal pain and fever; uterine tenderness on bimanual palpation. *Confirmed by:* **transvaginal ultrasound, cervical swabs and blood cultures.** *Management: OHCS* p244.
Endometrial proliferation due to oestrogen stimulation	*Suggested by:* heavy menstrual bleeding and irregular bleeding (dysfunctional uterine bleeding) and polyps. *Confirmed by:* 'cystic glandular hyperplasia' in specimen after *D&C.* *Management: OHCS* p244.
Pyometra (uterus distended by pus, associated with salpingitis or secondary to outflow blockage)	*Suggested by:* lower abdominal pain and fever; uterine tenderness on bimanual palpation. *Confirmed by:* **transvaginal ultrasound, cervical swabs and blood cultures.** *Management: OHCS* p244.
Haematometra due to imperforate hymen in the young, carcinoma, iatrogenic cervical stenosis after cone biopsy	*Suggested by:* lower abdominal pain and uterine tenderness on bimanual palpation. *Confirmed by:* no evidence of infection. **Transvaginal ultrasound** appearance. *Management: OHCS* p244.
Endometrial tuberculosis (also affects the Fallopian tubes with pyosalpinx)	*Suggested by:* infertility, pelvic pain, amenorrhoea, oligomenorrhoea. *Confirmed by:* **transvaginal ultrasound, cervical swabs** and +ve smear or **cultures for AFB.** *Management: OHCS* p244.

Ectopic pregnancy	*Suggested by:* abdominal pain or bleeding in a sexually active woman. Gradually increasing vaginal bleeding, shoulder-tip pain (diaphragmatic irritation) and pain on defecation and passing water (due to pelvic blood). Sudden severe pain, peritonism and shock with rupture.
	Confirmed by: **hCG** >6000iu/L and an intrauterine gestational sac not seen on pelvic ultrasound or if **hCG** 1000–1500iu/L and no sac is seen on **transvaginal ultrasound**.
	Management: OHCS p262–3.
Fibroids (uterine leiomyomata)	*Suggested by:* heavy and prolonged periods, infertility, pain, abdominal swelling, urinary frequency, oedematous legs and varicose veins, or cause retention of urine.
	Confirmed by: normal **hCG** and **transvaginal ultrasound** showing discrete lumps in the wall of the uterus or bulging out to lie under the peritoneum (sub-serosal) or under the endometrium (submucosal), pedunculated.
	Management: OHCS p276–7.
Acute salpingitis often associated with endometritis, peritonitis, abscess and chronic infection	*Suggested by:* being unwell, with pain, fever, spasm of lower abdominal muscles (more comfortable lying on back with legs flexed). Cervicitis with profuse, purulent, or bloody vaginal discharge. Cervical excitation and tenderness in the fornices bilaterally but worse on one side. Symptoms vague in subacute infection.
	Confirmed by: **laparoscopy**.
	Management: OHCS p286.
Chronic salpingitis (unresolved, unrecognised, or inadequately treated acute salpingitis) leading to fibrosis and adhesions, pyosalpinx or hydrosalpinx	*Suggested by:* pelvic pain, menorrhagia, secondary dysmenorrhoea, discharge, deep dyspareunia, depression. Palpable tubal masses, tenderness and fixed retroverted uterus.
	Confirmed by: **laparoscopy** to differentiate between infection and endometriosis.
	Management: OHCS p286.

Vaginal discharge

Some differential diagnoses and typical outline evidence

Excessive normal secretion	*Suggested by:* women of reproductive age, milky white or mucoid discharge.
	Confirmed by: normal investigations.
Bacterial vaginosis	*Suggested by:* fishy odour discharge, itching, irritation.
	Confirmed by: **high vaginal swab, wet saline microscopy shows presence of cells.**
	Management: OHCS p284.
Cervical erosions (ectropion)	*Suggested by:* no other obvious symptoms.
	Confirmed by: **speculum examination.**
	Management: OHCS p270.
Endocervicitis (gonococcus, chlamydia)	*Suggested by:* symptoms in partner of urethritis.
	Confirmed by: inflamed cervix on **speculum examination** and **endocervical swab** result.
	Management: OHCS p286–7.
Carcinoma of cervix	*Suggested by:* blood stained discharge, irregular vaginal bleeding, obstructive uropathy and back pain in late stage.
	Confirmed by: **cervical smear, cytology, colposcopy with biopsy.**
	Management: OHCS p272–3.
Foreign body	*Suggested by:* blood stained discharge, use of ring pessary, intrauterine contraceptive device, tampon.
	Confirmed by: speculum examination or colposcopy or hysteroscopy.
Endometrial polyp	*Suggested by:* blood stained discharge, intermenstrual spotting, post-menstrual staining.
	Confirmed by: **hysteroscopy.**
	Management: OHCS p274.

Trichomonas vaginitis	*Suggested by:* profuse greenish yellow frothy discharge, dysuria, dyspareunia.
	Confirmed by: protozoa and WBC on **smear**.
	Management: OHCS p284.
Gonococcal cervicitis	*Suggested by:* purulent discharge, lower abdominal pain, fever, cervix appears red and bleeds easily.
	Confirmed by: **gram stain of cervical or urethral exudates** shows intracellular gram-negative diplococci.
	Management: OHCS p270.
Monilia vaginitis	*Suggested by:* purulent discharge, intense pruritus vulvae.
	Confirmed by: hyphae or spores on **cervical smear**.
	Management: OHCS p284.
Chlamydia cervicitis	*Suggested by:* purulent discharge, lower abdominal pain, fever, cervix appears red and bleeds easily.
	Confirmed by: **endocervical swab**.
	Management: OHCS p270.

Psychiatric signs

Psychiatric signs

Psychiatric signs will have been noted to a large extent during the history and examination. The patient may have complained of 'anxiety' or 'depression', but in order for these diagnoses to be accepted by other doctors, a number of attributes have to be present, some of which are observed rather than reported by the patient.

General excessive anxiety

Some differential diagnoses and typical outline evidence

Generalised anxiety disorder	*Suggested by:* long history of fearful anticipation, irritability, sensitivity to noise, restlessness, poor concentration, worrying thoughts, insomnia, nightmares, depression, obsessions, depersonalisation, dry mouth, difficulty swallowing, tremor, dizziness, headache, parasthesiae, tinnitus, epigastric discomfort, excessive wind, frequent or loose motions, constriction/discomfort in the chest, difficulty breathing or hyperventilation, palpitations and awareness of missed beats, frequency or urgency of micturition, erectile dysfunction, menstrual problems. Panic attacks, depression and alcohol dependence.
	Confirmed by: evidence of no thyrotoxicosis, no hypoglycaemia, no Cushing's disease, no phaeochromocytoma.
	Management: OHCS p344.
Panic disorder	*Suggested by:* intense feeling of apprehension or impending disaster. Develops quickly and unexpectedly without a recognizable trigger. Shortness of breath and smothering, nausea, abdominal pain, depersonalization, choking, numbness, tingling, palpitations, flushes, trembling, shaking, chest discomfort, fear of dying, sweating, dizziness, faintness.
	Confirmed by: 4 symptoms of panic attack in one episode and 4 attacks in a month, or a persistent fear of attacks.
	Management: OHCS p344.
Alcohol withdrawal	*Suggested by:* recent heavy alcohol intake (usually super-imposed on habitually high intake). Visual hallucinations suggest 'delirium tremens'.
	Confirmed by: subsequent episodes in similar circumstances.
	Management: OHCM p254; *OHCS* p363.
Thyrotoxicosis	*Suggested by:* heat intolerance, tremor, nervousness, palpitation, frequent bowel movements, goitre.
	Confirmed by: ↓TSH, ↑FT4.
	Management: OHCM p304.

Hypoglycaemia	*Suggested by:* preceded by seconds or minutes by anxiety, fear, chest tightness, sweating, hunger, and darkening of vision. Usually in diabetic, usually on insulin.
	Confirmed by: ↓ blood sugar (<2mmol/L).
	Management: OHCM p820.
Phaeochromocytoma	*Suggested by:* abrupt episodes of anxiety, fear, chest tightness, sweating, headaches, and marked rises in BP.
	Confirmed by: catecholamines (↑VMA, ↑HMMA) or free metadrenaline ↑ in urine and blood soon after episode.
	Management: OHCM pp314, 822.

Anxiety in response to specific issues

Some differential diagnoses and typical outline evidence

Anorexia nervosa	*Suggested by:* intense fear of gaining weight, though underweight. Amenorrhoea in women for ≥3 mo. and diminished sexual interest. Bingeing and vomiting, purging or excessive exercise. Depression and social withdrawal, sensitivity to cold, delayed gastric emptying, constipation, low blood pressure, bradycardia, hypothermia. *Confirmed by:* (BMI <17.5kg/m^2) and many of above clinical features. *Management: OHCS* p348–9.
Bulimia nervosa	*Suggested by:* fear of gaining weight, recurrent episodes of binge eating, far beyond normally accepted amounts of food. Vomiting, use of laxatives, diuretics ± appetite suppressants. *Confirmed by:* normal menses and normal weight. *Management: OHCS* p348–9.
Somatization or hysteria alone or with depression, anxiety, schizophrenia and substance abuse	*Suggested by:* physical symptoms with preoccupation with bodily sensations combined with a fear of physical illness. *Management: OHCS* p334–5.
Somatization disorder (Briquet's syndrome)	*Suggested by:* long history of numerous unsubstantiated physical complaints with no adequate physical explanation and refusal to be reassured. *Management: OHCS* p641.
Simple phobia	*Suggested by:* symptoms and signs of generalised anxiety disorder. *Confirmed by:* inappropriate anxiety in the presence of particular circumstances e.g. enclosed spaces (claustrophobia), spiders (arachnophobia). *Management: OHCS* p346.
Social phobia	*Suggested by:* intense and persistent fear of being scrutinized or negatively evaluated by others resulting in fear and avoidance of social situations (e.g. meeting people in authority, using a telephone, speaking in front of a group). May fear most or specific social situations. *Management: OHCS* p346.

Agoraphobia	*Suggested by:* panic attacks in crowds or situations where escape is difficult. Staying at home, will not visit doctors. Also depression, depersonalisation and obsessional thoughts.
	Management: OHCS p346.
Post-traumatic stress disorder caused by experiencing or witnessing a traumatic event e.g. major accident, fire, assault, military combat	*Suggested by:* memories, nightmares (up to years after event), flashbacks, numbing of emotions, anxiety and irritability, insomnia, poor concentration, hyper-vigilance. Accompanying depression, anxiety and drug/alcohol abuse and dependence.
	Management: OHCS p347.

Depression

Some differential diagnoses and typical outline evidence
OHCS p336–43.

Major depression	*Suggested by:* depressed mood ± loss of interest in pleasure.
	Confirmed by: for example, the additional presence of ≥5 of the following 7 symptoms: (1) change in appetite or weight, (2) psychomotor agitation or retardation, (3) insomnia or hypersomnia, (4) sense of worthlessness or guilt, (5) fatigue or loss of energy, (6) recurrent thoughts of death, (7) poor concentration suicide.
	Management: OHCS p336–7.
Mild to moderate depression	*Suggested by:* depressed mood ± loss of interest in pleasure.
	Confirmed by: for example, the additional presence of <5 of the following 7 symptoms: (1) change in appetite or weight, (2) psychomotor agitation or retardation, (3) insomnia or hypersomnia, (4) sense of worthlessness or guilt, (5) fatigue or loss of energy, (6) recurrent thoughts of death, (7) poor concentration suicide.
	Management: OHCS p336–7.
Depression secondary or partly due to other conditions	*Suggested by:* history of any other illness that undermines self-confidence but especially anxiety disorders, alcohol abuse, substance abuse.
	Confirmed by: improvement when underlying condition alleviated.
	Management: OHCS p336–7.
Depression secondary or partly due to medication	*Suggested by:* history of taking beta blockers, alpha blockers, anticonvulsants, calcium channel blockers, corticosteroids, oral contraceptives, antipsychotic drugs, drugs used for Parkinson's disease (e.g. levodopa).
	Confirmed by: improvement when drug stopped or changed.
	Management: OHCS p336–7.
Seasonal affective disorder	*Suggested by:* 'Winter blues': depression of mood + increased ↑ sleep, ↑ food intake (with carbohydrate craving) and weight gain sometimes with opposite mood swings in summer.
	Management: OHCS p404.

Hallucinations or delusions or thought disorder

Hallucinations: visions, voices and sounds not apparent to others present.
Delusion: belief held despite evidence to the contrary.
Thought disorder: thoughts jumps from one idea to another in a bizarre way.

Some differential diagnoses and typical outline evidence

Mania and hypomania	*Suggested by:* persistent high or euphoric mood out of keeping with circumstances.
	Confirmed by: pressure of speech, no insight, overassertiveness, increased energy and activity, grandiose delusions, spending sprees, increased appetite, hallucinations, disinhibition, increased sexual desire, labile mood, elation, self-important ideas, diminished pain threshold, irritability, poor concentration, hostility when thwarted, diminished desire or need for sleep.
	Management: OHCS p354–5.
Bipolar disorder or manic depression	*Suggested by:* consists of episodes when the patient has mania (bipolar I) or hypomania (bipolar II) against a background of depression.
	Management: OHCS pp336–7, 354–5.
Acute schizophrenia	*Suggested by:* sufferer's apparent inability to distinguish between imaginary and external world.
	Confirmed by: at least one of the following Schneider first rank symptoms: somatic hallucinations, thought insertion ± withdrawal, thought broadcasting, primary delusions (in addition to thought delusions, passivity feelings, thought echo or hearing voices referring to the patient in the 3rd person).
Chronic schizophrenia	*Suggested by:* sufferer appearing unable to relate to external world with blunting of affect.
	Confirmed by: thought disorder and poverty of thought, apathy, inactivity, lack of volition, social withdrawal and loss of affect.
	Management: OHCS p356–61.

Confusion (global cognitive deficit)

(May be acute or chronic):

Some differential diagnoses and typical outline evidence

Acute confusional state (delirium) caused by infection, drugs, metabolic, alcohol or drug withdrawal, hypoxia, cardiovascular, intracranial lesion, thyrotoxicosis or hypothyroidism, carcinomatosis, epilepsy, nutritional deficiency	*Suggested by:* global cognitive deficit with onset over hours/days, fluctuating conscious level (typically worse at night), impaired memory (on recovery amnesia of the events is usual), disorientation in time and place, odd behaviour (may be underactive, drowsy ± withdrawn or hyperactive and agitated), disordered thinking, often slow and muddled ± delusions (e.g. accuse relatives of taking things), disturbed perceptions, hallucinations (particularly visual), mood swings. *Confirmed by:* outcome consistent with underlying cause and treatment. *Management: OHCS* p350–1.
Chronic confusion due to Alzheimer's disease (60%), vascular (multi-infarct) dementia, dementia with Lewy bodies	*Suggested by:* patient admitting to 'being a bit forgetful', but relatives complain of loss of short-term memory and inability to perform normally simple tasks or failure to cope at home or self-neglect. *Confirmed by:* no impairment of consciousness, clear history of progressive impairment of memory and cognition ± personality change, ± cerebral atrophy on CT brain scan. *Management: OHCS* p352–3.
Alzheimer's disease	*Suggested by:* features of dementia. *Confirmed by:* by absence of features of vascular (multi-infarct) dementia or Parkinsonism. *Management: OHCS* p352.
Vascular (multi-infarct) dementia	*Suggested by:* tends to occur with a stepwise progression of dementia with each subsequent infarct and pseudobulbar palsy. *Confirmed by:* by multiple lacunar infarcts or larger strokes cause on CT scan. *Management: OHCS* p374.
Lewy body dementia	*Suggested by:* fluctuating but persistent dementia with parkinsonism and hallucinations. *Confirmed by:* histology at post-mortem. *Management: OHCS* p648.

| Other neurode-generative diseases: Huntington's chorea, Bovine spongiform encephalopathy | *Suggested by:* other neuromuscular signs e.g. seizures, abnormal posture etc.

Confirmed by: clinical and post-mortem brain specimens. |

Neurological signs

Examining the nervous system

If there were no symptoms at all suggestive of neurological disease, it is usual to perform a quick examination of the nervous system, and if this examination is normal, then the nervous system is not examined further. There will have been an opportunity to note the patient's posture and gait in the consulting room (or as the patient moves around the bed on the ward). If the patient's face looks normal and moves normally during speech, then there is unlikely to be a cranial nerve abnormality. The patient is then asked to hold both arms out to assess posture, to perform a 'finger nose' test, to tap each hand on the other in turn, to 'unscrew doorknobs', to tap each foot on the floor (or the examiner's hand if in bed) and then to do a 'heel shin' test with each leg. Finally, reflexes are tested in the arms and legs. If all these are normal (and as emphasised already there are no symptoms of neurological disorder) then the nervous system is not examined further. If there is a symptom or sign of neurological disorder then the nervous system has to be examined carefully, perhaps beginning with the territory under suspicion.

Disturbed consciousness

Consciousness assessed using Glasgow coma scale (GCS) based on adding score for (a) best motor response (p510), (b) best verbal response (p512) and (c) eye opening (p512).

Some differential diagnoses and typical outline evidence

Probably no current brain damage	*Suggested by:* GCS = 15 (patient complying with all requests, oriented in time and place, opening eyes spontaneously).
	Confirmed by: neurological observation.
Probable minor brain injury	*Suggested by:* GCS of 13–15.
	Confirmed by: neurological observation or CT or MRI scan appearance.
Probable moderate brain injury	*Suggested by:* GCS of 9–12.
	Confirmed by: neurological observation or CT or MRI scan appearance.
Probable severe brain injury	*Suggested by:* GCS of 3–8.
	Confirmed by: neurological observation or CT or MRI scan appearance.
Probable very severe brain injury	*Suggested by:* GCS = 3 (no response to pain, no verbalisation and no eye opening).
	Confirmed by: neurological observation or CT or MRI scan appearance.

Best motor response

Comment: to be used to give GCS score.

Differential diagnosis

Carrying out verbal requests: score 6	*Confirmed by:* doing simple things that you ask. (Ignore grasp reflex.)
Localising response to pain: score 5	*Confirmed by:* purposeful movement in response to pressure on fingernail, supra-orbital ridges and sternum.
Withdraws to pain: score 4	*Confirmed by:* pulling limb away from painful stimulus.
Flexor response to pain 'decorticate posture': score 3	*Confirmed by:* flexion of limbs to painful stimulus.
Extensor response to pain 'decerebrate posture': score 2	*Confirmed by:* pain causing adduction and internal rotation of shoulder and pronation of forearm.
No response to pain: score 1	*Confirmed by:* no response to painful stimulus.

Best verbal response

Comment: to be used to give GCS score.

Differential diagnosis

Oriented: score 5	*Confirmed by:* knowing own name, the place, why there, year, season and month.
Confused conversation: score 4	*Confirmed by:* conversation but does not know name, not the place, not why there, nor year, season or month.
Inappropriate speech: score 3	*Confirmed by:* no conversation but random speech or shouting.
Incomprehensible speech: score 2	*Confirmed by:* moaning but no words.
No speech at all: score 1	*Confirmed by:* silence.

Eye opening

Comment: to be used to give GCS score.

Differential diagnosis

Spontaneous eye opening: score 4	*Confirmed by:* eyes open and fixing on objects.
Eye opening in response to speech: score 3	*Confirmed by:* response to specific request or a shout.
Eye opening in response to pain: score 2	*Confirmed by:* response to pain.
No eye opening at all: score 1	*Confirmed by:* no response to pain.

Speech disturbance

Inability to converse can be due to disturbance in any part of the process due to deafness, poor attention, receptive dysphasia, motor dysphasia, dysarthria, dysphonia, or aphonia or combinations of these.

Some differential diagnoses and typical outline evidence

Deafness due to ear disease or 8th cranial nerve lesions	*Suggested by:* no reaction to speech or noises (e.g. startling). *Confirmed by:* features of ear disease.
Inattention due to dementia, depression etc.	*Suggested by:* normal reaction (e.g. startling) to noise or speech but no interest in source of noise or speech. *Confirmed by:* features of causal condition e.g. dementia or depression.
Sensory dysphasia due to lesion's in Wernicke's area	*Suggested by:* inability to understand or comprehend speech (as if a foreign language is being spoken to patient). Worse for vocabulary or language acquired later in life. *Confirmed by:* CT or MRI scan showing lesion in Wernicke's area in dominant temporal lobe.
Motor dysphasia (or aphasia) due to lesion in dominant frontal-parietal lobe	*Suggested by:* inability to find words or names of things (nominal dysphasia). *Confirmed by:* CT or MRI scan showing lesion in Broca's area in frontal lobe.
Dysarthria (or anarthria) due to cerebellar connections, upper or lower motor neurone lesion	*Suggested by:* inability to coordinate speech with slurring, mumbling, failure to initiate or sustain speech. *Confirmed by:* associated features of weakness or in coordination of oral muscles.
Dysphonia (or aphonia) due to vocal cord dysfunction	*Suggested by:* hoarseness, voice loss or weakness, inability to cough properly. *Confirmed by:* indirect laryngoscopy (using mirror) to show vocal cord dysfunction or paresis.

Dysarthria

Difficulty with articulation and inco-ordination of speech muscles.

Some differential diagnoses and typical outline evidence

Cortical cerebral lesion (due to bleed, infarction or tumour)	*Suggested by:* slow, stiff speech (and dysphasia if extensive lesion in dominant hemisphere i.e. most dextrous hand is also affected) and other 'cortical' signs. *Confirmed by:* CT or MRI scan of brain.
Internal capsule cerebral lesion (due to bleed, infarction or tumour)	*Suggested by:* slow, stiff speech and other internal capsule signs (e.g. spastic hemiparesis). *Confirmed by:* CT or MRI scan of brain.
Upper motor neurone brain stem (pseudobulbar palsy due to ischaemia, motor neurone disease, MS)	*Suggested by:* slow stiff nasal quality, slurred) and other brain stem signs (e.g. spastic hemiparesis, dysphagia). *Confirmed by:* MRI scan of brain stem.
Lower motor neurone brain stem (bulbar) palsy (due to ischaemia, motor neurone disease, 'polio' syringobulbia, MS)	*Suggested by:* nasal ('Donald Duck' quality) and other brain stem signs (e.g. spastic hemiparesis, dysphagia). *Confirmed by:* MRI scan of brain stem.
Extrapyramidal dysarthria (due to Parkinson's disease)	*Suggested by:* difficulty in initiating speech which is slow with other signs of Parkinsonian syndrome. *Confirmed by:* response to dopaminergic drugs.
Cerebellar lesion (due to MS, ischaemia, tumour, hereditary ataxias)	*Suggested by:* staccato, undulating, broken flow, slurred and other cerebellar signs (e.g. ataxia). *Confirmed by:* MRI scan of cerebellum.
Drug effect (e.g. alcohol, sedatives)	*Suggested by:* dysarthria (slurred) and other drug effects. *Confirmed by:* response to removal of drug.

Absent sense of smell

This is not tested routinely but ask the patient if there is anything abnormal about their smell or taste. Tested using bottles with familiar essences.

Some differential diagnoses and typical outline evidence

Coryza (common cold)	*Suggested by:* running nose, fever, headache, sporadic perhaps with contact history.
	Confirmed by: history and nasal speculum examination.
Nasal allergy	*Suggested by:* running nose, fever, headache, recurrent and recognizable precipitant.
	Confirmed by: history and nasal speculum examination.
Skull fracture	*Suggested by:* history of facial or head injury.
	Confirmed by: history or skull X-ray in acute phase.
Frontal lobe tumour	*Suggested by:* personality change, features of dementia, recent epilepsy.
	Confirmed by: CT or MRI scan of brain.
Kallman's syndrome	*Suggested by:* delayed puberty or poor secondary sexual characteristics and libido, infertility. Primary amenorrhoea in ♀.
	Confirmed by: low oestrogens or testosterone and low FSH and LH.

Abnormal ophthalmoscopy appearance

Start with high positive (+) numbers for the eye surface and use the lowest light level possible. Look for the red reflex and zoom in to the eye until the red reflex fills the field of view. Examine the retina by rotating down to negative (−) numbers. Start with the disc, found by looking towards the patient's midline, and then follow the four main arteries out and back. Examine the macula by asking the patient to look at the light.

Some differential diagnoses and typical outline evidence

Corneal opacity in quiet eye (old ulcer due to past trauma, trachoma—tropical countries)	*Suggested by:* grey opacity in the clear cornea without dilated blood vessels gradual loss of vision. *Confirmed by:* absence of staining with fluoresceine. *Management:* OHCS p432.
Cataract (due to ageing (75%), diabetes, trauma, steroids, radiation, intra-uterine rubella or toxoplasmosis, or rubella, hypocal-caemia, etc.)	*Suggested by:* history of gradual onset of visual blurring and lens opacity visible during the red reflex examination with the ophthalmoscope. Usually >65 years or history of underlying condition (often already known and cataract develops later). *Confirmed by:* ophthalmoscopical appearance. *Management:* OHCS p442.
Optic nerve swelling or (eventually) atrophy (due to papillitis from multiple sclerosis, or papilloedema or optic nerve in-farction in temporal arteritis and retinal artery occlusion)	*Suggested by:* raised pink optic disc with blurred margins ± distended capillaries, and adjacent streak haemorrhages progressing to pale white disc with pale margins. Gradual loss of vision after initial disturbance. *Confirmed by:* visual field charting. Ophthalmoscopical appearance. *Management:* OHCS p438.
Peripheral retinal damage (laser therapy for diabetic retinopathy)	*Suggested by:* irregular pale patches of depigmentation with central black areas of pigment clumping. *Confirmed by:* ophthalmoscopical appearance and history.

Age-related macular degeneration (usually senile)	*Suggested by:* gradual loss of central vision, large, central yellowish white scar or haemorrhage when patient looks at ophthalmoscope light.
	Confirmed by: ophthalmoscopical appearance.
	Management: OHCS p438.
Retinal vein occlusion	*Suggested by:* sudden vision loss often in upper or lower half only.
	Confirmed by: extensive superficial retinal haemorrhages following the nerve fibre layer which may be in only the upper or lower half of the retina.
	Management: OHCS pp435–6.
Retinal artery occlusion	*Suggested by:* sudden loss of vision. May be total or partial upper or lower field.
	Confirmed by: in the first few days retinal pallor. Later a white thready thin artery.
	Management: OHCS pp435–6.
Primary optic atrophy (prior inflammation not seen— due to multiple sclerosis or optic nerve infarction)	*Suggested by:* gradual visual loss in a quiet eye and pale disc with sharp margins.
	Confirmed by: ophthalmoscopical appearance of pale white featureless disc and may have thin thready vessels.
	Management: OHCS p438.
Glaucoma	*Suggested by:* gradual loss of vision, deeply cupped disc.
	Confirmed by: ophthalmoscopical appearance of deep cupping with visible cribriform plate and nasal displacement of vessels. Loss of peripheral field. Raised intraocular pressure.
	Management: OHCS pp430, 440.
Retinitis pigmentosa	*Suggested by:* loss of peripheral and night vision.
	Confirmed by: visual field charting. Pale disc, thin thready blood vessels and fine star shaped pigment without patches of depigmentation. Visual field charting.
	Management: OHCS p444.
Choroidoretinitis	*Suggested by:* gradual loss of vision or blurring (in acute phases), and 'patchy' visual loss—scotoma.
	Confirmed by: visual field charting showing irregular patchy areas of visual loss. Corresponding areas in the eye of irregular depigmentation with dense areas of pigment in the centre. Tests results for underlying cause: CXR, serology, sputum, lung biopsy.
	Management: OHCS p438.

Ophthalmoscopy appearance in the diabetic

Red-free or green light of ophthalmoscope very useful for retinopathy.
NB serial visual acuity measurements to detect early maculopathy.

Some differential diagnoses and typical outline evidence

'Diabetic' cataract	*Suggested by:* gradual visual loss in a diabetic.
	Confirmed by: ophthalmoscopical appearance.
	Management: OHCS pp446–7.
'Diabetic' glaucoma	*Suggested by:* pale, deeply cupped disc with sharp margins.
	Confirmed by: ophthalmoscopical appearance and visual field test. Raised intraocular pressure.
	Management: OHCS p440.
Diabetic microaneurysm and bleeding into retina	*Suggested by:* **dots** (micro-aneurysms or deep haemorrhages) and **blots or flames** (deep and superficial haemorrhages).
	Confirmed by: regular retinal photography for progress.
	Management: OHCS pp446–7.
Venous irregularity preceding haemorrhage	*Suggested by:* localised widening of veins (e.g. sausage-shaped).
	Confirmed by: regular retinal photography for progress.
	Management: OHCS pp446–7.
Diabetic hard exudates	*Suggested by:* round and small pale area (after a single serous leak), circular with central red dot (indicating a continuous leak) enlarging circle with time.
	Confirmed by: regular retinal photography for progress.
	Management: OHCS pp446–7.
Diabetic macular exudates (leading to visual loss)	*Suggested by:* star-shaped pallor (as the exudates follow the radial nerve fibre arrangement) and loss of visual acuity.
	Confirmed by: regular retinal photography for progress.
	Management: OHCS pp446–7.

Diabetic soft exudates (nerve fibre infarct preceding new vessels)	*Suggested by:* pale grey area with indistinct margins.
	Confirmed by: regular retinal photography for progress.
	Management: OHCS pp446–7.
Diabetic new vessel formation (leads to haemorrhage)	*Suggested by:* 'frond' growing forwards into the vitreous (seen by adjusting focus) or like a net growing on the surface of the retina, arising from disc or larger peripheral veins.
	Confirmed by: 3-dimensional clinical appearance.
	Management: OHCS pp446–7.
Retinal haemorrhage and detachment	*Suggested by:* subhyaloid haemorrhage obscuring underlying vessels, often forming 'nest shape'—flat top and round bottom.
	Confirmed by: 3-dimensional clinical appearance.
	Management: OHCS p444.
Vitreous haemorrhage	*Suggested by:* sudden loss of vision in a diabetic and a poor red reflex on ophthalmoscopy.
	Confirmed by: retinal photography.
	Management: OHCS p434.
Retinal vein occlusion	*Suggested by:* sudden vision loss often in upper or lower half only.
	Confirmed by: extensive superficial retinal haemorrhages following the nerve fibre layer which may be in only the upper or lower half of the retina.
	Management: OHCS pp435–6.

Ophthalmoscopy appearances in the hypertensive

Some differential diagnoses and typical outline evidence

Grade I hypertensive retinopathy	*Suggested by:* raised blood pressure on 3 occasions typically >90mmHg diastolic or >140mmHg systolic.
	Confirmed by: segmental narrowing and tortuosity of arteries.
	Management: OHCS pp448–9.
Grade II hypertensive retinopathy	*Suggested by:* moderately raised blood pressure on 3 occasions typically >100mmHg diastolic or >160mmHg systolic.
	Confirmed by: segmental narrowing and tortuosity of arteries and arteriovenous nipping.
	Management: OHCS pp448–9.
Grade III hypertensive retinopathy	*Suggested by:* severely raised blood pressure on 3 occasions typically >120mmHg diastolic or >180mmHg systolic.
	Confirmed by: segmental narrowing and tortuosity of arteries and arteriovenous nipping and haemorrhages and exudates.
	Management: OHCS pp448–9.
Grade IV hypertensive retinopathy	*Suggested by:* severely raised blood pressure typically >140mmHg diastolic or >200mmHg systolic.
	Confirmed by: segmental narrowing and tortuosity of arteries and arteriovenous nipping and haemorrhages and exudates and papilloedema.
	Management: OHCS pp448–9.

Loss of central vision and acuity only

Visual acuity is tested in each eye with a Snellen chart at 6 metres: 6/6 = 100% acuity and 6/60 = 10% acuity (letters normally read at 60 metres only readable at 6 metres). Fields are tested by facing patient 1 metre away and patient closing matching eyes. Wag your finger, moving in from the periphery horizontally and diagonally, changing hands. Test for scotoma with red marker-pen top, moving horizontally and asking for change of colour and disappearance. The rate of onset is important, sudden loss of vision is an emergency.

Acute onset of visual loss:

Optic nerve swelling or (eventually) atrophy (due to papillitis from multiple sclerosis, or papilloedema or optic nerve infarction in temporal arteritis and retinal artery occlusion)	*Suggested by:* raised pink optic disc with blurred margins ± distended capillaries, and adjacent streak haemorrhages progressing to pale white disc with pale margins. Gradual loss of vision after initial disturbance.
	Confirmed by: visual field charting. Ophthalmoscopical appearance.
	Management: OHCS p434.
Temporal/giant cell or cranial arteritis	*Suggested by:* scalp tenderness, jaw claudication, loss of temporal arterial pulsation, sudden loss of vision, ↑↑ESR.
	Confirmed by: **temporal artery biopsy** (may be done shortly after starting prednisolone).
	Management: OHCM pp424–5.
Retinal artery occlusion	*Suggested by:* sudden loss of vision. May be total or partial upper or lower field.
	Confirmed by: in the first few days retinal pallor. Later a white thready thin artery.
	Management: OHCS p435.
Retinal vein occlusion	*Suggested by:* sudden vision loss often in upper or lower half only.
	Confirmed by: extensive superficial retinal haemorrhages following the nerve fibre layer which may be in only the upper or lower half of the retina.
	Management: OHCS p435.
Vitreous haemorrhage	*Suggested by:* sudden loss of vision in a diabetic and a poor red reflex on ophthalmoscopy.
	Confirmed by: retinal photography.
	Management: OHCS p435.

Gradual onset of visual loss:

Cataract (due to ageing (75%), diabetes, trauma, steroids, radiation, intra-uterine rubella or toxoplasmosis, or rubella, hypocal-caemia, etc.)	*Suggested by:* gradual onset of visual blurring and lens opacity visible during the red reflex examination with the ophthalmoscope. Usually >65 years or history of underlying condition (often already known and cataract develops later). *Confirmed by:* opthalmoscopical appearance. *Management:* OHCS pp442–3.
Macular degeneration (age-related)	*Suggested by:* gradual loss of central vision, large, central yellowish white scar or haemorrhage when patient looks at ophthalmoscope light. *Confirmed by:* ophthalmoscopical appearance. *Management:* OHCS p438.
Choroidoretinitis	*Suggested by:* gradual loss of vision, or blurring (in acute phases), and 'patchy' visual loss—scotomata. *Confirmed by:* visual field charting showing irregular patchy areas of visual loss. Corresponding areas in the eye of irregular depigmentation with dense areas of pigment in the centre. Tests results for underlying cause: CXR, serology, sputum, lung biopsy. *Management:* OHCS p438.
Glaucoma	*Suggested by:* gradual loss of vision, deeply cupped disc. *Confirmed by:* ophthalmoscopical appearance of deep cupping with visible cribriform plate and nasal displacement of vessels. Loss of peripheral field. Raised intraocular pressure. *Management:* OHCS pp440–1.
Primary optic atrophy (prior inflammation not seen—due to multiple sclerosis or optic nerve infarction)	*Suggested by:* gradual visual loss in a quiet eye and pale disc with sharp margins. *Confirmed by:* ophthalmoscopical appearance of pale white featureless disc and may have thin thready vessels. *Management:* OHCS p438.

Peripheral visual field defect

An upper or lower half defect is due to ocular pathology. Lesions between eye and chiasm cause unilateral defects but those from chiasma to brain are homonymous, i.e. affecting same area in each eye.

Some differential diagnoses and typical outline evidence

Psychogenic field defect	*Suggested by:* 'TUNNEL' vision' (same diameter at all distances). Normal optic disc, visual acuity and colour vision.
	Confirmed by: no progression on follow up.
Retinitis pigmentosa	*Suggested by:* funnel vision with good visual acuity in light with inability to navigate around objects and virtually blind in the dark.
	Confirmed by: pale atrophic disc, thin thready vessels and asterisk or reticular type pigment in the retina without pale patches of depigmentation. Visual field charting.
	Management: OHCS p444.
Choroiditis (choroido-retinitis) (due to TB, sarcoid toxoplasmosis, toxacara)	*Suggested by:* gradual loss vision or blurring (in acute phases), grey—white raised patch on retina, vitreous opacities, muddiness in the anterior chamber, then white patch with pigmentation around on retina (choroidoretinal scarring).
	Confirmed by: tests results for underlying cause: CXR, serology, sputum, lung biopsy.
	Management: OHCS p438.
Optic chiasm lesion (due to pituitary tumour, cranio-pharyngioma, aneurysm)	*Suggested by:* bitemporal hemianopia (or sometimes bitemporal upper quadrantinopia from tumour pushing up).
	Confirmed by: visual field charting. CT or MRI scan appearance.
	Management: OHCS pp428–9.
Optic tract lesion (due to middle cerebral artery thrombosis of contralateral side)	*Suggested by:* homonymous hemianopia.
	Confirmed by: visual field charting. MRI scan appearance.
	Management: OHCS p428–9.

Visual cortex lesion (due to posterior cerebral artery occlusion, tumour)	*Suggested by:* homonymous hemianopia or occasionally quadrantanopia. May have macular sparing (visual acuity normal). Funnel vision if bilateral.
	Confirmed by: visual field charting. CT or MRI scan appearance.
	Management: OHCS pp428–9.

Ptosis

Drooping of one or both upper eyelids.

Some differential diagnoses and typical outline evidence

Oculomotor (3rd nerve) lesion due to pituitary tumour, intra-cavernous or posterior communicating artery aneurysm, meningioma, tentorial pressure cone diabetes mellitus, syphilis and brain stem ischaemia	*Suggested by:* ptosis, diplopia, and squint maximal on looking up and in; but therefore in total loss eye looks down and out. **Dilated pupil (except in diabetes mellitus, syphilis and brain stem ischaemia when pupil not dilated);** other cranial nerve lesions that form pattern (see p548). *Confirmed by:* CT or MRI scan appearance. *Management: OHCS* pp442–4.
Horner's syndrome due to neck trauma or tumours, cervical rib, Pancoast tumour (in lung apex) syringo-myelia (in cervical spine), lateral medullary syndrome (in brain stem), hypothalamic lesion	*Suggested by:* ptosis and constricted (miotic) pupil, recessed globe of the eye and diminished sweating on same side of face. *Confirmed by:* history of trauma or onset over week or months suggestive of tumour, or years suggestive of MS or syrinx. Other cranial nerve signs that form a pattern of cervical plexus lesion or brain stem lesion. X-ray of upper chest, ribs or neck. CT of neck or upper chest or MRI scan of brain stem. *Management: OHCS* p424.
Myasthenia gravis	*Suggested by:* bilateral partial ptosis worsening as day progresses. *Confirmed by:* eyes begin to droop after 15 minutes of upgaze. +ve Tensilon test (edrophonium results in improvement in ptosis). *Management: OHCM* p400.

Myopathy (dystrophia myotonica)	*Suggested by:* bilateral partial ptosis with evidence of weakness in other muscle groups. Frontal balding, inability to release hand grip.
	Confirmed by: biopsy histology of other affected muscle.
	Management: OHCS p398.
Congenital ptosis	*Suggested by:* unilateral or bilateral partial ptosis present since birth. Compensatory head posture.
	Confirmed by: absence of other neurological signs.
	Management: OHCM p80.

Large (mydriatic) pupil with no ptosis

Some differential diagnoses and typical outline evidence

Holmes–Adie pupil due to ciliary ganglion degeneration	*Suggested by:* dilated pupil (often widely) that only reacts slowly to light by constricting in well-lit room after 30 minutes. Reacts to accommodation. Usually unilateral. Absent knee jerks. Usually in females.
	Confirmed by: benign outcome with no action necessary.
	Management: OHCS p424.
Traumatic iridoplegia	*Suggested by:* **history of direct trauma.** Dilated, fixed irregular pupil that does not accommodate nor react to light.
	Confirmed by: slit lamp examination of anterior eye chamber.
Drug effect due to cocaine, amphetamines, tropicamide, atropine	*Suggested by:* bilateral pupil dilation.
	Confirmed by: drug history and resolution with withdrawal.
Severe brain stem dysfunction (or death)	*Suggested by:* bilateral pupil dilation with no reaction to light, comatose, long tract pyramidal signs.
	Confirmed by: absent corneal reflex response, no vestibulo-ocular reflexes, no cranial motor response to stimulation, no gag reflex, insufficent respiratory effort when PCO_2 >6.7kPa to prevent further ↑ of PCO_2 and ↓PO_2.
	Management: OHCM p816.

Small (miotic) pupil with no ptosis

Some differential diagnoses and typical outline evidence

Argyll Robinson pupil (due to syphilis and diabetes mellitus, rarely)	*Suggested by:* unilateral, small, irregular pupil that 'accomodates' by constricting when focusing on near finger but does not react to light. *Confirmed by:* syphilis serology or fasting blood glucose ≥7mmol/L and random GTT glucose ≥11.0mmol/L. *Management: OHCS p424.*
Anisocoria normal variation	*Suggested by:* unilateral, small, miotic pupil that reacts normally to light and accommodation. *Confirmed by:* no change with time, benign outcome with no action necessary.
Age-related miosis due to autonomic degeneration	*Suggested by:* bilateral, small, miotic pupils that react normally to light and accommodates normally. *Confirmed by:* discovery in old age, no change with time, benign outcome with no action.
Drug effect due to opiates, pilocarpine	*Suggested by:* bilateral, small pupils. Not reacting to light. *Confirmed by:* drug history and resolution with withdrawal.
Pontine haemorrhage	*Suggested by:* bilateral, small, miotic pupils that react to light. Patient comatose, bilaterally or unilaterally hyper-reflexic and high or fluctuating temperature. *Confirmed by:* evolution of signs to localise to brain stem. MRI scan. *Management: OHCS p354.*

Squint and diplopia: ocular palsy

Elicited by asking the patient to follow the examiner's finger and asking if this results in 'seeing double' and looking for development of a convergent or divergent squint. Cover test: Fix focus in the distance and alternately cover either eye in quick succession. As cover is lifted observe the eye. If the uncovered eye now moves in, this indicates a divergent squint. If the eye moves out, this indicates a convergent squint.

Some differential diagnoses and typical outline evidence

Oculomotor (3rd nerve) paresis intracavernous or posterior communicating artery aneurysm, meningioma, tentorial pressure cone, diabetes mellitus, syphilis and brain stem ischaemia.	*Suggested by:* ptosis, diplopia and squint maximal on looking up and in; but therefore in total loss eye looks down and out. **Dilated pupil (except in diabetes mellitus, syphilis and brain stem ischaemia when pupil not dilated).** *Confirmed by:* other cranial nerve lesions that form pattern (see p548), skull X-ray P-A and lateral, CT or MRI scan appearance. *Management: OHCS* pp422–3.
Trochlear (4th cranial nerve paresis)	*Suggested by:* diplopia and squint maximal on looking down and in. Double vision for reading and walking down stairs. *Confirmed by:* other cranial nerve lesions that form pattern (see p548). MRI scan appearance. *Management: OHCS* pp422–3.
Abducent (6th cranial) nerve paresis	*Suggested by:* **double vision looking in direction of the affected muscle.** Head turn in direction of affected muscle. *Confirmed by:* other cranial nerve lesions that form pattern (see p548). MRI scan appearance. *Management: OHCS* pp422–3.
Myasthenia gravis, Graves disease, orbital cellulitis or tumour	*Suggested by:* diplopia and squint in all directions of gaze. *Confirmed by:* CT or MRI scan of orbit or +ve Tensilon test (edrophonium results in less diplopia and squint in myasthenia).

| Internuclear ophthalmoplegia | *Suggested by:* impaired conjugate gaze (slowness of adducting eye and nystagmus in abducting eye). |
| due to lesion in the medial longitudinal bundle usually due to multiple sclerosis or sometimes vascular | *Confirmed by:* other signs of brain stem lesion. |

Loss of facial sensation

Some differential diagnoses and typical outline evidence

Ophthalmic branch of trigeminal nerve lesion	*Suggested by:* absent corneal reflex (present corneal reflex excludes lesion) with diminished touch and pain sensation in upper face above the line of the eye.
	Confirmed by: other cranial nerve lesions that form pattern (see p548). MRI scan appearance.
Maxillary branch of trigeminal nerve lesion	*Suggested by:* diminished touch and pain sensation in mid face between line of mouth and line of eye.
	Confirmed by: other cranial nerve lesions that form pattern (see p548). MRI scan appearance.
Mandibular branch of trigeminal nerve lesion	*Suggested by:* diminished touch and pain sensation in lower face below line of mouth.
	Confirmed by: other cranial nerve lesions that form pattern (see p548). MRI scan appearance.

Jaw muscle weakness

Some differential diagnoses and typical outline evidence

Motor branch of trigeminal nerve (5th cranial): *lower* motor neurone type on same (ipsilateral) side.	*Suggested by:* weakness of jaw movement. Deviation of jaw when opening against resistance and poor contraction of masseter on clenching. **Decreased** jaw jerk. *Confirmed by:* other cranial nerve lesions that form pattern (see p548). MRI scan appearance.
Motor branch of trigeminal nerve (5th cranial): *upper* motor neurone type on other (contra-lateral) side.	*Suggested by:* weakness of jaw movement. Deviation of jaw when opening against resistance and poor contraction of masseter on clenching. **Increased** jaw jerk *Confirmed by:* other cranial nerve lesions that form pattern (see p548). MRI scan appearance.

Facial muscle weakness

Distinguish between upper (forehead muscles movement preserved) and lower (forehead movement weak) motor neurone type.

Some differential diagnoses and typical outline evidence

Facial nerve palsy (7th cranial): *upper motor neurone type* other (contralateral) side due to internal capsule lesion—cerebrovascular accident, tumour	*Suggested by:* **able** to raise eyebrows and close eye but **unable** to grimace nor smile symmetrically; other cranial nerve lesions that form pattern (see p548). *Confirmed by:* MRI scan. *Management: OHCM* p356.
Facial nerve palsy (7th cranial): *lower motor neurone type* on same (ipsilateral) side (see below for causes)	*Suggested by:* inability to raise eyebrows nor close eye (rolls upwards to hide iris revealing the white of the eye) nor grimace nor smile symmetrically; other cranial nerve lesions that form pattern (see p548). *Confirmed by:* MRI scan. *Management: OHCS* p574.
Bell's palsy	*Suggested by:* lower motor neurone 7th nerve palsy. Prior ache behind ear. No other physical signs (NB corneal reflex present and no deafness or vertigo). *Confirmed by:* above clinical features. *Management: OHCM* pp388–9; *OHCS* p574.
Ramsey Hunt syndrome	*Suggested by:* lower motor neurone 7th nerve palsy. Taste diminished on same side. Vesicles in external auditory meatus. *Confirmed by:* above clinical features.
Facial nerve palsy from parotid swelling	*Suggested by:* lower motor neurone 7th nerve palsy. Swelling in mid face on same side. *Confirmed by:* above clinical features and MRI scan. *Management: OHCS* p574.

Cerebello-pontine lesion (e.g. tumour)	*Suggested by:* lower motor neurone 7th nerve palsy. Associated 5th (loss of corneal reflex) and 7th cranial nerve lesion.
	Confirmed by: above clinical features. MRI scan appearance.
	Management: OHCM pp386–7.
Cholesteatoma	*Suggested by:* lower motor neurone 7th nerve palsy. Also deafness and vertigo.
	Confirmed by: above clinical features. MRI scan appearance.
	Management: OHCS p539.
Facial nerve palsy from demyelination	*Suggested by:* lower motor neurone 7th nerve palsy. Other focal neurological signs and symptoms disseminated in time and space.
	Confirmed by: above clinical features. MRI scan appearance.
Facial nerve palsy from brain stem ischaemia	*Suggested by:* lower motor neurone 7th nerve palsy. Signs of adjacent dysfunction e.g. nystagmus, long tract signs e.g. spastic hemiparesis.
	Confirmed by: above clinical features. MRI scan appearance.

Loss of hearing

Inability to hear whispering or ticking watch, and test with tuning fork held near ear (testing air and bone conduction together).

Some differential diagnoses and typical outline evidence

8th nerve con-duction defect on side X due to wax, foreign body, otitis externa, recurrent otitis media, injury to tympanic membrane, otosclerosis, cholesteatoma	*Suggested by:* forehead vibration heard louder on side X than on side Y (Weber's test) and mastoid vibration on side X louder than for air (Rinne's test). *Confirmed by:* auroscope appearance, formal audiometry and other cranial nerve lesions that form pattern (see p548). MRI scan appearance. *Management: OHCS pp550–1.*
Sensorineural (8th cranial) lesion on side Y due to old age, noise trauma, Paget's disease, Menier's disease, drugs, viral infections (e.g. measles), congenital rubella, meningitis, acoustic neuroma, meningioma	*Suggested by:* forehead vibration heard louder on side X than on side Y (Weber's test) and mastoid vibration same for both sides (Rinne's test). *Confirmed by:* other cranial nerve lesions that form pattern (see p548), formal audiometry and MRI scan appearance. *Management: OHCS pp550–1.*

Abnormal tongue, uvula and pharyngeal movement

9th, 10th (not 11th) and 12th cranial nerve lesions.

Some differential diagnoses and typical outline evidence

Glossopharyngeal (9th cranial) nerve lesion	*Suggested by:* loss of gag reflex and taste on posterior 1/3 of tongue; other cranial nerve lesions that form pattern (see p548).
	Confirmed by: MRI scan.
Vagus (10th cranial) nerve lesion due to jugular foramen lesion, bulbar palsy	*Suggested by:* deviation of uvula away from affected side when saying 'ah'; nasal regurgitation of water. Dysarthria; other cranial nerve lesions that form pattern (see p548).
	Confirmed by: MRI scan.
Lower motor neurone hypoglossal (12th cranial) nerve lesion on same (ipsilateral) side of deviation	*Suggested by:* deviation of tongue to side of lesion on protrusion. Fasciculation and wasting; other cranial nerve lesions that form pattern (see p548).
	Confirmed by: MRI scan.
Upper motor neurone hypoglossal (12th cranial) nerve lesion on other (contralateral) side of deviation	*Suggested by:* deviation of tongue to one side on protrusion. Small stiff tongue and cortical or internal capsule signs.
	Confirmed by: CT or MRI scan.

Multiple cranial nerve lesions

Some differential diagnoses and typical outline evidence

Pituitary tumour	*Suggested by:* optic tract or chiasm lesion. 3rd cranial nerve lesion.
	Confirmed by: CT or MRI scan appearance.
Anterior communicating artery aneurysm due to pituitary tumour or cerebral artery aneurysm	*Suggested by:* optic nerve lesion, 3rd and 4th cranial nerve lesions.
	Confirmed by: CT or MRI scan appearance.
Posterior carotid artery aneurysm	*Suggested by:* 4th and 5th cranial nerve lesions.
	Confirmed by: CT or MRI scan appearance.
Gradenigo's syndrome (lesion in petrous temporal bone)	*Suggested by:* 5th and 6th cranial nerve lesions.
	Confirmed by: MRI scan appearance.
Facial canal lesion e.g. cholesteatoma	*Suggested by:* 7th, 8th cranial nerve lesions alone (no 5th or 6th).
	Confirmed by: CT or MRI scan appearance.
Cerebello-pontine angle lesion e.g. tumour	*Suggested by:* 5th, 7th and 8th ± 6th cranial nerve lesions.
	Confirmed by: CT or MRI scan appearance.
Jugular foramen syndrome	*Suggested by:* 9th, 10th and 11th cranial nerve lesions.
	Confirmed by: MRI scan appearance.
Lateral medullary syndrome	*Suggested by:* vertigo, nystagmus, 5th cranial nerve lesion, Horner's syndrome, contralateral spinothalamic loss on trunk.
	Confirmed by: above clinical features. MRI scan appearance.

Weber's syndrome	*Suggested by:* ipislateral 3rd cranial nerve lesion and contralateral hemiparesis.
	Confirmed by: above clinical features. MRI scan appearance.

Odd posture of arms and hands at rest

Some differential diagnoses and typical outline evidence

Internal capsule lesion or pre-central gyrus and connections, or lower pyramidal tract (upper motor neurone)	*Suggested by:* arms flexed at elbow and wrist and weak. Increased tone and reflexes. Upper motor neurone facial weakness. *Confirmed by:* brain CT or MRI scan appearance.
T1 anterior root lesion	*Suggested by:* **claw hand**, wasting of all small muscles of the hand. Loss sensation of ulnar 1.5 fingers and ulnar border of forearm. *Confirmed by:* Nerve conduction study result.
Ulnar nerve lesion (below elbow)	*Suggested by:* **claw hand,** wasting of hypothenar eminence and dorsal guttering esp first. Weakness of finger abduction and adduction. Loss sensation of ulnar 1.5 fingers.
Radial nerve lesion (or C7 anterior root lesion)	*Suggested by:* **wrist drop**. Inability to extend wrist and grip. Loss sensation over 1st dorsal interosseous muscle. *Confirmed by:* Nerve conduction study result.

Fine tremor of hands

Elicited by asking patient to hold arms out straight in front and placing sheet of paper to rest on them (to amplify fine tremor).

Some differential diagnoses and typical outline evidence

Thyrotoxicosis	*Suggested by:* fine tremor, anxiety, tachycardia, sweating, weight loss, goitre, increased reflexes.
	Confirmed by: ↑ FT4 or FT3 and ↓↓ TSH.
	Management: OHCM p304.
Anxiety state	*Suggested by:* fine tremor, anxiety, tachycardia, sweating, weight loss, goitre, increased reflexes.
	Confirmed by: normal thyroid function tests. Improvement with sedation, psychotherapy etc.
Alcohol withdrawal	*Suggested by:* fine or coarse tremor, history of high alcohol intake and recent withdrawal, anxiety.
	Confirmed by: improvement with sedation, etc.
	Management: OHCM p254.
Sympathomimetic drugs	*Suggested by:* fine tremor, drug history.
	Confirmed by: improvement with withdrawal of drug.
Benign essential tremor	*Suggested by:* usually coarse tremor, long history, no other symptoms or signs.
	Confirmed by: normal thyroid test results. Improvement with beta blocker.

Coarse tremor of hands

Elicited by asking patient to hold arms out straight in front and extending wrists (for asterixis or flap), then asking the patient to touch their own nose and then the examiner's finger with arm extended, repetitively (for intention tremor).

Some differential diagnoses and typical outline evidence

Hepatic failure	*Suggested by:* flapping tremor (asterixis) aggravated when wrists extended. Spider naevi. Jaundice.
	Confirmed by: abnormal liver function tests and prolonged prothrombin time.
	Management: OHCM p230.
Carbon dioxide retention	*Suggested by:* flapping tremor (asterixis), aggravated when wrists extended. Muscle twitching, bounding pulse, warm peripheries.
	Confirmed by: blood gases show $\uparrow$ pCO$_2$.
	Management: OHCM p192.
Cerebellar disease	*Suggested by:* intention tremor (past pointing) when patient attempts to touch examiner's finger.
	Confirmed by: MRI scan.
Parkinsonism due to Parkinson's disease, drug-induced (chlorpromazine, haloperidol, metoclopramide, prochlorperazine); multisystem atrophy, Alzheimer's disease; postencephalitis, normal-pressure hydrocephalus	*Suggested by:* **resting** coarse tremor, ('pill-rolling'); 'lead-pipe rigidity'; expressionless face, paucity of movement, small hand writing, rapid shuffling ('festinant') gait with small steps.
	Confirmed by: clinical findings e.g. persistent blinking when forehead tapped (e.g. 'glabellar tap'). Clinical improvement with appropriate treatment.
	Management: OHCM pp382–3.
Benign essential tremor	*Suggested by:* usually coarse tremor, long history, no other symptoms or signs.
	Confirmed by: normal thyroid test results. Improvement with beta blocker.

Wasting of some small muscles of hand

Inter-metacarpal grooves are prominent due to muscle wasting.

Some differential diagnoses and typical outline evidence

Median nerve palsy usually due to carpal tunnel syndrome	*Suggested by:* wasting of thenar eminence. Weakness of thumb flexion, abduction and opposition. **Unable** to lift thumb with palm upwards but **able** to press with index finger. Loss of sensation over palmar aspect of radial 3.5 fingers of hand.
	Confirmed by: nerve conduction study results.
Ulnar nerve lesion from elbow (high) to wrist (low)	*Suggested by:* wasting of hypothenar eminence. **Able** to lift thumb with palm upwards but **unable** to press with index finger. Weakness of finger abduction and adduction. Loss of sensation in ulnar aspect 1.5 fingers of hand. Claw hand (in lower lesions).
	Confirmed by: nerve conduction study results.
T1 lesion: anterior horn cell or root lesion	*Suggested by:* wasting of all small muscles of hand. **Unable** to lift thumb with palm upwards but **unable** to press with index finger.
	Confirmed by: nerve conduction study results. MRI scan appearance around T1 level.
Motor neurone disease	*Suggested by:* **signs of T1 lesion**, prominent fasciculation, spastic paraparesis, wasted fasciculating tongue, no sensory signs.
	Confirmed by: clinical presentation and absence of structural abnormality on MRI scan appearance.
	Management: OHCM p394.
Syringomyelia	*Suggested by:* **signs of T1 lesion**, fasciculation **not** prominent, burn scars, dissociated sensory loss, Horner's syndrome, nystagmus. History over months to years.
	Confirmed by: MRI scan appearances.
	Management: OHCM p404.
Any prolonged systemic illness	*Suggested by:* global muscle wasting, general weight loss.
	Confirmed by: improvement in muscle wasting if primary disease treatable.

Cervical spondylosis compressing nerve root	*Suggested by:* **signs of T1 lesion**, neck pain and stiffness, and referred pain.
	Confirmed by: MRI scan showing root canal compression.
	Management: OHCM p396.
Tumour compressing nerve root	*Suggested by:* **signs of T1 lesion**, referred pain. Progressing over months.
	Confirmed by: MRI scan showing root canal compression.
Brachial plexus lesion	*Suggested by:* **signs of T1 lesion** and history of trauma to shoulder area or birth injury.
	Confirmed by: nerve conduction study results.
Cervical rib	*Suggested by:* **signs of T1 lesion** aggravated by movement or posture.
	Confirmed by: X-ray: presence of cervical rib. Relief by surgery.
Pancoast tumour (OHCM p732)	*Suggested by:* **signs of T1 lesion**, Horner's syndrome, features of lung cancer (clubbing, chest signs, lymph nodes etc.).
	Confirmed by: CXR and CT scan appearances.

Wasting of arm and shoulder

Loss of rounded contour of deltoid and biceps muscle. Fasciculation is localised twitching of muscle. Note facial expression.

Some differential diagnoses and typical outline evidence

Progressive muscular atrophy	*Suggested by:* bilateral wasting of hand, arm and shoulder girdle with fasciculation.
	Confirmed by: EMG results.
	Management: OHCM p398.
Motor neurone disease (amyotrophic lateral sclerosis) with anterior horn cell degeneration	*Suggested by:* initially unilateral wasting of shoulder abductor and biceps. Weakness of speech, swallowing. No sensory signs.
	Confirmed by: EMG results.
	Management: OHCM p394.
Primary muscle disease	*Suggested by:* bilateral wasting of shoulder abductor and biceps.
	Confirmed by: EMG findings or muscle biopsy.
	Management: OHCM p398.

Abnormalities of arm tone

Elicited by supporting elbow in one hand and asking patient to allow you to flex and extend arm at the elbow without assistance.

Some differential diagnoses and typical outline evidence

Cerebellar lesion	*Suggested by:* **tone diminished**, no wasting. Diminished reflexes. Past pointing, truncal ataxia, nystagmus.
	Confirmed by: CT or MRI scan appearance of cerebellum.
Primary muscle disease	*Suggested by:* **tone diminished** with wasting ± fasciculation.
	Confirmed by: EMG findings or muscle biopsy.
	Management: OHCM p398.
Upper motor neurone	*Suggested by:* **tone increased**. Brisk reflexes below lesion.
	Confirmed by: CT or MRI scan of brain or spinal cord.
Parkinson's disease	*Suggested by:* **tone increased** with cogwheel effect (superimposed tremor). Poor facial movement, shuffling hesitant 'festinant' gait, coarse temor.
	Confirmed by: Response to drug therapy.
	Management: OHCM pp382–4.

Weakness around the shoulder and arm without pain

Elicited by asking the patient to flex and extend wrist and elbow against resistance and to abduct, adduct, flex and extend shoulder against resistance, comparing both sides.

Some differential diagnoses and typical outline evidence

C4–5 root lesion	*Suggested by:* weakness of abduction at the shoulder only (not elbow or wrist).
	Confirmed by: nerve conduction studies and MRI scan of neck.
C5–6 root lesion Erb's palsy	*Suggested by:* weakness of flexion at the shoulder and elbow but not wrist. Arm externally rotated and adducted behind back (note porter's tip position). History of birth trauma.
	Confirmed by: nerve conduction studies and MRI scan of neck.
C7 root lesion	*Suggested by:* wrist drop or weakness of grip and extension at the **elbow and wrist.**
	Confirmed by: nerve conduction studies and MRI scan of neck.
Radial nerve lesion	*Suggested by:* wrist drop or weakness of grip and extension at the wrist but **not** at the elbow.
	Confirmed by: nerve conduction studies and history of trauma.
C8-T1 root lesion (Klumpke's paralysis)	*Suggested by:* arm held in adduction, paralysis/paresis of the small muscles of the hand, loss of sensation over ulnar border of the hand. History of birth trauma.
	Confirmed by: nerve conduction studies and MRI scan of neck.

Incoordination (on rapid wrist rotation or hand tapping)

Comment: this is often used as a 'screening' test (i.e. if normal you can discount any significant neuromuscular condition of the upper limbs in the absence of other symptoms or signs.

Some differential diagnoses and typical outline evidence

Upper motor neurone paresis	*Suggested by:* spastic weakness (i.e. with increased tone) in upper limb.
	Confirmed by: CT scan of brain or MRI scan of neck.
Lower motor neurone paresis	*Suggested by:* flaccid weakness (i.e. with decreased tone) in upper limb.
	Confirmed by: nerve conduction studies and MRI scan of neck.
Ipsilateral cerebellar lesion	*Suggested by:* decreased tone, past pointing, diminished reflexes.
	Confirmed by: CT or MRI scan of cerebellum.
Loss of proprioreception	*Suggested by:* loss of joint position sense and vibration sense.
	Confirmed by: nerve conduction studies.

Muscle wasting

Comment: has to be assessed in context of the bulk of other muscles.

Some differential diagnoses and typical outline evidence

Adjacent bone, joint or muscle disease	*Suggested by:* wasting with pain and limitation of movement. Visible swelling or deformity of bone or joint.
	Confirmed by: X-ray of affected part. EMG.
Lower motor neurone lesion	*Suggested by:* wasting and fasciculation. Tone decreased. Weakness and diminished reflexes.
	Confirmed by: nerve conduction studies.
Muscle disease	*Suggested by:* wasting. Tone decreased. Weakness and diminished reflex.
	Confirmed by: EMG.
	Management: OHCM p398.

Weakness around one lower limb joint

These weaknesses may point strongly to one nerve root lesion. Test by asking the patient to perform the movement against your resistance.

Some differential diagnoses and typical outline evidence

L1/2 root lesion or femoral nerve	*Suggested by:* weakness of hip flexion alone.
	Confirmed by: X-ray of lumbar spine and sacrum. Nerve conduction studies. MRI scan where lesion localised clinically.
L2/3 root lesion or obturator nerve	*Suggested by:* weakness of hip adduction alone.
	Confirmed by: X-ray of lumbar spine and sacrum. Nerve conduction studies. MRI scan where lesion localised clinically.
L3/4 root lesion or femoral nerve	*Suggested by:* weakness of knee extension alone.
	Confirmed by: X-ray of lumbar spine and sacrum. Nerve conduction studies. MRI scan where lesion localised clinically.
L4/5 root lesion or tibial nerve	*Suggested by:* weakness of foot dorsiflexion and inversion at the ankle.
	Confirmed by: X-ray of lumbar spine and sacrum. Nerve conduction studies. MRI scan where lesion localised clinically.
L5/S1 root lesion or common peroneal nerve	*Suggested by:* weakness of knee flexion alone.
	Confirmed by: X-ray of lumbar spine and sacrum. Nerve conduction studies. MRI scan where lesion localised clinically.
S1/2 root lesion or sciatic nerve	*Suggested by:* weakness of toe flexion alone.
	Confirmed by: X-ray of lumbar spine and sacrum. Nerve conduction studies. MRI scan where lesion localised clinically.
Lateral popliteal nerve palsy (usually traumatic)	*Suggested by:* flaccid 'foot drop' with weakness of eversion and dorsiflexion of the foot and a sensory loss over lateral aspect of leg.
	Confirmed by: nerve conduction study result.

Bilateral weakness of all foot movements

Some differential diagnoses and typical outline evidence

Guillain–Barré syndrome.	*Suggested by:* onset over days, preceding viral illness.
	Confirmed by: high CSF protein. Progressive course then variable recovery.
	Management: OHCM p727.
Lead poisoning	*Suggested by:* gradual onset over weeks to months.
	Confirmed by: nerve conduction studies, and history of exposure.
Porphyria	*Suggested by:* onset over months to years. Usually known to have porphyria.
	Confirmed by: EMG and ↑urine or faecal porphobilinogens.
	Management: OHCM p708.
Charcot–Marie–Tooth disease	*Suggested by:* onset over years. Associated with foot drop and peroneal atrophy upper limbs affected later.
	Confirmed by: EMG.
	Management: OHCM p720.

Spastic paraparesis

Bilateral lower limb paresis with increased tone. This is a *medical emergency* if acute.

Some differential diagnoses and typical outline evidence

Prolapsed disc (anteriorly thus compressing spinal cord)	*Suggested by:* sudden onset often associated with change in spinal posture.
	Confirmed by: MRI scan appearance.
	Management: OHCM p350.
Traumatic vertebral displacement or fracture	*Suggested by:* sudden onset associated with violent injury.
	Confirmed by: MRI scan appearance.
Collapsed vertebra (due to secondary carcinoma or myeloma)	*Suggested by:* sudden onset over minutes or hours. Other symptoms suggestive of neoplasia over months.
	Confirmed by: nerve conduction studies. MRI scan appearance.
Spondylitic bone formation compressing spinal cord	*Suggested by:* onset over months to years. Often past history of spondylitic back pain.
	Confirmed by: MRI scan appearance.
	Management: OHCM p396.
Multiple sclerosis affecting spinal cord	*Suggested by:* this and other intermittent neurological symptoms disseminated in site and time.
	Confirmed by: MRI scan appearance.
	Management: OHCM pp384–5.
Infective space occupying lesion e.g. TB or abscess	*Suggested by:* onset over days or weeks with fever from low grade to spiking.
	Confirmed by: MRI scan and findings at surgery, histology and microbiology.

Glioma or ependymoma in spinal cord	*Suggested by:* gradual onset over months.
	Confirmed by: MRI scan and findings at surgery, histology.
Parasaggital cerebral meningioma or other tumour	*Suggested by:* gradual onset over months.
	Confirmed by: MRI scan and findings at surgery, histology.

Hemiparesis (affecting arm and leg)

(See OHCM pp332–3 and 354–9)

Some differential diagnoses and typical outline evidence

Occlusion of upper branch of middle cerebral artery with infarction including Broca's area	*Suggested by:* expressive dysphasia and contralateral lower face and arm weakness. *Confirmed by:* MRI or CT scan appearance.
Occlusion of perforating branch of middle cerebral artery with lacunar infarction	*Suggested by:* hemiparesis alone with subsequent spasticity (or receptive dysphasia alone or hemi-anaesthesia alone). *Confirmed by:* MRI or CT scan appearance.
Total middle cerebral artery territory infarction (usually embolic)	*Suggested by:* contralateral flaccid hemiplaegia (with little subsequent spasticity) and hemi-anaesthesia with deviation of head to side of lesion. Also homonymous hemianopia with aphasia if dominant hemisphere affected or 'neglect' if non-dominant hemisphere affected. *Confirmed by:* MRI or CT scan appearance.
Posterior cerebral artery infarction	*Suggested by:* contralateral homonymous hemianopia or upper quadrantinopia, mild contralateral hemiparesis and sensory loss, ataxia and involuntary movement, memory loss, dyslexia, and ipsilateral 3rd nerve palsy. *Confirmed by:* MRI or CT scan appearance.
Anterior cerebral artery infarction	*Suggested by:* paresis of contralateral leg, rigidity, perseveration, grasp reflex in opposite hand, urinary incontinence and dysphasia if in dominant hemisphere. *Confirmed by:* MRI or CT scan appearance.

Disturbed sensation in upper limb

Elicit by testing touch (a piece of cotton wool), heat (a cold metal object), and pain (pin prick with a sterile needle) in each dermatome distribution. Note any discrepancy between these modalities of sensation. In the palm, examine the radial 3.5 fingers and the ulnar 1.5 fingers. Test joint position sense (by holding digits at their sides) and vibration with a tuning fork over bony prominences. Then use a two pointed device (2-point discrimination), placing objects into the patients hand and asking to guess what they are with eyes closed e.g. a 20 pence piece (stereognosis) and drawing figures on the palm (graphaesthesia). Consider if you have discovered any of the patterns described below.

Some differential diagnoses and typical outline evidence

Contralateral cortical (pre-central gyrus) lesion	*Suggested by:* astereognosis, diminished 2-point discrimination and graphaesthesia.
	Confirmed by: CT or MRI scan of brain.
Peripheral neuropathy	*Suggested by:* Loss of touch and pinprick sensation worse in hand, progressing upwards.
	Confirmed by: Nerve conduction studies.
Spinothalamic tract damage (no dorsal column loss) due to syringomyelia in cervical cord	*Suggested by:* loss of pinprick and temperature sensation, normal or disturbed touch but normal joint position and vibration sense in hand.
	Confirmed by: Nerve conduction studies. MRI of cervical cord.
Cervical or thoracic nerve root lesion	*Suggested by:* loss of sensation in dermatome distribution in hand or forearm or upper arm.
	Confirmed by: nerve conduction studies. X-ray and MRI scan of neck.
Peripheral nerve lesions in arm	*Suggested by:* loss of sensation localised to the forearm, upper arm or radial 3.5 fingers or ulnar 1.5 fingers in the palm.
	Confirmed by: nerve conduction studies.

Diminished sensation in arm dermatome

Some differential diagnoses and typical outline evidence

C5 posterior root lesion	*Suggested by:* loss of sensation of **lateral aspect of upper arm.**
	Confirmed by: nerve conduction studies. MRI scan appearance.
C6 posterior root lesion	*Suggested by:* loss of sensation of **lateral forearm and thumb.**
	Confirmed by: nerve conduction studies. MRI scan appearance.
C8 posterior root lesion	*Suggested by:* loss of sensation of **palmar and dorsal aspect of ulnar 1.5 fingers** *and* the ulnar border of the wrist.
	Confirmed by: nerve conduction studies. MRI scan appearance.
T1 posterior root lesion	*Suggested by:* loss of sensation of **ulnar border of the forearm.**
	Confirmed by: nerve conduction studies. MRI scan appearance.
T2 posterior root lesion	*Suggested by:* loss of sensation of **inner aspect of upper arm and breast.**
	Confirmed by: nerve conduction studies. MRI scan appearance.

Diminished sensation in the hand

Some differential diagnoses and typical outline evidence

Median nerve lesion due to carpal tunnel syndrome, 'pill', pregnancy, hypothyroidism, acromegaly, rheumatoid arthritis or nerve trauma	*Suggested by:* loss of sensation of **palmar aspect of radial 3.5 fingers** (in carpal tunnel syndrome, also discomfort in forearm and tingling if front of wrist tapped). If nerve severed, wasting of thenar eminence and thumb opposition. *Confirmed by:* X-ray wrist and elbow. Nerve conduction studies, and thyroid function tests, rheumatoid factor etc.
Ulnar nerve lesion to compression of deep palmar branch from trauma or ulnar groove at elbow from trauma or osteoarthritis	*Suggested by:* loss of sensation of **palmar and dorsal aspect of ulnar 1.5 fingers** *but not* the ulnar border of the wrist. *Confirmed by:* nerve conduction studies. X-ray wrist and elbow.
Radial nerve lesion due to local compression (e.g. arm left hanging over chair)	*Suggested by:* loss of sensation of **dorsal aspect of radial 3.5 fingers**. *Confirmed by:* nerve conduction studies.
C7 posterior root lesion due to cervical osteophytes	*Suggested by:* loss of sensation of **middle finger alone**. *Confirmed by:* nerve conduction studies. MRI scan appearances.
C8 posterior root lesion due to cervical osteophytes	*Suggested by:* loss of sensation of **palmar and dorsal aspect of ulnar 1.5 fingers** *and* the ulnar border of the wrist. *Confirmed by:* nerve conduction studies. MRI scan appearances.

Disturbed sensation in lower limb

Look for specific patterns as indicated below.

Some differential diagnoses and typical outline evidence

Contralateral cortical (pre-central gyrus) lesion	*Suggested by:* graphaesthesia.
	Confirmed by: CT or MRI scan of brain.
Peripheral neuropathy (due to diabetes mellitus, carcinoma, vitamin B$_{12}$ deficiency, drugs therapy, heavy metal or chemical exposure	*Suggested by:* loss of touch and pinprick sensation worse in foot (e.g. stocking distribution), progressing upwards.
	Confirmed by: nerve conduction studies. MRI scan appearance.
Spinothalamic tract damage (no dorsal column loss) due to contralateral hemisection of the cord	*Suggested by:* loss of pinprick and temperature sensation, normal or disturbed touch but normal joint position and vibration sense in foot.
	Confirmed by: nerve conduction studies. MRI of cervical cord.
Dorsal column loss due to vitamin B$_{12}$ deficiency, ipsilateral hemisection of the cord, rarely tabes dorsalis	*Suggested by:* loss of joint position and vibration sense in foot. Pinprick and temperature sensation normal.
	Confirmed by: nerve conduction studies. B$_{12}$ levels.
L1 posterior root lesion	*Suggested by:* loss of sensation in **inguinal region**.
	Confirmed by: nerve conduction studies. X-ray of lumbar spine and sacrum.

L2/3 posterior root lesion	*Suggested by:* loss of sensation in **anterior thigh**.
	Confirmed by: nerve conduction studies. X-ray of lumbar spine and sacrum.
L4/5 posterior root lesion	*Suggested by:* loss of sensation in **anterior shin**.
	Confirmed by: nerve conduction studies. X-ray of lumbar spine and sacrum.
S1 posterior root lesion	*Suggested by:* loss of sensation in **lateral border of foot**.
	Confirmed by: nerve conduction studies. X-ray of lumbar spine and sacrum.

Brisk reflexes

Some differential diagnoses and typical outline evidence

Thyrotoxicosis	*Suggested by:* brisk reflexes in all limbs with normal **flexor** plantar responses.
	Confirmed by: ↑FT4 and ↓↓TSH levels.
	Management: OHCM p304.
High level pyramidal tract lesion (cervical cord, brain stem, bilateral internal capsule or diffuse bilateral cortical lesion)	*Suggested by:* brisk reflexes in all limbs with **extensor** plantar responses. *Confirmed by:* normal FT4 and TSH levels. MRI scan appearances.
Contralateral pyramidal tract lesion in internal capsule, primary cortex, brain stem or cervical cord	*Suggested by:* unilateral brisk reflexes in upper and lower limb. *Confirmed by:* MRI of brain or cervical cord.

Diminished reflexes

Some differential diagnoses and typical outline evidence

Sensory neuropathy	*Suggested by:* diminished reflexes most marked peripherally. Normal muscle power. Normal **flexor** plantar responses.
	Confirmed by: nerve conduction studies.
Motor neuropathy	*Suggested by:* diminished reflexes, muscle wasting, fasciculation and weakness.
	Confirmed by: nerve conduction studies and normal electromyography.
Primary muscle disease	*Suggested by:* diminished reflexes, muscle wasting and weakness. No fasciculation.
	Confirmed by: nerve conduction studies and abnormal electromyography and muscle biopsy.
	Management: OHCM p398.
Cerebellar disease	*Suggested by:* unilateral brisk reflexes in upper and lower limb.
	Confirmed by: CT and MRI of brain posterior fossa.
Posterior root lesion in C7/C8	*Suggested by:* loss of **triceps** jerk.
	Confirmed by: MRI of disc space.
Posterior root lesion in C5/C6	*Suggested by:* Loss of **biceps** jerk.
	Confirmed by: MRI of disc space.
Posterior root lesion in L3/L4	*Suggested by:* Loss of **knee** jerk.
	Confirmed by: MRI of disc space.
Posterior root lesion in S1/S2	*Suggested by:* Loss of **ankle** jerk.
	Confirmed by: MRI of disc space.

Gait abnormality

Some differential diagnoses and typical outline evidence

Somatomization 'functional' cause	*Suggested by:* **bizarre gait with exaggerated delay on affected limb**. No other physical signs of a lesion.
	Confirmed by: patience and careful follow-up.
Contralateral pyramidal tract lesion (in cerebral hemisphere, internal capsule, brain stem or spinal cord)	*Suggested by:* **stiff leg swung in arc**. Other motor (± sensory) localising signs indicating level of lesion.
	Confirmed by: CT scan or MRI of probable site.
Parkinsonism	*Suggested by:* **shuffling festinant gait**, paucity of facial expression and movement, stiffness, tremor, etc.
	Confirmed by: response to treatment by dopamine agonist drugs etc.
	Management: OHCM p382.
Cerebellar lesion (tumour, ischaemia etc.)	*Suggested by:* **wide based gait**, inability to stand with feet together, falling to one side (truncal ataxia). Loss of tone and reflexes on same side as lesion.
	Confirmed by: MRI of posterior fossa of brain.
Dorsal column loss or peripheral neuropathy (due to Vitamin B_{12} deficiency, etc.)	*Suggested by:* **bilateral stamping, high stepping gait**, unsteadiness made worse by closing eyes (positive Rombergism).
	Confirmed by: nerve conduction studies and response to treatment of cause (if found).
Bilateral upper motor neurone lesion (usually in spinal cord)	*Suggested by:* **'scissors' or 'wading through mud' gait**. Bilateral leg weakness and brisk reflexes.
	Confirmed by: MRI of clinically probable site of lesion.

Pelvic girdle and proximal muscle weakness (e.g. due to hereditary muscular dystrophy	*Suggested by:* **waddling gait (hip tilts down when leg lifted)**. Hypotonic limb weakness and poor reflexes. *Confirmed by:* electromyography.
Joint, bone or muscle lesion	*Suggested by:* **hobbling with minimal time spent on affected limb**. Tenderness and limited range of movement. *Confirmed by:* X-rays and response to treatment or resolution of cause.
Lateral popliteal nerve palsy	*Suggested by:* **unilateral stamping, high stepping gait with foot drop**. Flaccid weakness around ankle. Loss of sensation of lateral lower leg. *Confirmed by:* nerve conduction studies.
Drug effect	*Suggested by:* wide based gait, nystagmus, past pointing. History of alcohol intake or other drug. *Confirmed by:* raised alcohol or other drug level, improvement with withdrawal.

Difficulty in rising from chair or squatting position

Some differential diagnoses and typical outline evidence

Polymyositis	*Suggested by:* muscle wasting, weakness and poor reflexes.
	Confirmed by: electromyography and muscle biopsy.
	Management: OHCM p420.
Carcinomatous neuromyopathy	*Suggested by:* muscle wasting, weakness and poor reflexes. Evidence of cancer (usually late stage).
	Confirmed by: electromyography and evidence of carcinomatosis.
Thyrotoxicosis	*Suggested by:* weight loss, tremor, sweating, anxiety, loose bowels. ↑ T3 or T4 and ↓↓ TSH.
	Confirmed by: response to treatment of thyrotoxicosis.
	Management: OHCM p304.
Diabetic amyotrophy	*Suggested by:* long history of diabetes mellitus.
	Confirmed by: nerve conduction studies and muscle biopsy.
Cushing's syndrome	*Suggested by:* facial and truncal obesity with limb wasting.
	Confirmed by: high midnight cortisol etc., and response to treatment.
	Management: OHCM pp310–11.
Osteomalacia	*Suggested by:* ↓ calcium and ↑ alkaline phosphatase.
	Confirmed by: response to treatment with calcium and vitamin D.
	Management: OHCM p700.

Hereditary dystrophy	*Suggested by:* evidence of primary muscle disease and family history.
	Confirmed by: muscle biopsy.
	Management: OHCM p398.

Pathology tests

Asymptomatic microscopic haematuria

This is detected on routine urine dipstick testing.

Some differential diagnoses and typical outline evidence

Menstruation	*Suggested by:* history of current, recent or imminent periods and no urinary symptoms.
	Confirmed by: –ve on repeating in mid-cycle.
Urinary tract infection	*Suggested by:* fever, frequency or dysuria, Nitrites ↑, leucocytes ↑ on 'dipstick'!
	Confirmed by: MSU microscopy and culture, response to antibiotics. US scan for possible anatomical abnormality.
	Management: OHCM pp262–3.
Recent urethral trauma	*Suggested by:* recent urethral catheterisation.
	Confirmed by: history, no infection in MSU.
Bleeding diathesis	*Suggested by:* bruising, anticoagulant therapy.
	Confirmed by: abnormal platelet and clotting screen.
Calculus or tumour anywhere in renal tract	*Suggested by:* persistent x3 microscopic haematuria.
	Confirmed by: urinalysis, renal ultrasound, IVU, then cystoscopy by urologist.
	Management: OHCM pp264–5.
Glomerulonephritis 1° or 2°s to SLE, SBE, etc.	*Suggested by:* persistent x3 microscopic haematuria, associated proteinuria, hypertension.
	Confirmed by: urine microscopy, renal ultrasound, immunoglobulins, complement, ANA, ANCA positive blood cultures/response to antibiotics.
	Management: OHCM pp268–9.
Nephritis 2°s to NSAIDs etc.	*Suggested by:* persistent x3 microscopic haematuria, taking NSAID or other suspicious drug.
	Confirmed by: urine microscopy, renal ultrasound, improvement on stopping suspected drug, IVU, etc.
	Management: OHCM pp280–1.

Asymptomatic proteinuria

Total protein excretion is usually <50mg/24 hours of which albumin alone is normally <30mg/24 hours. Abnormal proteinuria is regarded as >150mg/24 hours.

Some differential diagnoses and typical outline evidence

Postural or orthostatic proteinuria	*Suggested by:* specimen from ambulant person <40 years.
	Confirmed by: protein testing negative on early morning urine specimen.
Non-specific febrile illness	*Suggested by:* known febrile illness.
	Confirmed by: normal when illness resolved.
Urinary tract infection	*Suggested by:* fever. Nitrites ↑, leucocytes ↑, blood ↑ on 'dipstick' test.
	Confirmed by: MSU microscopy and culture. US scan abdomen for possible anatomical abnormality.
	Management: OHCM p262.
Glomerulonephritis 1° or 2°s to SLE, etc.	*Suggested by:* proteinuria >1g/24 hours, persistent x3 microscopic haematuria, hypertension.
	Confirmed by: urine microscopy, renal ultrasound, immunoglobulins, complement, ANA, ANCA etc.
	Management: OHCM pp268–9.
Nephritis 2°s to NSAIDs etc.	*Suggested by:* proteinuria >1g/24 hours, taking NSAID or other suspicious drug.
	Confirmed by: urine microscopy, renal ultrasound, improvement on stopping suspected drug, IVU, etc.
	Management: OHCM pp280–1.
Nephrotic syndrome due to minimal change GM, diabetes mellitus etc.	*Suggested by:* proteinuria >3g/24 hours.
	Confirmed by: serum albumin low (<30g/L) and oedema and ↑ cholesterol and ↑ triglycerides.
	Management: OHCM p270.

Glycosuria

Almost always indicates diabetes and blood sugar has to be tested, but consider other possibilities.

Some differential diagnoses and typical outline evidence

Diabetes mellitus	*Suggested by:* fatigue or other unexplained symptoms, thirst, polydipia, polyuria.
	Confirmed by: fasting blood glucose ≥7.0mmol/L on two occasions OR fasting; random or glucose tolerance test (GTT) glucose ≥11.1mmol/L once only with symptoms.
	Management: OHCM pp292–5.
Renal glycosuria	*Suggested by:* patient well, or, renal disease.
	Confirmed by: glycosuria when blood sugar shown to be normal on glucose tolerance test.

Raised urine or serum bilirubin

OHCM pp222–3.

Some differential diagnoses and typical outline evidence

Hepatocellular jaundice (due to hepatitis or very severe liver failure) (see p602)	*Suggested by:* jaundice with *dark* stools and dark urine. Also raised urine urobilinogen (you can check this immediately).
	Confirmed by: raised serum bilirubin and raised urine urobilinogen. Highly abnormal liver function tests. Normal bile ducts but abnormal liver parenchyma on Ultrasound scan.
Obstructive jaundice due to intrahepatic causes (drugs, hepatitis, etc.) or extrahepatic (stones, tumours, etc.) (see p604)	*Suggested by:* Jaundice with *pale* stools and dark urine. Also NO raised urinary urobilinogen.
	Confirmed by: Raised plasma bilirubin but markedly raised alkaline phosphatase, otherwise slightly abnormal liver function tests. Dilated bile ducts on ultrasound scan.

Hepatocellular jaundice

Suggested by: jaundice with *dark* stools and dark urine.

Confirmed by: raised serum bilirubin and raised urine urobilinogen. Highly abnormal liver function tests. Normal bile ducts on ultrasound scan.

Some differential diagnoses and typical outline evidence

Acute (viral) hepatitis A	*Suggested by:* tender hepatomegaly.
	Confirmed by: presence of hepatitis A IgM antibody suggests acute infection.
	Management: OHCM p576.
Acute hepatitis B	*Suggested by:* history of iv drug user, blood transfusion, needle punctures, tattoos, tender hepatomegaly.
	Confirmed by: presence of HBsAg in serum.
	Management: OHCM p576.
Acute hepatitis C	*Suggested by:* history of transfusion or other blood products. Tender hepatomegaly.
	Confirmed by: presence of anti-HCV antibody and antigen.
	Management: OHCM p576.
Alcoholic hepatitis	*Suggested by:* history of drinking, presence of spider naevi and other signs of chronic liver disease.
	Confirmed by: AST:ALT ratio >2, liver biopsy.
	Management: OHCM p223.
Drug-induced hepatitis e.g. paracetamol (dose dependent), halothane (independent)	*Suggested by:* drug history, recent surgery.
	Confirmed by: improvement after stopping the offending drug.
	Management: OHCM p223.
Primary hepatoma	*Suggested by:* weight loss, abdominal pain, RUQ mass.
	Confirmed by: ultrasound/CT liver, liver biopsy, ↑alpha-fetoprotein.
	Management: OHCM pp242, 243.
Right heart failure	*Suggested by:* ↑JVP, hepatomegaly, ankle oedema.
	Confirmed by: CXR, echocardiogram.
	Management: OHCM pp136–9.

Obstructive jaundice

Suggested by: jaundice with *pale* stools and dark urine.

Confirmed by: raised urine and serum bilirubin but NO raised urobilinogen in urine. Markedly raised alkaline phosphatase, otherwise slightly abnormal liver function tests. Dilated bile ducts on ultrasound scan.

Management: OHCM p443.

Some differential diagnoses and typical outline evidence

Common bile duct stones	*Suggested by:* pain in RUQ ± Murphy's sign.
	Confirmed by: ultrasound liver/biliary ducts.
	Management: OHCM pp484, 485.
Cancer of head of pancreas	*Suggested by:* painless jaundice, palpable gall-bladder (*Courvoisier's law*), weight loss.
	Confirmed by: CT pancreas, ERCP or MRCP.
	Management: OHCM p248.
Sclerosing cholangitis	*Suggested by:* progressive fatigue, pruritus.
	Confirmed by: serum alkaline phosphatase, no gall-stones, ERCP (beading of the intra- and extra-hepatic biliary ducts).
	Management: OHCM p238.
Primary biliary cirrhosis	*Suggested by:* scratch marks, non-tender hepatomegaly, ± splenomegaly, xanthelasmata and xanthomas, arthralgia.
	Confirmed by: +ve anti-mitochondrial antibody, ↑↑serum IgM, liver biopsy.
	Management: OHCM p238.
Drug-induced e.g. oral contraceptive pill, phenothiazines, anabolic steroids, erythromycin	*Suggested by:* drug history.
	Confirmed by: symptoms recede when offending drug is discontinued.
	Management: OHCM p223.
Pregnancy (last trimester)	*Suggested by:* jaundice during pregnancy and severe itching.
	Confirmed by: resolution following delivery.

Alcoholic hepatitis/ Cirrhosis	*Suggested by:* history of drinking, presence of spider naevi and other signs of chronic liver disease.
	Confirmed by: liver biopsy.
	Management: OHCM p254.
Dubin–Johnson syndrome (see OHCM p722)	*Suggested by:* intermittent jaundice, and associated pain in the right hypochondrium. No hepatomegaly.
	Confirmed by: normal alkaline phosphatase, normal LFT. Urinary bilirubin raised. Pigment granules on liver biopsy.

Hypernatraemia

Some differential diagnoses and typical outline evidence

Hypertonic plasma with hypervolaemia (e.g. excess IV saline) or hypovolaemia (e.g. diabetic polyuria or diabetes insipidus)	*Suggested by:* little hypotonic fluid orally or intravenously and thirsty, high volume of urine with low sodium content (e.g. in diabetic polyuria). *Confirmed by:* plasma osmolality high and urine osmolality higher (unless diabetes insipidus). *Management:* OHCM p690.
Diabetes inspidus with hypovolaemia	*Suggested by:* drinking excessively and passing large volumes of urine (polydipsia and polyuria). Thirsty. *Confirmed by:* plasma osmolality high and urine osmolality low. *Management:* OHCM p326.
Primary hyperaldosteronism due to adrenal hyperplasia or Conn's sydrome with adrenal tumour	*Suggested by:* normal fluid intake, blood pressure elevated. Serum potassium ↓. *Confirmed by:* plasma renin activity low and aldosterone levels high. CT or MRI scan appearance. *Management:* OHCM p314.

Medical Books Department (ER)
Academic Division
Oxford University Press
Great Clarendon Street
Oxford OX2 6DP
UK

Reader's comments card

Help us to make the *Oxford Handbook of Clinical Diagnosis* even better!

Send this card, or a letter, with your comments, to:

Medical Books Department (ER),
Oxford University Press,
Great Clarendon Street,
Oxford, OX2 6DP, UK

email: elizabeth.reeve@oup.com

or submit your comments online at the
Oxford Handbooks website:
www.oup.co.uk/medicine/handbooks

Where relevant, please give references
to back up points.

1: Are you currently a medical student/junior doctor/specialist registrar/nurse/midwife/other (specify)?

2: What do you like/dislike about the *Oxford Handbook of Clinical Diagnosis*?

3: Please list any words you have not been able to find in the index.

4: Would you like to add any further suggestions or comments?

Personal details (optional):

Name: .... Position. ....

Address: ....

.... Post/Zip Code: .... Country: ....

email: ....

Medical specialties/subjects of interest: ....

We may wish to send you information by post or email on OUP products or services including news and special offers on Oxford Handbooks. Please tick here if you do not wish to be included on our mailing list. ☐

Hyponatraemia

Also usually indicates hypotonicity—low plasma osmolality.

Some differential diagnoses and typical outline evidence

Hypotonic with hypovolaemia due to excess renal or non-renal loss	*Suggested by:* excessive diuretic therapy, history of renal tubular disease, diarrhoea, vomit, fistula, burns, small bowel obstruction, blood loss.
	Confirmed by: response to removal or treating of cause, iv saline with careful monitoring of U&E in severe cases.
	Management: OHCM pp690, 691.
Hypotonic with normovolaemia	*Suggested by:* history of severe hypothyroidism or glucocorticoid deficiency.
	Confirmed by: response to treating cause, balancing fluid intake.
	Management: OHCM pp690, 691.
Hypotonic with hypervolaemia	*Suggested by:* history of water overload, cardiac failure, cirrhosis, renal failure, glucocorticoid deficiency, inappropriate ADH secretion.
	Confirmed by: response to treating cause, reducing fluid intake.
	Management: OHCM pp690, 691.
Syndrome of inappropriate antidiuretic hormone secretion	*Suggested by:* serum sodium usually <120mmol/L. Confusion, progressing to coma, mild oedema.
	Confirmed by: urine osmolality > serum osmolality despite serum osmolality being low (<270mmol/L). Urine sodium >20mmol/L usually.
	Management: OHCM 690.

Hyperkalaemia

Some differential diagnoses and typical outline evidence

Drug effect: potassium administration or other drug effect	*Suggested by:* potassium supplements, blood transfusion, ACE inhibitor, spironolactone, amilioride, triamterene, etc.
	Confirmed by: normal potassium when drug reduced or stopped.
Metabolic acidosis, renal failure, diabetic ketoacidosis	*Suggested by:* usually obvious illness and severe metabolic disturbance pH↓ and plasma HCO_3↓.
	Confirmed by: response to treatment of metabolic disturbance.
Addison's disease	*Suggested by:* fatigue, blood pressure low, pigmented buccal mucosa and palmar creases Na↓, K↑.
	Confirmed by: random and 9am cortisol↓, ACTH↑, and poor response to synacthen stimulation. Response to iv hydrocortisone and Normal saline.
	Management: OHCM p312.
Recent blood transfusion	*Suggested by:* history.
	Confirmed by: fall of potassium after few hours.
Spurious result due to haemolysis in specimen bottle	*Suggested by:* laboratory reporting haemolysis in specimen bottle.
	Confirmed by: normal potassium when repeated with no delay in delivery to lab.

Hypokalaemia

OHCM p692.

Some differential diagnoses and typical outline evidence

Diuretic therapy	*Suggested by:* taking thiazide or loop diuretic (fondness of liquerice of Pernod drink).
	Confirmed by: normal potassium after stopping diuretic.
Beta-agonist treatment	*Suggested by:* taking high doses of beta-agonist usually in nebuliser for acute asthmatic attack in hospital.
	Confirmed by: normal potassium after stopping drug.
Vomiting e.g. pyloric stenosis	*Suggested by:* history of severe vomiting with poor fluid intake.
	Confirmed by: normal potassium without subsequent need for replacement when cause of vomiting treated.
Chronic diar-rhoea, purgative abuse, intestinal fistula, villous adenoma of rectum	*Suggested by:* history of severe diarrhoea or mucous loss.
	Confirmed by: normal potassium without need for further replacement when cause treated subsequently.
Primary hyper-aldosteronism due to adrenal hyperplasia or Conn's syndrome with adrenal tumour	*Suggested by:* normal fluid intake, blood pressure ↑. Serum potassium ↓.
	Confirmed by: plasma renin activity low and aldoster-one levels high. CT or MRI scan appearance.
	Management: OHCM p314.
Renal tubular defect	*Suggested by:* recovery phase from renal failure, recent pyelonephritis, associated myeloma, heavy metal poisoning.
	Confirmed by: test for renal concentrating ability.
	Management: OHCM p684.

Hypercalcaemia

Present when specimen taken without a venous cuff and calcium result was corrected for albumin concentration (see *OHCM* p696).

Some differential diagnoses and typical outline evidence

Bone metastases from breast, bronchus, kidney, thyroid, ovary, colon	*Suggested by:* normal phosphate and high alkaline phosphatase .
	Confirmed by: secondaries on bone scan.
Thiazide diuretics	*Suggested by:* mild hypercalcaemia, drug history, normal phosphate and alkaline phosphatase.
	Confirmed by: normal calcium when drug stopped.
Primary (or tertiary) hyperparathyroidism	*Suggested by:* low phosphate and high alkaline phosphatase (3° after years of 2° hyper-parathyroidism).
	Confirmed by: plasma parathyroid levels high with high calcium.
	Management: OHCM p308.
Myeloma	*Suggested by:* normal phosphate and alkaline phosphatase.
	Confirmed by: Bence-Jones protein in urine. Protein electrophoresis. Secondaries on bone scan.
	Management: OHCM p666.
Sarcoidosis	*Suggested by:* high phosphate and alkaline phosphatase. Bilateral hilar shadows on chest X-ray.
	Confirmed by: histology, ↑ vitamin D levels and ↑ ACE levels.
	Management: OHCM p198.
Vitamin D excess	*Suggested by:* drug history and ↑ phosphate.
	Confirmed by: normal calcium when drug stopped.
Thyrotoxicosis	*Suggested by:* mildly ↑ calcium, T4 ↑ or T3 ↑ and TSH very ↓. Normal phosphate and alkaline phosphatase.
	Confirmed by: response to treatment of thyrotoxicosis.
	Management: OHCM p304.

| Ectopic parathyroid hormone due to lung cancer usually | *Suggested by:* ↓ phosphate and ↑ alkaline phosphatase. |
| | *Confirmed by:* plasma parathyroid levels ↑ with high calcium presence of underlying neoplasm. |

Hypocalcaemia

Present when specimen taken without a venous cuff and corrected for albumin concentration. (see *OHCM* p695).

Some differential diagnoses and typical outline evidence

Vitamin D deficiency—due to dietary deficiency or 1, 25(OH)₂D abnormality	*Suggested by:* diet history, ↓ phosphate and ±↑ alkaline phosphatase.
	Confirmed by: 1, 25(OH)₂ vit D, normal calcium after adequate treatment with vitamin D.
	Management: OHCM p700.
Hypoparathyroidism (transient or permanent after thyroid surgery, auto immune disease, radiations)	*Suggested by:* recent neck surgery ± ↑phosphate.
	Confirmed by: parathyroid hormone ↓ or normal in presence of calcium↓.
	Management: OHCM p308.
Chronic renal failure	*Suggested by:* ±↑ phosphate, ±↑ creatinine, ±↑ alkaline phosphatase normochromic anaemia.
	Confirmed by: improvement with control of renal failure and phosphate levels.
	Management: OHCM p274.
Pseudohypo-parathyroidism	*Suggested by:* short stature, obesity, round face, short metacarpals, ±↑ phosphate.
	Confirmed by: plasma parathyroid levels ↑ with calcium ↓ or normal.
Pancreatitis	*Suggested by:* abdominal pain and tenderness, phosphate normal or ↓normal alkaline phosphatase.
	Confirmed by: ↑↑ serum amylase and ultrasound scan of abdomen.
	Management: OHCM pp478–9.
Fluid overload	*Suggested by:* history and ↓ phosphate and normal alkaline phosphatase.
	Confirmed by: normalisation with correction of fluid balance.
Rhabdomyolysis	*Suggested by:* muscle pains, phosphate↑.
	Confirmed by: CPK↑↑, ± creatinine↑.
	Management: OHCM p281.

Raised alkaline phosphatase

Some differential diagnoses and typical outline evidence

Paget's disease	*Suggested by:* deformity of skull or tibia typically, ↑↑alkaline phosphatase.
	Confirmed by: bone deformity especially of skull and tibia and urinary hydroxyproline ↑.
	Management: OHCM p698.
Vitamin D deficiency due to dietary deficiency	*Suggested by:* diet history, ↓ phosphate and ↑ alkaline phosphatase.
	Confirmed by: 1,25 (OH)$_2$ vit D level ↓ and normal calcium after oral vitamin D and calcium supplement.
	Management: OHCM p700.
Bone metastases from breast, bronchus, kidney, thyroid, ovary, colon	*Suggested by:* normal phosphate ↑calcium and ↑alkaline phosphatase.
	Confirmed by: secondaries on bone scan.
Primary or tertiary hyperparathyroidism	*Suggested by:* low phosphate and ↑ alkaline phosphatase after years of 2° hyperparathyroidism.
	Confirmed by: plasma parathyroid levels high with high calcium.
Cholestasis	*Suggested by:* jaundice with *pale* stools and *dark* urine. Bilirubin (i.e. conjugated and thus soluble) in urine.
	Confirmed by: ↑ urine and serum bilirubin but NO ↑ urobilinogen in urine. ↑↑ alkaline phosphatase, otherwise slightly abnormal liver function tests.
	Management: OHCM pp222–3.

Raised serum urea and creatinine

Some differential diagnoses and typical outline evidence

High protein load due to GI bleed catabolism, sepsis etc.	*Suggested by:* ↑ blood urea and normal creatinine or urea/creatinine ratio strongly in favour of urea. *Confirmed by:* recovery when catabolism or GI bleeding stops. *Management: OHCM* p272.
Pre-renal failure due to hypovolaemia due to low fluid intake, or high fluid loss of any cause	*Suggested by:* ↑ blood urea and creatinine. History of fluid imbalance with fluid loss exceeding intake. Urea/creatinine ratio in favour of urea. *Confirmed by:* improvement with restoration of fluid volume. *Management: OHCM* p272.
Chronic renal failure due to pyelonephritis, glomerulo nephritis, interstitial nephritis, diabetes mellitus, renovascular disease, analgesic nephropathy, hypertension, etc.	*Suggested by:* ↑ blood urea and creatinine and not rising rapidly over days. ↓Hb, small renal size on US scan, etc. *Confirmed by:* renal biopsy appearance. *Management: OHCM* pp276–7.
Acute tubular necrosis, severe hypotension, nephrotoxins (NSAIDs aminoglycosides, amphoteracin B etc.)	*Suggested by:* raised blood urea and creatinine and rising rapidly over days. Hb normal. Recent acute illness with hypotension and oliguria (fall in urine output <1ml/kg/hr). ↑K^+, etc. US scan: normal kidney size and no obstructive uropathy. *Confirmed by:* no improvement when normovolaemic and renal biopsy. *Management: OHCM* p272.
Obstructive post-renal failure	*Suggested by:* raised blood urea and creatinine and rising. Hb normal. Fall in urine output. *Confirmed by:* US scan showing dilatation of renal calyces or ureters. Improvement in renal function with bladder or ureteric catheterisation or nephrostomy. *Management: OHCM* p272.

Low haemoglobin

Some differential diagnoses and typical outline evidence

Microcytic anaemia (see p624)	*Suggested by:* history of blood loss or familial microcytic anaemias (esp. in Mediterranean origin).
	Confirmed by: ↓Hb and ↓MCV.
Macrocytic anaemia (see p626)	*Suggested by:* FH of pernicious anaemia, medication or alcohol.
	Confirmed by: ↓Hb and ↑MCV.
	Management: OHCM p632.
Normocytic anaemia (see p628)	*Suggested by:* history of chronic intercurrent illness e.g. pancytopenia chronic renal failure.
	Confirmed by: ↓Hb and MCV normal.

Microcytic anaemia

Usually accompanied by low mean corpuscular haemoglobin concentration

Some differential diagnoses and typical outline evidence

Iron deficiency anaemia	*Suggested by:* history of blood loss (e.g. history of heavy periods, passing blood rectally), or poor diet.
	Confirmed by: ↓serum iron, ↓ferritin and total iron binding capacity ↑.
	Management: OHCM pp624–6.
Thalassaemia: α, β, inter-media, and variants	*Suggested by:* FH, Mediterranean origin. MCV very low for degree of anaemia.
	Confirmed by: Film: target and nucleated cells. Hb electrophoresis shows ↑HbF or ↑HbA2.
	Management: OHCM p642.
Sideroblastic anaemia rarely congenital or acquired due to alcohol lead poisoning, etc.	*Suggested by:* history of chronic intercurrent illness e.g. chronic renal failure.
	Confirmed by: ↑serum iron, ↑ferritin and total iron binding capacity normal.
	Management: OHCM p626.

Macrocytic anaemia

Some differential diagnoses and typical outline evidence

B_{12} deficiency: pernicious anaemia (PA), intestinal malabsorption	*Suggested by:* associated auto-immune disease e.g. primary hypothyroidism, vitilgo, etc. Hb ↓, WBC and Plts low.
	Confirmed by: ↓serum B_{12} (folate often ↓too, due to anorexia) but PA diagnosed in absence of general malabsorption.
	Management: OHCM p634.
Folate deficiency	*Suggested by:* poor diet, pregnancy, lactation, general malabsorption
	Confirmed by: ↓folate but serum B_{12} normal.
	Management: OHCM p632.
Antifolate drugs	*Suggested by:* phenytoin typically, barbiturates and similar, methotrexate and similar.
	Confirmed by: response to high dose folic acid treatment or stopping drug (serum folate may be normal).
Alcohol abuse	*Suggested by:* history of abuse and poor diet.
	Confirmed by: response to abstention (serum folate may be normal).
	Management: OHCM p254.
Hepatitis and liver disease	*Suggested by:* abnormal liver enzymes.
	Confirmed by: normal (or high) B_{12} and poor response to folic acid.
	Management: OHCM pp232, 576.
Hypothyroidism	*Suggested by:* ↓T4 and ↑TSH.
	Confirmed by: normal B_{12} and response to treatment with thyroxine.
	Management: OHCM p306.
Haemolysis (due to reticulosis)	*Suggested by:* urobilinogen in urine.
	Confirmed by: reticulocytes on blood film.
	Management: OHCM pp636–8.

Myelodysplasia	*Suggested by:* hepato- or splenomegaly.
	Confirmed by: bone marrow examination, normal B_{12} and folate.
	Management: OHCM pp624–6.

Normocytic anaemia

Some differential diagnoses and typical outline evidence

Anaemia of chronic disease (e.g. rheumatoid arthritis, hypogonadism, etc.)	*Suggested by:* associated chronic disease. *Confirmed by:* iron, B_{12}, normal. Folate often ↓, ferritin often ↑ from inflammation.
Chronic renal failure	*Suggested by:* high creatinine and urea. *Confirmed by:* response to erythropoietin treatment only. *Management:* OHCM p274.
'Anaemia of pregnancy'	*Suggested by:* pregnant state. *Confirmed by:* persistence despite folic acid and iron supplements, resolution after birth.
Hypothyroidism	*Suggested by:* ↓T4 and ↑TSH. *Confirmed by:* normal B_{12} and response to treatment with thyroxine. *Management:* OHCM p306.
Haemolysis (due to reticulosis)	*Suggested by:* urobilinogen in urine. *Confirmed by:* reticulocytes on blood film. *Management:* OHCM p636.
Bone marrow failure	*Suggested by:* pancytopenia. *Confirmed by:* bone marrow examination. *Management:* OHCM p662.

Very high ESR or CRP

An ESR (erythrocyte sedimentation rate) or CRP (C-reactive protein) which is just above normal is non-specific as it is associated with any cause of inflammation including infection—but an ESR near 100 or above is a good lead.

Some differential diagnoses and typical outline evidence

Severe bacterial infection e.g. osteomyelitis empyema, peritonitis	*Suggested by:* high fever, leucocytes ↑↑.
	Confirmed by: positive bacterial culture from blood and/or site of infection and response to antibiotics and/or surgical drainage.
Giant cell arteritis	*Suggested by:* localized headache especially over temple, late loss of vision, ± muscle pain and stiffness in shoulder area.
	Confirmed by: vessel wall inflammation on biopsy.
	Management: OHCM p424.
Bacterial endocarditis	*Suggested by:* fever, changing heart murmurs, nail splinter haemorrhages.
	Confirmed by: bacterial growth from several blood cultures, echocardiogram may show vegetations.
	Management: OHCM p152.
Myeloma	*Suggested by:* bone pain or fractures. Bence-Jones protein in urine and monoclonal protein band on electrophoresis.
	Confirmed by: myeloma cells on bone marrow examination.
	Management: OHCM p666.
Prostatic carcinoma	*Suggested by:* bone pain, few urinary symptoms.
	Confirmed by: sclerotic changes in pelvic bones and raised prostatic-specific antigen (PSA) and prostatic biopsy.
	Management: OHCM p498.

Chest X-ray appearances

The general approach

1. Use good viewing conditions—preferably a light box in a dark area.
2. Check the patient's name, gender, age and address to ensure correct identity.
3. Check if the film is marked P-A (X-rays passing from posterior to anterior in a standard way) or A-P (X-rays passing from anterior to posterior). A-P views are done when the patient is ill, using a portable X-ray tube—these will often be semi-erect films with suboptimal exposure factors. This projection magnifies the mediastinum so A-P films should not be used to assess cardiac size or hilar configuration.
4. Check which sides are marked left and right and whether the cardiac apex is on the left (if not, the patient may have dextrocardia).
5. Check the patient's positioning. Are the sterno-clavicular joints equidistant from the spinous processes of the vertebral column? If not then the patient was rotated. Rotation causes asymmetry of shoulder girdle muscles projected over the lung fields. The side which has the less space between the end of the clavicle and spinous process has more muscle projected over the lung fields and should be whiter than the other side. Be cautious in the interpretation of a rotated chest radiograph.
6. Can you see the vertebral column through the heart shadow? If not, then it is 'under-penetrated' (the X-ray beam was too weak). This means that normal lung tissue will look abnormally opaque (white).
7. If the lungs appear dark, the vertebral column can be seen very clearly and the heart shadow is vague, it was over-penetrated and abnormalities may be missed.
8. Is the diaphragm between the $5^{th}/6^{th}$ anterior rib ends? If it is higher, then the patient did not take a deep breath, and interpretation of the appearance of the lungs and mediastinum will be suboptimal. If the diaphragm is flattened then emphysematous changes are likely.
9. Having considered the technical issues, is there anything that strikes you immediately? Check for foreign bodies, e.g. endotracheal tubes, chest drains, etc. A striking radio-opaque (white) or lucent (dark) area is likely to be a good lead.
10. After noting the obvious finding, or if there is nothing dramatic, assess the X-ray systematically, as there could well be more subtle abnormalities.
11. Compare the lung fields in the lower zones, mid zones and upper zones and check 'behind' the heart.
12. Look at the superior mediastinum, the hilum, the heart, the cardio-phrenic angles, the diaphragms and the costo-phrenic angles.
13. Lastly, look at the ribs, the shoulders, the overlying soft tissue from the neck down to the upper abdomen. Note artefacts from skin folds, hair and clothing, especially braids and buttons.

14. Initially, try to look at the film without considering the clinical setting (otherwise there is a tendency to miss obvious things which do not fit in with your differential diagnosis), then look again with the clinical setting in mind.

15. Remember to compare any chest film with an abnormality with any previous X-rays. Progression over time will often hold the key to the correct diagnosis.

This brief account only includes some common X-ray features of some common diagnoses. Get the X-rays formally reported by a radiologist urgently if you do not recognise a sign and the patient is unwell. Remember that all radiation exposures have to be justified by clinical benefit to comply with IR(ME)R (Ionising Radiation Medical Exposure) Regulations.

Abnormal chest X-ray appearances

Many chest X-ray appearances may be recognisable immediately as indicating a specific diagnosis but if not, classify an appearance into one of the leads on the following pages and then approach the lead systematically.

Area of uniform lung opacification (whiteness) with a well-defined border

This typically occurs when there is abnormal substance (liquid, cells, pus, blood) in the alveolar spaces next to an anatomical border (e.g. a fissure) causing a sharp border definition. The silhouette sign consists of loss of normal demarcation between white tissue and darker lung due to latter's abnormal opacification. The position of this sign can help localise an affected lobe as follows: loss of a diaphragm silhouette $\Rightarrow$ (implies) lower lobe consolidation; loss of right (R) heart border silhouette $\Rightarrow$ R middle lobe consolidation; loss of left heart border silhouette $\Rightarrow$ lingular segment consolidation; loss of upper R mediastinal border silhouette $\Rightarrow$ R upper lobe consolidation. A veil-like shadow over the whole left hemithorax $\Rightarrow$ left upper lobe opacification.

Some differential diagnoses and typical outline evidence

Consolidation due to lobar pneumonia	*Suggested by:* well demarcated uniform whiteness, with a straight border (due to containment by fissural pleura) **with no volume loss** ± air bronchograms. Background of bronchial breathing, fever, ↑neutrophils, productive cough.
	Confirmed by: resolution on antibiotics and clearing of opacification after 6 weeks.
	Management: OHCM pp172–6.
Collapsed lobe due to bronchial obstruction from carcinoma, mucus plugs, foreign body, misplacement of endo-bronchial tube	*Suggested by:* dense, well demarcated whiteness with straight borders (due to containment by fissures **with volume loss.** Background picture suggestive of cause (e.g. cachexia, monophonic wheeze and central soft tissue opacity in carcinoma or inhalation of foreign body, recent endotracheal intubation, etc).
	Confirmed by: resolution following appropriate treatment for intraluminal cause, bronchoscopy and biopsy for carcinoma.
	Management: OHCM p182.
Pulmonary infarction	*Suggested by:* wedge-shaped regions of opacification peripherally ± atelectasis and pleural effusion. Background history of pleuritic chest pain haemoptysis and breathlessness.
	Confirmed by: CT pulmonary angiogram (V/Q is only helpful when the chest X-ray is completely normal).
	Management: OHCM p194.

Dense pulmonary fibrosis	*Suggested by:* parenchymal opacification (i.e. reticulonodular shadowing), usually with volume loss, often shrunken against apical pleura. Background history of previous TB exposure, radiation, extrinsic allergic alveolitis, chronic sarcoid, ankylosing spondylitis, pneumoconiosis etc.
	Confirmed by: no change on longstanding followup.
	Management: OHCM pp202–3.
Pleural effusion: transudate due to heart failure, or exudate due to tumour/ pneumonia, etc.	*Suggested by:* homogeneus dense area of opacification obscuring the hemidiaphragm in erect position, less dense superiorly with concave meniscus. No air bronchogram. Shift with change of position ± interfissural or subpulmonary loculation. Background of stony dullness to percussion. Absent breath sounds.
	Confirmed by: aspiration of fluid in diagnostic tap, ± ultrasound to differentiate from consolidation.
	Management: OHCM pp196, 748, 750, 751.
Empyema	*Suggested by:* large, lentiform pleural opacification. Background of spiking temperature.
	Confirmed by: pleural tap (pus cells, pH↓, bacteria present).
	Management: OHCM pp176, 196–7.
Pneumonectomy	*Suggested by:* dense white area over entire lung with ipsilateral displacement of mediastinal structures.
	Confirmed by: history of pneumonectomy.
Complete lung collapse	*Suggested by:* dense white area over entire lung, trachea and heart shifted well to affected side, dullness to percussion, TVF↑, absent breath sounds.
	Confirmed by: CT thorax and complete obstruction of main bronchus or bronchoscopy.

Round opacity (or opacities) > 5mm in diameter

Beware skin/rib lesions or artefact from hair, braids or clothing which can mimic intrathoracic pathology.

Some differential diagnoses and typical outline evidence

Carcinoma of bronchus	*Suggested by:* solitary opacity with irregular or lobulated or spiculed, border ± hilar enlargement and destructive bone changes in ribs and other features of metastases. Background of cough, haemoptysis, cachexia. *Confirmed by:* tissue diagnosis via bronchoscopy or CT guided biopsy. *Management: OHCM pp182–3.*
Pulmonary metastasis	*Suggested by:* multiple rounded opacities ± background history of neoplasia or lymphoma. *Confirmed by:* CT scan appearance ± biopsy. *Management: OHCM pp438–1.*
'Rounded pneumonia' or lung abscess	*Suggested by:* round opacity in child, cavitating thick rimmed lesion in adult. Background of raised inflammatory markers, neutrophilia and cough, pyrexia, spiking (in abscess). *Confirmed by:* sputum microscopy, culture and sensitivity resolution following appropriate antibiotic therapy. *Management: OHCM pp172, 176.*
TB granuloma	*Suggested by:* coin lesion ± cavitation in upper lobe. Background history of TB exposure, lymphadenopathy. *Confirmed by:* CT scan appearance. AFB on smear or culture. *Management: OHCM pp564–8.*
Rheumatoid nodule	*Suggested by:* peripherally positioned, multiple soft tissue nodules ± cavitatation. Background history of rheumatoid arthritis. *Confirmed by:* CT scan appearance and +ve rheumatoid serology. *Management: OHCM p414.*

Histoplasmosis	*Suggested by:* coin lesion ± cavitation in upper lobe. Patient from USA, Africa or HIV positive.
	Confirmed by: CT scan appearance. Yeast-like organisms in sputum. Positive complement fixation test.
	Management: OHCM p612.
Wegener's granuloma	*Suggested by:* multiple rounded opacities ± cavitatation with background of proteinuria, skin lesions, etc.
	Confirmed by: biopsy of lung lesion or kidney.
	Management: OHCM p738.
Klebsiella pneumonia	*Suggested by:* multiple cavitating opacities especially in the upper lobes in an elderly person.
	Confirmed by: growth of klebsiella on blood culture and response to cefuroxime.
	Management: OHCM pp174, 539.
Hydatid cyst	*Suggested by:* opacity in a lower lobe with dark cavity ± daughter cysts within large cyst. Water lily sign may be seen. Patient from endemic area in contact with working sheep dogs.
	Confirmed by: CT scan appearance. Positive complement fixation test or ELISA.
	Management: OHCM pp494, 616.
Pulmonary A-V malformation	*Suggested by:* other symptoms or signs ± occasional haemoptysis
	Confirmed by: CT thorax showing feeding blood vessel on contrast enhanced scan.
Benign tumours	*Suggested by:* no other symptoms and no change over 6 months.
	Confirmed by: excision and histology.

Multiple 'nodular' shadows and 'miliary mottling'

These are round lesions 2–5mm in diameter of variable density, from small and soft in miliary (<2mm) mottling to larger and calcified in old chickenpox.

Some differential diagnoses and typical outline evidence

Metastases	*Suggested by:* low density nodules more profuse in the lower lung zones ± mediastinal widening and other manifestations of malignancy e.g. lytic lesions in ribs. Background history of malignancy, e.g. thyroid or renal cell carcinoma. Anorexia and weight loss.
	Confirmed by: Imaging, tissue diagnosis.
	Management: OHCM pp438–41.
Miliary tuberculosis	*Suggested by:* innumerable grain-like low density discrete nodules with background history of TB contact.
	Confirmed by: AFB on sputum, culture of bone marrow or biopsy specimens from pleura, lung, liver or lymph nodes.
	Management: OHCM pp564–8.
Sarcoidosis	*Suggested by:* low density nodules more profuse in the peri-hilar and mid lung zones. Bilateral hilar ± paratracheal lymph node enlargement. Background of rash, uveitis, etc.
	Confirmed by: histology showing non-caseating granuloma with no acid-fast bacilli, ↑ serum ACE.
	Management: OHCM p198.
Past chickenpox	*Suggested by:* dense opacities suggesting calcification. No current symptoms. Past history of adult chickenpox.
	Confirmed by: no change over months on serial rays.
	Managed with no action.
Mitral stenosis with pulmonary hypertension	*Suggested by:* dense opacities due to calcification. Background of tapping left ventricular impulse (palpable 1st heart sound).
	Confirmed by: other clinical findings, ECG findings, echocardiogram and cardiac catheterisation.
	Management: OHCM p146.

Pneumoconiosis *Suggested by:* discrete opacities mainly in upper lobe. Background of employment history of >10 years (coal mining, metal mining, quarrying).

Confirmed by: Comparison with previous CXR. HR-CT scan.

Management: OHCM p202.

Diffuse poorly defined hazy opacification

Some differential diagnoses and typical outline evidence

Pulmonary oedema: (cardiogenic or fluid overload or both)	*Suggested by:* symmetrical haziness more florid in a perihilar distribution, fluffy alveolar opacities ± confluence, (if fluid is in air spaces), Kerley B lines or peri-bronchial cuffing (if in interstitium), or effusion (if in pleural space). Background history of fluid overload ± heart disease ± abnormal ECG, fine crackles in lung bases.
	Confirmed by: ventricular dysfunction on echocardiogram if cardiogenic and response to diuretics or vasodilators.
	Management: OHCM pp136–8.
Acute respiratory distress syndrome (ARDS)	*Suggested by:* symmetrical diffuse poorly defined opacities which become confluent. Acutely ill patient with severe hypoxia. Normal heart size, history of precipitating cause (e.g. smoke inhalation, aspiration, drug exposure, fat/ amniotic fluid emboli, viral infection, DIC), no signs of LVF.
	Confirmed by: (1) acute onset, (2) bilateral infiltrates, (3) PCWP <19mmHg or no CCF, (4) P_aO_2:FiO_2 < 200, in the presence of good LV function. Often fatal and no response treatment.
	Management: OHCM pp190–1.
Infective infiltration: due to viral pneumonia, gram negative organisms	*Suggested by:* region of patchy pulmonary infiltrate ± air bronchogram ± pleural effusion. Background of cough, sputum, raised inflammatory markers, neutropenia (viral) or neutrophilia (bacterial).
	Confirmed by: positive cultures or resolution following appropriate antibiotics.
	Management: OHCM pp172–5.
Alveolar cell carcinoma	*Suggested by:* region of poorly defined opacification which may contain air bronchogram. Background of progressive breathlessness, copious watery productive cough. No resolution with antibiotic therapy.
	Confirmed by: sputum cytology, lung biopsy.
	Management: OHCM p182.
Lung haemorrhage	*Suggested by:* region of poorly defined opacification ± air bronchogram. Background history of trauma/contusion or Good Pastures syndrome.
	Confirmed by: swift resolution, CT appearances + renal biopsy (for Good Pastures syndrome).

Increased linear markings

Indicates thickening of the interstitial tissues.

Some differential diagnoses and typical outline evidence

Pulmonary fibrosis: cryptogenic or idiopathic, chronic bronchitis, extrinsic allergic alveolitis, asbestosis, sarcoidosis, collagen vascular disease, pneumoconiosis	*Suggested by:* increased interstitial markings with background of exposure history and X-ray features of above conditions. *Confirmed by:* typical appearances on HR-CT. Lung biopsy. *Management:* OHCM pp202–3.
Interstitial fluid = pulmonary oedema	*Suggested by:* smooth thickening of the interlobular septa (Kerley B lines) with background lung crackles. *Confirmed by:* rapid resolution following diuretic therapy or correct fluid balance or dialysis. *Management:* OHCM pp136–8 and p786.
Metastatic cells = lymphangitis carcinomatosis	*Suggested by:* irregular thickening of the interlobular septa (Kerley B lines) with background of other features of malignancy. *Confirmed by:* HR-CT, lung biopsy or progressive malignant disease. *Management:* OHCM p439.
Bronchiectasis	*Suggested by:* tram lines and rings with background of cough with high volume of sputum (± foul and purulent (if super-added infection). *Confirmed by:* HR-CT. *Management:* OHCM pp178–9.

Symmetrically dark lungs

Some differential diagnoses and typical outline evidence

Chronic obstructive pulmonary disease	*Suggested by:* long narrow heart and chest, flat diaphragms, ribs horizontal, 7th rib visible anteriorly and 11th rib visible posteriorly. Prominent pulmonary arteries with peripheral pruning (in pulmonary hypertension). Large thin rimmed dark areas with no lung markings—bullae. Background history of smoking.
	Confirmed by: Lung function tests showing fixed obstructive deficit $FEV_1 < 80\%$, $FEV_1/FVC < 70\%$.
	Management: OHCM pp188, 189.
Asthma	*Suggested by:* hyperexpanded lungs. No loss of lung markings. Background history of asthma.
	Confirmed by: peak flow improvement following appropriate treatment.
	Management: OHCM pp184–7.

Single dark lung

Some differential diagnoses and typical outline evidence

Pneumothorax	*Suggested by:* visible lung edge with absence of lung markings peripheral to this. Central mediastinum. Beware skin folds which may mimic a lung edge. Background of sudden onset of breathlessness.
	Confirmed by: convincing appearances on an expiration film.
	Management: OHCM p798.
Tension pneumothorax (medical emergency)	*Suggested by:* visible lung edge with absence of lung markings peripheral to this, mediastinal shift away from the black lung. Background of acute progressive dyspnoea, tachycardia, low BP.
	Confirmed by: relief when needle or catheter inserted and re-expansion of lung when chest tube inserted later.
	Management: OHCM p798.
Bulla	*Suggested by:* loss of lung markings inside lucent, thin rimmed circular region. Background history of COPD.
	Confirmed by: Comparison with previous CXR, CT thorax.
Mastectomy	*Suggested by:* no breast shadow.
	Confirmed by: history of mastectomy.

Abnormal hilar shadowing

Check that the film is not rotated—this can give false positive. Compare with old films if possible for duration of abnormality.

Some differential diagnoses and typical outline evidence

Metastatic lymphadenopathy ± primary bronchial carcinoma	*Suggested by:* unilateral hilar opacity ± lung opacity or bilateral hilar opacity ± evidence of metastatic deposits e.g. lytic rib lesions. Background history of neoplasia.
	Confirmed by: bronchoscopy ± CT staging. Sputum cytology showing cancer cells.
Hodgkin's or non-Hodgkin's lymphoma	*Suggested by:* bilateral hilar shadows, ± parenchymal opacification. Background of anaemia, lymph node enlargement elsewhere.
	Confirmed by: histology with Reed–Sternberg cells in Hodgkin's or without in non-Hodgkin's.
	Management: OHCM pp658, 660.
Primary tuberculosis with hilar node (primary complex) or viral infection	*Suggested by:* unilateral hilar mass (lymphadenopathy) and poorly defined opacificaiton in peripheral lung field, often with paratracheal nodal enlargement. Background of clinical features of TB or viral infection.
	Confirmed by: CT scan showing no tumour. Acid-fast bacilli on ZN stain and culture growth from sputum after up to 12 weeks for TB. Resolution on specific anti-TB therapy.
	Management: OHCM pp 566, 567.
Prominent pulmonary artery due to embolus	*Suggested by:* smooth non-lobular appearance tapering off peripherally with dark peripheral lung fields.
	Confirmed by: CT pulmonary angiogram.
	Management: OHCM p194.
Prominent pulmonary arteries due to pulmonary hypertension	*Suggested by:* bulky bilateral hila with outline suggestive of prominent pulmonary arteries, tapering off peripherally with dark peripheral lung fields ± widening of upper mediastinum (SVC) ± bulging right heart border.
	Confirmed by: CT pulmonary angiogram.
	Management: OHCM p204.

Sarcoidosis	*Suggested by:* bilateral hilar convex shadows, possibly with other lung changes of sarcoid. Background of rash, uveitis, etc.
	Confirmed by: histology showing non-caseating granuloma with no acid-fast bacilli.
	Management: OHCM p198.

Upper mediastinal widening

Some differential diagnoses and typical outline evidence

Retrosternal goitre	*Suggested by:* superior mediastinal mass shadow extending from the neck.
	Confirmed by: clinical examination, ultrasound, or radioisotope scan.
Hodgkin's or non-Hodgkin's lymphoma or metastatic lymphadeno-pathy	*Suggested by:* dense often multi-nodular masses causing mediastinal widening.
	Confirmed by: CT scan appearance, mediastinoscopy or surgical removal showing histology.
	Management: OHCM pp658, 660.
Thymoma	*Suggested by:* clearly outlined opacity (calcification in 20%). Background features of myasthenia gravis (in 30%).
	Confirmed by: CT scan appearance and histology from mediastinoscopy or surgical removal.
Teratoma: benign or malignant	*Suggested by:* anterior mediastinal opacification, rarely with calcification e.g. in teeth.
	Confirmed by: CT scan appearance ± fat, hair, teeth and histology from mediastinoscopy or surgical removal.
Kinked or aneurysmal aorta	*Suggested by:* opacification continuous with descending aorta shadow.
	Confirmed by: CT scan appearance.

Abnormal cardiac shadow

Some differential diagnoses and typical outline evidence

Left ventricular failure	*Suggested by:* large heart mainly to left of mid-line (with central trachea), linear upper lobe opacities (veindilation) and fluffy lung opacities centrally more than peripherally.
	Confirmed by: echocardiogram showing poor contraction of left ventricle.
	Management: OHCM pp136–8.
Pulmonary hypertension	*Suggested by:* prominent right heart border (of right ventricle), upwardly rounded apex and bilateral prominence of hila. Background of loud pulmonary valve closure ± history of P.E.
	Confirmed by: tall R waves in V1 to V3 on ECG and right axis deviation.
	Management: OHCM p204.
Cardiomyopathy	*Suggested by:* generally large heart with clear borders (indicating poor contraction). Background history of predisposing condition e.g. chronic alcohol abuse, amyloid, leukaemia, rheumatoid arthritis etc.
	Confirmed by: echocardiogram showing low ejection fraction.
	Management: OHCM p156.
Pericardial effusion	*Suggested by:* large globular cardiac outline and clear borders (indicating little or no contraction).
	Confirmed by: echocardiogram.
	Management: OHCM p158.
Atrial septal defect	*Suggested by:* unusually convex right heart border, upwardly rounded cardiac apex and bilateral prominence of hila.
	Confirmed by: echocardiogram.
	Management: OHCM p160.

Mitral stenosis	*Suggested by:* large heart, enlarged left atrium (rounded opacity behind the heart which 'splays' the carinal angle) ± calcification in position of mitral valve and dense nodules due to haemosiderosis. History of rheumatic heart disease.
	Confirmed by: echocardiogram and cardiac catheterisation.
	Management: OHCM p146.
Left ventricular aneurysm	*Suggested by:* bulge in left ventricular border ± calcification. Background history of IHD ± myocardial infarction.
	Confirmed by: echocardiogram.
	Management: OHCM p124.
Mediastinal emphysema	*Suggested by:* gas around the mediastinal contour, ± surgical emphysema. Background history of acute asthma, OGD, oesophageal rupture, etc., signs of surgical emphysema.
	Confirmed by: CT thorax.
Hiatus hernia	*Suggested by:* circular shadow behind the heart, ± air/fluid level, absent gastric bubble. Intermittent appearance on previous CXR.
	Confirmed by: barium swallow, endoscopy.
	Management: OHCM p216.

Thinking about diagnosis

Understanding and explaining diagnostic conclusions

The roles and responsibilities of doctors and others are always changing but what characterises medical training is its breadth. It is therefore the medical members of the team who are responsible for understanding the overall situation and ensuring that appropriate action is taken for the patient's care. In order to convey this understanding to patients, nurses, other doctors and examiners, analyse the overall situation in your mind first. The important practical information is what is to be done in terms of treatments, tests and further observations. Before trying to explain to others what you imagine is wrong, think of what is wrong in the form of diagnoses and then consider the facts that form the evidence for the diagnoses.

After assessing a patient you write out the history, examination, diagnoses, proposed tests and treatments, then sign and date your account. You might use memory jogging devices as explained in Chapters 1 and 2 or read up what you are about to do. After deciding what you are going to do, consider the diagnostic indication for each action and check that it is already in your list. You can explain your conclusions by creating a 'current past medical history'.

Take each diagnosis in turn and reconsider the evidence for it. This has to include the presenting complaint (if there was one) because the diagnosis may not become 'final' until this has been resolved to the patient's satisfaction. Choose the smallest combination of findings that would convince a listener. 'Evidence' is a matter of convention and you have to be aware of what listeners expect to hear in order for them to be convinced of your opinion. It is often not possible to use strict diagnostic criteria in day to day clinical practice and if they do not apply, the examples in Chapters 3 to 14 of this book can guide you. If there are any findings that can be markers of progress then mention these because their response to a specific treatment may be a useful later as evidence for the diagnosis.

Test results are 'objective' in that they are less prone to false positives from closed, over-zealous direct questions or a physical examination. They are not necessarily better predictors of treatment response than symptoms and signs if these are elicited well. You should specify the dates (and times if relevant) of all the findings used as 'evidence'. ECG traces and X-ray images preserve the original result. By contrast, the original evidence for past or long established diagnoses may have been lost and the original symptoms forgotten. They may have to be indicated as 'not known'. Management decisions can be thought of under a third sub-heading.

Current past medical history or 'Medical History':

- *Acute follicular tonsillitis (meningitis unlikely)*
  Evidence: **severe sore throat, sweats and severe malaise for 2 days**. Bilaterally swollen tonsils, large and red with small white patches. WCC 18.33×10^9/L, neutrophils 90%.
  Management: throat swab sent. Start penicillin V 500mg qds po, paracetamol 1gr qds po and review with bacteriology.

- *Probable Type II diabetes mellitus*
  Evidence: glycosuria +, random blood sugar 8.4mmol/L.
  Management: for fasting blood sugar when current acute illness resolved. 'Healthy diet' meanwhile.

- *Controlled thyrotoxicosis*
  Evidence: presented 2 months ago with **anxiety, weight loss**, abnormal thyroid function tests in Osler Hospital.
  Management: continue taking Carbimazole, 5mg daily po.

- *Anxiety about meningitis*
  Evidence: voiced severe concerns during history.
  Management: details of this summary explained to patient and that penicillin would be effective also against meningitis.

- *Inadequate home care*
  Evidence: lives alone with no friends nearby.
  Management: assist patient to contact family.

During case presentations (and in hospital discharge summaries), the information is given in the same order as the original history and examination. However, if you have considered the links between the actions, diagnoses and findings beforehand (mentally or on paper), then you will be able to emphasise the important positive and negative features and be better prepared to respond to questions, which should be about the headings and sub-headings in the 'Current past medical history' on the previous page (p657). The same preparation will also be needed for examiners, patients and relatives and when handing over care to colleagues.

Current past medical histories of this kind that explain the links between symptoms, treatment and diagnoses can be typed out and read by patients, relatives, medical staff and other members of the team who are expected to understand a doctor's overall analysis (e.g. during handover of care). Readers of such a past medical history would be able to ask if they did not understand the meaning of any terms and they would be able to raise issues in a more informed way, especially for informed consent.

Discovering and justifying diagnoses

You may have noticed that there are two different thought processes involved in the diagnostic and clinical decision-making process. The first is the process of arriving at the diagnosis and the second is explaining and checking the diagnosis. It is very important to recognise this difference. The process of discovering the diagnosis is done in as systematic a way as possible but the urgency of the situation or disruptive events means that a planned sequence has to be abandoned frequently. In general practice, much will be known about the patient already, for example the past medical history, drug history, recent blood pressure etc. However, it is always important to pay careful attention to, and to take a careful history of, the presenting complaints. With experience in any speciality highly predictive combinations of features are usually recognised quickly as a pattern.

Diagnoses are arrived at in the form of imagined processes with different degrees of certainty. These diagnoses, some tentative, others more certain, will suggest tests to clarify the situation, and treatments to try to reverse or divert their course. This first thought process will thus depend on the imagination of the individual diagnostician combined with different types of thought process ranging from rapid pattern recognition for familiar issues to a more tentative approach when on unfamiliar territory. Students will always be on unfamiliar territory when they start and no doctor can become familiar with every situation. Doctors who see lots of patients will come across unfamiliar problems more often. It is this that makes medical practice a constant challenge. Because of this, a more methodical checking process is also needed.

Explanation

The second thought process is the one required to explain a diagnostic opinion to others, especially nurses who have responsibility for making sure that things are done properly for the patient. The purpose of the diagnostic process is to identify patients who will respond to specific treatments, but the immediate purpose is to suggest what should be done and to give an explanation to the patient and the rest of the team as to why. If this explanation is to be transparent, then it has to be based on facts with dates that are linked clearly to the corresponding diagnosis and management. The explaining process is a mirror image of the first process. The first begins by eliciting findings and then progressing via imagination to action. The explanation starts with the treatment and diagnosis and the latter is 'substantiated' by pointing to findings with dates. The findings are usually kept to a minimum by only mentioning a sufficient number to convince the listener, for example, the diagnostic criteria.

Diagnostic criteria

Diagnostic criteria are conventions which allow diagnoses to be made in a consistent way so that different doctors can agree about what to imagine and what to do. These criteria vary in complexity and may be based on symptoms, physical signs or test results in various combinations. For example, it is generally accepted that 'chronic bronchitis' will be present if a patient has a cough with grey sputum for 'most' days for more than 3 months of the year in at least 2 successive years. In logical terms, this is a 'sufficient' criterion because if a patient had a cough every morning for 2 months of the year for 5 years and smoked, it would not satisfy the criterion to the letter, but most would accept that such a patient would have underlying chronic bronchitis. A criterion is definitive if it is assumed that all those with the criterion will be declared to have the diagnosis and no patients without the criterion are to be declared to have the diagnosis; otherwise it is a 'sufficient criterion'. Note that criteria are man-made 'boxes'. Criteria are useful to maintain consistent standards of practice and for making comparisons between treatment and other populations in research. However, when the term 'chronic bronchitis' is used we imagine a persistently inflamed bronchial mucosa with loss of ciliary function and susceptibility to recurrent infection and progressive lung damage.

'Working' diagnoses and 'final' diagnoses

Many patients have symptoms, physical signs and tests results that do not satisfy diagnostic criteria. Some diagnostic criteria are not easily accessible; for example they depend on histology or an appearance at major surgery. We may thus have to begin treatment when there are no recognised criteria. For example, most antibiotics are prescribed for a 'chest infection' before it is confirmed by culturing bacteria. However, when we decide to treat, we always assume that if a randomised controlled trial were to be done on such a group of patients, then more would benefit from treatment than placebo (but we would think so with more confidence when there is a diagnostic criterion). If we are asked to explain why we have chosen that particular treatment then we could say that we imagine the presence of the disease process for the time being. This is called a 'working diagnosis'. It is equivalent to a scientific hypothesis during an experiment. If the patient gets better in the expected way and if there was no practical purpose for doing further tests then we would then assume that we were 'correct'. This would be called a 'final diagnosis'. It would be the same as a hypothesis becoming a 'scientific theory' because there is no immediate intention to do another experiment to test it.

In both cases, we would be citing an imagined process knowing that it was 'theoretical' and not 'proven' (i.e. by direct observation of everything being imagined). In the case of a treatment, we would not have been able to 'prove' that the patient would not have got better anyway without the treatment. In order to 'prove' this, we would have to do the impossible by turning the clock back and not giving the treatment in order to see what happens. It should also be remembered that even if diagnostic criteria are present, this does not guarantee a response to treatment. Diagnostic criteria are there for consistency between different doctors' diagnoses and they also allow randomised trials to be done and the knowledge to be shared. Thus, if the diagnostic criteria were chosen carefully to be valid in terms of predicting outcome, then more patients would respond to treatment (and fewer to placebo in a clinical trial) when using the criterion than when not using it. If we stray away from such published clinical trial criteria when giving treatments, then we have to accept that we are guessing treatment response by 'extrapolating' and not basing it on formal documented experience in that clinical trial.

If the patient failed to respond to the treatment that might lead to a 'final diagnosis', then we would carry out further tests in order to discover if there is evidence for some other diagnosis or to look for further evidence for the original diagnosis that simply did not respond to the treatment. This further evidence might be a successful response to some other treatment that could work for the original working diagnosis. The practical purpose of a diagnosis from the patient's point of view is to predict the outcomes of a distressing complaint with or without treatment. Sophisticated technology is there to improve the validity of diagnostic criteria in terms of their ability to predict what will happen to the patient's symptoms. A diagnosis represents imagination that includes clinical findings and test results, so it can never be proven to be 'true' in its entirety by a single test. The number of detailed imaginary models (e.g. at the molecular level) under the umbrella term of the diagnosis is limited only by the human imagination.

Science is concerned with imaginative theories or models that can be tested against observed facts, documented and then shared with others. If no aspect of a theory can be tested by any form of observation then it cannot be the subject of scientific study. The process of imagining more models of disease (and discarding some of them because they do not fit the facts) results in scientific models becoming more detailed. One effect of this is that diagnoses may become subdivided, e.g. myocardial infarction (MI) has become subdivided into 'ST elevated MI' responsive to thrombolysis and 'non-ST elevated MI' which is not. So a working or final diagnosis is simply the title to a model, hypothesis or theory that explains and connects the combination of pre-treatment 'facts' (e.g. chest pain with ST elevation) to an outcome of treatment with or without a treatment (e.g. lowering of raised ST segments after thrombolysis).

Dynamic diagnoses

It is important to understand that clinical diagnosis is not a static classification system based on diagnostic criteria or their probable presence. It is a dynamic process.

Diagnostic algorithms classify patients by following a logical pathway which relies on interpreting components of diagnostic criteria. Other systems use findings such as symptoms and physical signs to predict the probable presence of diagnostic criteria. These methods can be regarded as 'diagnosing' a snap-shot of what is happening at a particular time. However, the diagnostician who is helping a patient will be trying to imagine the presence of a dynamic process that changes with time. This could be over seconds, minutes, hours, days, weeks, months or years and the response in terms of investigation and treatment has to be timed appropriately.

There may be several processes taking place at the same time, some progressing over years, (e.g. atheromatous changes), some over minutes to hours (e.g. a thrombosis in a coronary artery), some over minutes or seconds (e.g. ventricular tachycardia) and others instantaneously (e.g. such as a cardiac arrest). This means that a diagnostic process leading to treatment may have to happen repeatedly and for a number of diagnoses at the same time. It might be more appropriate to think of the process as one of 'feed-back' control. In this way the doctor would be acting as an external control mechanism to assist those of the patient who are failing. After the initial history and examination, the feed-back information may come from electronic monitoring, nursing observations, ward rounds, hospital clinic or primary care follow up.

The mechanisms of interest to the diagnostician are of three types. The first type is those that control the 'internal milieu' by keeping temperature, tissue perfusion, blood gases and biochemistry constant. The second type is those mechanisms that control the body's structure by effecting repair in response to any damage. The third type is those that control the 'external milieu' of day to day living. They are all interdependent. If one mechanism fails then it may unmask other weaknesses by causing other failures. It may not be enough to treat the main failure. It is often necessary also to treat the causes and consequences as they may be unable to recover on their own. For example, a coronary thrombosis may be treated with thrombolysis, but any resulting rhythm abnormalities may need to be treated and also the causative risk factors (e.g. smoking) that could result in recurrence. So when we explain our diagnostic thought processes, it helps to think of each diagnosis as a subheading with its own evidence and decision as on p657.

When you take a history and examine a new patient, the process may take about an hour. If the patient is acutely ill, then there may have to be a quick life-saving diagnosis and treatment with a reassessment every few minutes until the patient is stable. The presenting complaint and a quick examination may also suggest a minor complaint such as a viral sore throat that is best managed by simple measures and for the patient to return in a few days if necessary. What all these diagnostic approaches have in common is a cycle of evidence gathering, working diagnosis (with or without a diagnostic criterion) and management. The management may involve tests, treatments and their results which produce further evid-ence, a revised diagnosis and further management.

The probability of any diagnosis being confirmed with diagnostic criteria or becoming the final diagnosis by responding to treatment may not be very high initially. However, you can reassure the patient that the follow-up process will allow further attempts to take place until you 'get it right'. In many cases the problem will resolve spontaneously before you can arrive at any diagnosis that suggests a treatment. In other cases you may have to observe the patient closely as the mystery disease progresses so that new evidence becomes available. In this way, uncertainty may be overcome by cycles of follow up and review.

Explaining a diagnosis

The patient may already be imagining with some trepidation what might be happening and may have been asked already at the end of the presenting complaint for his or her opinion about this. The words and images used by the patient can be used as a starting point to lead him or her to your opinion of what is happening. However, by referring to a mental explanatory summary as in p657, anchor this explanation in 'facts' by recalling and agreeing what the patient complained of originally and describing the smallest combination of findings (e.g. chest pain for 2 hours and abnormal ECG findings) that indicate what should be done (e.g. thrombolysis). Ideally, this small combination should be a diagnostic criterion.

Ask what the patient understands if they use words such as 'heart attack' or 'coronary'. Describe what you understand by using analogies that can connect the process to any possible treatments (e.g. that a clot is forming in a small blood vessel, causing pain coming from the heart muscle and that the clot needs dissolving). The details of the imagined process can be as detailed or basic as you choose from imagining what happens to platelet biochemistry in the thrombus adjacent to an atheromatous plaque (more appropriate for a scientific meeting) to a more basic 'model' that likens the clot to a jelly that dissolves in warm water. However, relate this imagery to 'clinical scientific facts' by explaining the actual or approximate result of a trial (e.g. that a high proportion avoided a full heart attack with thrombolysis but fewer did so without the treatment).

A patient may be too ill to be able to hold a discussion (or may even be unconscious). Many patients would prefer to listen and only ask the occasional question and for a relative or friend to hold the conversation. (This has to be agreed so as not to breach a duty of confidentiality.) There is an advantage in having several family members who can support each other, so that fewer questions will be forgotten. It may also help to have a nurse or other member of staff present to support and raise issues on behalf of the patient. Much of the discussion will be forgotten and members of a group will be able to fill in the gaps for each other in their own later discussions. If the patient is too ill to consent to treatment, then this can be discussed and agreed with the next of kin in the presence of other family members. Such shared responsibility may avoid later feelings of individual blame or guilt if things do not go well.

Risk and uncertainty

Diagnosis means 'seeing through' the findings by imagining other hidden phenomena. Prognosis is 'seeing into the future'. Some patients apparently claim that they were told 'You have only got 6 months to live' and that this proved to be wrong. But people do understand that the future is not certain. Try to discuss uncertainty in a clear and logical way by using frequencies. Although uncertainty is a psychological phenomenon, it is based on the mind's response to external experience. For example, we might know that a diabetic patient arriving in the clinic was one of a group of 590 diabetics who took part in a clinical trial of which 59 (10%) developed nephropathy within 2 years. If this patient arrived in a clinic after the trial had finished (but without knowing if he was given placebo or treatment) then before looking in the records, our degree of 'belief' that this patient was one of those who had developed nephropathy would also be 59/590 = 10% (i.e. without knowing the type of treatment).

The effect of treatment on prognosis

If a new patient arrived in the clinic with the same features as the previous one in the trial and asked about the effect of treatment on the risk of developing 'kidney trouble', then on the basis of the same study above we could say that his risk would be 19/119 (24.4%) if he did not take treatment, but 9/124 (7.3%) if he took the maximum treatment dose. If all we could do were to guess a risk, then we could also explain this by saying that 'Of 100 people like you about 25 would have nephropathy without treatment and about 7 with treatment'. This would induce the appropriate sense of certainty in that patient's mind. However, it might create more pessimism and anxiety in some than in others.

Explaining prognosis by using a diagnosis

If a patient was told that there was a 7% chance of developing kidney disease needing intensive treatment, or 7% of chance of dialysis or a 7% risk of death, the psychological impact of the 7% risk of would be different for each outcome. The patient would wish to know what life would be like for the first two and what sort of death to expect with the third. Some patients might already be prone to anxiety and depression and would envisage each outcome with more fear than others. Also, such a patient would 'believe in his mind' that the risk of a poor outcome was higher than actual experience had shown. For example, one patient might become convinced that he would certainly die within 2 years. Another patient might be recklessly optimistic and refuse to take any sensible action. Most patients would fall between these extremes. The pessimists may need to be encouraged with more optimism than usual and the reckless warned more strongly. This can be reinforced with appropriate counselling. In some cases patients might need anti-depressants or other treatment if they are psychologically unwell.

Many patients recognise that it is not possible to say whether they will be in the 93% who do well or the 7% who do not. They also know that more information may become available that will change the probability but whatever that probability, the fundamental principle is that it is not possible to know which group they will belong to at any time. Some assume that this will be a matter of luck; others will think it as God's will. Religious beliefs allow patients to face what may happen rationally as a result of natural events. Many will do this by putting the future out of their mind and concentrating on what they have to do to optimise their chances. After all, this is what we all do when we are healthy and there-fore not self-conscious about our health, but nevertheless avoid danger in day to day life even when crossing a street. Being told probabilities about our fate in the forthcoming weeks, months or years and trying to ponder their meaning is a very new phenomenon in terms of human experience. Many would regard knowledge of their future from a 'crystal ball' as a curse. Most patients respond philosophically especially when their risks are compared with the chances of survival of children, their mothers and young men in areas of poverty and conflict.

Different types of certainty

The term 'probability' itself creates uncertainty because it has many meanings. The easiest to understand is a degree of certainty equal to some observed frequency. For example, if we know that 6/9 people in a room are diabetic, then if we approach one of these people, then we simply adopt a degree of belief of 6/9 or 0.677 that the person is diabetic. This is known as a 'mathematical probability'. It is important to distinguish it from an 'estimated frequency probability' based on sampling from a source population. We can illustrate this concept by 'creating' a box full of cards by 'sampling' a person from the original room with 9 people, asking if he or she was diabetic, returning the patient to the room and then writing the answer on a card and placing in the box. We could repeat the process a large number of times and then count the proportion of cards with 'diabetes' written on them. This should approximately 6/9 = 67.7%. This would be an 'estimated probability' based on sampling. Different samples might give different results. If the number in the original room was very large, then returning them would have little effect on the estimate, which is what is assumed to happen when conducting research on 'samples' of patients.

Confusion often arises when the term 'probability' is used when what is meant is an 'estimated' probability which has been arrived at by combining sampling methods and mathematical assumptions. These are untested assumptions, so that the 'probabilities' are 'subjective' or theoretical. For example if nephropathy is found in 40% of a sample of diabetics, and retinopathy in 50% of a different sample, then we might 'estimate' that both occurred in 40% × 50% = 20% by assuming that nephropathy and retinopathy only occur together by chance. The concept of probability and its relationship to observed frequencies is fundamental to providing general scientific evidence for the type knowledge in this handbook.

Explaining a treatment by using a diagnosis

Treatments are often advised and accepted at face value. The doctor may be busy and the patient may not wish to hold things up and assume that something would have been said if the treatment was not effective and safe. The patient might thus need to be invited to ask for an explanation. (Do you have any questions about the treatment?) By asking the questions, the patient and supporters influence how detailed the explanation becomes. The explanation has 4 components:

1. What the treatment entails (e.g. a drug regimen or surgery)
2. How the treatment is imagined to affect the underlying process
3. How often it is successful compared to no treatment or other treatments
4. How often adverse effects occur (including financial costs)

If the treatment does have potential for serious adverse effects e.g. surgery or use of a potentially toxic drug, then the patient's formal written informed consent may be needed. It is then important to test if the explanation has been understood by asking the patient to repeat it. If the patient is unable to do so, then this suggests that there is 'incapacity' in legal terms to give consent. The next of kin or other legal representative may have to give consent on behalf of the patient. (The need for this may be obvious, e.g. if the patient is a young child or is an adult with known mental incapacity.)

If the patient and supporters ask for a detailed explanation this might be based on the processes described for the diagnosis. In the case of the diabetic, we might explain that high blood sugar 'weakens' blood vessel walls and lowering the blood pressure as well as the sugar reduces the risk of serious damage, including the damaged blood vessels in the kidney that might result in 'nephropathy'. We might then say that 'Of 100 people like you about 25 would have nephropathy without treatment and about 7 with treatment'. We might also say that as the patient has no contraindications, then the frequency of side effects in such patients is low and it generally accepted that it should be given. However, we may describe what these may be (e.g. see p139 of *OHCM* for the details in the case of an ACE inhibitor).

You may be pressed for more information, perhaps because a supporter has a medical background and is very anxious about what is happening. You might even be asked rarely to describe a supporting trial result and how relevant that trial done elsewhere is to the patient. You may thus say that the study was described in detail and that the patients and methods were similar to those locally. The original study showed a difference of response between the full dose and placebo of 24.4% − 7.3% = 17.1%. You might explain that the number of patients in the study were such that if it was done again with the same number of patients, there was a 95% chance that a series of repeat studies done in the same way would show a difference between treatment and placebo in the range between 8.2% and 26.1% (when the difference in the original study was 17.1%). It would thus seem unnecessary to repeat the study locally.

Give the patient a fact sheet if possible. Fact sheets for drugs are included in the packaging. Pharmacists will often provide excellent counselling, check that the patient has understood a previous explanation and will contact the doctor if there are any concerns. There are special counselling services for informed consent in some situations e.g. for HIV testing or organ donation. They use methods to avoid biased advice from someone who may have a vested interest. A tool called 'Decision Analysis'[1,2] has also been used to explore how a decision is affected by a patient's opinions and feelings regarding different combinations of outcomes with and without treatment and thus to explain the decision in a transparent way.

1 Llewelyn H., Hopkins A. eds. (1993). Analysing how we reach clinical decisions. Royal College of Physicians of London, London.
2 Dowie J., Elstein A. eds. Professional judgement: a reader in clinical decision making. Cambridge: Cambridge University Press.

The validity of the diagnostic criterion as a treatment indication

Pay careful attention to the patient's diagnosis when considering if a treatment is expected to be of benefit. It does not matter how powerful a treatment might be, it will not work if it is given to the wrong patients and may indeed do more harm than good by causing adverse effects with no prospect of benefit. The role of a doctor is to decide which patients will benefit from a specific treatment or advice and this is done by arriving at a diagnosis. For this reason, the explanation given for a treatment is bound up with the diagnosis. This applies to the explanation for how the treatment changes the imagined underlying process and to the pragmatic result of a clinical trial comparing the response to treatment with that of something else. So, a perfectly 'valid' diagnostic criterion will identify all those and only those patients who will respond to a treatment.

If only a proportion of patients respond to a treatment then it is better to subdivide the diagnosis to identify those who do and those who do not respond. For example only a proportion of patients suffering from a myocardial infarction benefit from thrombolysis. However, more patients with ST elevation do so (suggesting that the infarction is in the process of taking place but not yet complete). The 'diagnosis' of myocardial infarction has thus been subdivided into 'ST-elevated myocardial infarction' with a high response rate to thrombolysis and 'non-ST elevated myocardial infarction' which identifies those who are not very responsive and who are thus not offered the treatment. The ability of a diagnostic criterion to predict treatment response is known as its 'validity'. The most 'valid' test result for an 'evolving myocardial infarction' would be the one that identified all those and only those who responded to thrombolysis.

If a 'gold standard' test (i.e. diagnostic criterion) is based on a measurement, another factor that needs determining is the best cut-off point. For example, the upper limit of the normal range for the albumin excretion rate is 20µg/min based on samples taken from healthy laboratory volunteers. This cut-off point is also used to decide if a diabetic patient has 'incipient nephropathy' by assuming that all those above this level are at significantly increased risk of nephropathy e.g. within 2 years. However, if only a small proportion of patients with an initial AER between 20–40µg/min develop nephropathy (e.g. as shown in the Figure, opposite) then nephropathy will be 'incipient' for a very few only. If the risk of nephropathy rises rapidly above 40µg/min, this might be a more suitable cut-off point for 'incipient nephropathy'.[1] Thus empirical evidence should be sought for the validity of a diagnostic criterion and not just choosing a cut-off point on theoretical grounds e.g. two standard deviations above the logarithmic mean.

The 'particular evidence' regarding a 'particular' patient's diagnosis throughout this hand-book is presented as 'Suggested by' and 'Confirmed by'. 'Suggested by' introduces features that make it probable that the diagnosis will be 'Confirmed by' another set of tests, which are thus worth doing. The confirming features usually indicate that some specific advice or treatment should be given. However, in urgent cases, treatment may begin sooner, when the danger of avoiding delay is greater than giving it prematurely and unnecessarily. In other cases, the result of treatment may be the only practical confirmatory test. So, if the treatment can be stopped when the initial response is not promising, then this is referred to as a 'therapeutic' gold standard test. This is done sometimes in a 'double-blind crossover manner: the so-called 'N of 1 trial'. The design is 'double-blind' so that neither the patient nor doctor knows what treatment is being taken until the trial of therapy is complete, when they both decide if the preliminary response is worth pursuing with continuous treatment.

A perfectly valid diagnostic criterion would identify all those and only those with a presenting complaint who would respond to a particular treatment by their presenting complaint resolving, not returning and leaving them with perfect health. The perfect treatment given to those with a perfect diagnostic criterion would cause no adverse effects and cause all those with a presenting complaint and diagnostic criterion to get better, who would not otherwise get better without that treatment.

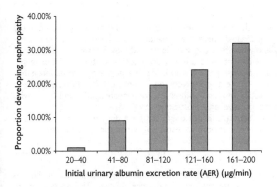

Proportion of patients developing diabetic nephropathy 2 years after initial AER value as shown

1 Llewelyn DEH., Garcia-Puig J. (2004) How different urinary albumin excretion rates can predict progression to nephropathy and the effect of treatment in hypertensive diabetics. *JRAAS*, **5**; 141–5.

The effect of sensitivity, prevalence and incidence on diagnosis

If the patient is asked 'open' questions, important symptoms may be remembered and minor ones may be forgotten. If the patient is asked 'closed' questions then fewer symptoms may be missed but spurious positive responses may be given, perhaps to agree with the doctor. Similarly, if a detection process is made more sensitive, e.g. by calling a smaller colour change on the urine dipstick paper 'positive' then it may result in more spurious false positive results so that the test will not be very 'specific'. However, if the process is modified to make it more specific by only calling a larger colour test change on the urine dipstick 'positive' then it may be less sensitive.

If a sensitive screening test is negative, the patient is usually reassured that no further tests need be done. However, if for example a sensitive urine test for microalbuminuria is positive, then three 24 hour urine collections may have to be done to see if incipient diabetic nephropathy is actually present. The simple arithmetic of how preliminary findings in this book are interpreted is important. (*Read this intricate page slowly.*)

The *Venn diagram* opposite represents 20 diabetic patients in a waiting-room of which 9 are known to have 'incipient nephropathy'. There are 12 patients with a 'positive dipstick test'. There are 8 patients with incipient nephropathy who are 'dipstick positive' and these are enclosed in the overlapping circles. There are 7 patients who have no incipient nephropathy and who are 'dipstick negative' and they fall outside both circles. There are 4 patients who are 'dipstick positive' with no incipient nephropathy and a single patient who is 'dipstick negative' with incipient nephropathy. These numbers are also represented in the usual *2×2 table*, which also show the totals with and without incipient nephropathy and those who are 'dipstick positive' and 'dipstick negative'.

The term 'sensitive' is not only used for a detection process but also for the proportion of positive test results when the 'gold standard' test is positive. In the above example, the 'sensitivity' was 8/9 and it is shown near the top of the '*Mind Map*' on p677. This map shows the relationship between the 8 logical propositions that can be based on a Venn diagram. Read the line representing 'sensitivity' from right to left as: 'If there is incipient nephropathy then 8/9 are dipstick positive'. The obverse of this is false negative rate: 'If there is nephropathy then 1/9 are dipstick negative'. The converse to the 'sensitivity' is the 'predictiveness', which is read from left to right as: 'If the dipstick is positive then 8/12 have nephropathy'. The 'negative predictiveness' is at the bottom of the map, which is read as 'If the dipstick is negative then 7/8 have no nephropathy'. The converse is read in the reverse direction and is called the 'specificity': 'If there is no nephropathy then 7/11 are dipstick negative'. Finally, the obverse of the specificity is the false positive rate: 'If there is no nephropathy then 4/11 are dipstick positive'. The 'prevalence' of incipient nephropathy in the population studied is 9/20 and the prevalence of 'dipstick positive' patients is 12/20 (note that there are 4 prevalences).

Groups of patients with preliminary findings and diagnostic criteria

Venn diagram

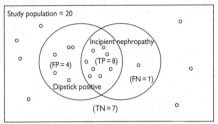

TP = true positives, FP = false positives, FN = false negatives, TN = true negatives

2 x 2 Table

	Nephropathy	No nephropathy	Totals
Dipstick positive	**8(TP)**	4(FP)	12
Dipstick negative	1(FN)	7(TN)	8
Totals	**9**	11	20

Sensitivity = TP/(TP + FN) = 8/9
Predictiveness = TP/(TP + FP) = 8/12

Specificity = TN/(TN + FP) = 7/11
Negative predictiveness = TN/(TN + FN) = 7/8

The arithmetic representation of the 'converse' relationship is called 'Bayes theorem':

Prevalence of × Sensitivity ÷ Prevalence of nephropathy		dipstick positive)	= Predictiveness
9/20	× 8/9 ÷	12/20	= **8/12**

The nature of the population can have a profound effect on the predictive performance of the findings in this book and you must be alert to this in different settings e.g. general practice, accident and emergency departments, and hospital clinics. The above group might be the patients in a diabetic follow-up clinic waiting room. If another waiting room contained many new diabetic patients, then the prevalence of incipient nephropathy might be lower (e.g. 4/20). Also, the severity of the nephropathy in new cases might be less, so that fewer would test positive with a dipstick (e.g. the 'sensitivity' might be 2/4). If the 20 patients all had normal protein urine tests the year before, this 'prevalence' of a new result would be the 'incidence' per year. If the incidence of a newly dipstick positive result was 8/20, the predictiveness in this new setting would be less at 2/8:

$$4/20 \quad \times \quad 2/4 \quad \div \quad 8/20 \quad = \quad \textbf{2/8}$$

'Mind map'

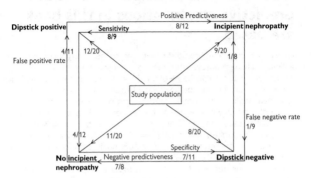

'The lead': the principle on which predictive combinations in this book are based

Unless the presenting complaint happens to be a diagnostic criterion, a clinical finding is always interpreted in combination with other findings. These combinations may be recognised immediately as a highly predictive 'pattern'. If not, they can be assembled logically by using one component as a 'lead' and using the others to make up a combination that identifies a group of patients within which all but one of the differential diagnoses is improbable. Each page in Chapters 3–14 of this book is based on the concept of a 'lead' that is usually predictive of a limited list of differential diagnoses. The suggestive and confirmatory findings on each page can be used to confirm one diagnosis by making the other causes of the lead improbable (or not possible if the findings are diagnostic criteria). The principle behind the logic of 'following up leads' is as follows.

If a 24 year old man presents with acute abdominal pain which is local-ised in the right lower quadrant (RLQ pain) and is accompanied by guard-ing, then this pattern of findings would be recognisable immediately as suggesting probable appendicitis. This 'working' diagnosis might be 'con-firmed' during a laparotomy by seeing the 'definitive' finding of a red swollen appendix and treated with appendicectomy with resolution of the pain so that the diagnosis becomes 'final'.

The same combination of findings can also be assembled 'logically' be-cause right lower quadrant pain (RLQP) would be a good short lead due to appendicitis (e.g. in 40/100 of hypothetical patients with the lead), 'non-specific abdominal pain' ('NSAP', e.g. in 60/100). 'Guarding' occurs commonly in appendicitis but rarely in those with the diagnosis of 'NSAP', which means that the probable diagnosis is appendicitis. This 'verbal reasoning' can also be analysed numerically (*for those who are interested*).

This logic depends on a 'lead' giving a finite number of possibilities to consider. It also depends on the principle that the low 'sensitivity' of one infrequent finding gives an upper limit for the frequency of occurrence of a combination that includes that finding. So, if guarding occurs in 5% × 60 = 3 of those with NSAP then guarding with RLQP must occur in 3 patients or fewer (as RLQP may subdivide the group of 3 who have guarding). Care must be taken with the rest of the logic, however. If guarding occurs in 50% and RLQP also occurs in 50% of those with appendicitis it is just possible that each finding occurs in different halves of those with appendicitis and that these findings never occur together in those with appendicitis. Under these circumstances it would be wrong to assume that most patients with RLQP and guarding had appendicitis. However, if guarding and RLQP both occurred in 90% of those with appendicitis, then even if they occur together as infre-quently as possible, both have to occur in at least 80% (i.e. in at least 80% × 40 = 32 of the original 100 patients). Therefore appendicitis must occur in at least 32/(32 + 3) = 91% of those with RLQP and guarding.

It is commonly assumed that findings such as guarding and RLQP occur together by chance in conditions such as appendicitis. This can be used to give an estimate of the 'likelihood' of finding the combination of findings in patients with a diagnostic criterion (or the 'sensitivity' of the combination). Thus the likelihood of getting 'RLQP with guarding' in those with appendicitis would be estimated to be 90% x 90% = 81%.

In practice, this reasoning process is done informally and little thought is given to the underlying rigorous logical principles or frequencies. Also, once a diagnostic criterion is discovered, then this 'by definition' does not occur in the other conditions and 'eliminates' them completely. The 'probability' of the diagnosis then becomes 100% irrespective of nature of the preceding findings. Thus many findings discovered in the early part of the diagnostic process are often not mentioned when better evidence becomes available later (even if the better evidence does not give 100% certainty). Better later evidence is assumed to give a good estimate of the probability for the 'total evidence'. This small bit of powerful evidence is often called the 'relevant' or 'central' evidence. However, the patient's original presenting complaint is always relevant.

Discussions with patients and relatives

Patients and relatives usually ask questions spontaneously or request an appointment for time to be set aside to do this. Some may be too shy and need encouragement to do so; otherwise this important aspect of care will be omitted. Informed consent is also based on similar questions and discussion. The patient has to ask the questions for the process to be effective (i.e. the process has to be 'patient centred'). However, there is some basic information that has to be covered. Ask the patient and relatives to describe their understanding by going over the type of headings in the 'Current past medical history' on p657 (which is also in a similar format to the pages in Chapters 3–14 of this book).

Ask patient or supporters to state the original problem as they saw it. This will be the presenting complaint. Ask what the patient and relatives understand was the cause (the primary diagnosis or differential diagnoses). Ask if they know what findings suggested or confirmed this (i.e. the evidence), what treatments have been given and then ask how the original symptoms have responded. If there is time, ask about all the other treatments, why they are taking them (i.e. the other diagnoses), what the original symptoms were (presenting complaints) or other markers of response (e.g. the blood pressure) and how they have responded. Ask if they are satisfied and if there are any outstanding problems that are not yet resolved.

You can check the answers systematically against the headings in your mind's eye. If the patient and relatives do not remember something, invite them to ask questions and answer by using words similar to their own. Patients and relatives might welcome reading a typewritten 'Current past medical history' of the presenting complaints, diagnoses, evidence and decisions as on p657 and to use it to help them ask further questions. It might also be helpful for such a handover summary to be given to nurses and other staff. The questions and answers can cover diagnostic ideas such as imagined mechanisms, working and final diagnoses and prognosis. Discussion of tests can cover the concepts of 'gold standards' (sufficient or definitive criteria), screening, leads and combinations. Discussion of treatments should also cover explanations of imagined mechanisms, benefits and adverse effects.

If you need to ask for informed consent, then explain the purpose of the proposed test or treatment against the background of your review of what has happened already by pointing out at which diagnosis or suspected diagnosis the proposed procedure is directed. Ideally, this should be done in the presence of a colleague such as a nurse and also a relative or friend of the patient. Describe the benefits to be gained and the adverse effects, emphasising the most frequent and serious. Again, use a framework such as that described on p657. The same approach applies to tests if one of the test's results leads to a treatment, because the 'package' of 'test and treatment' are analysed just like a treatment alone. In many cases, the patient would simply ask what the doctor would do in the patient's place or wish for a spouse, child, parent, or other family member. The patient may then choose the same option as the doctor's family.

Ask the patient to repeat what you have said, invite questions and be prepared to answer them in as much detail as the patient requires. In many cases the patient will wish to ask very few questions, accept what you have said at face value and choose what you would wish for in that situation. However, if the patient is not able to repeat what you have said clearly and with understanding, then this raises a question of capability to provide informed consent. You may then have to turn to the next of kin or some other legal representative. The same principles apply to admitting and discharging the patient from hospital. Both actions have potential benefits and hazards and the patient and relatives should understand and agree to what is being proposed. For many actions there is no formal signed consent but the patient's actions of concordance (e.g. extending an arm for blood to be taken or coming into hospital) imply such consent.

Transparency and replication

Doctors have to work closely with patients, relatives, other doctors and members of other disciplines. They frequently hand over care to others who have to understand what is happening, and if they agree, to continue with the plan. There is little place in all this for mystery and obscurity, which may arouse suspicion about the doctor's motives or competence. The 'Current past medical history' on p657 is based on the structure of the pages in Chapters 3 to 14. It provides a structure for providing concise information when explaining things to patients or handing over care to colleagues, by anticipating the questions that they should be asking.

An experienced doctor given answers to such questions would know quickly if the evidence did not 'add up'. You can check with the patient to see if the presenting complaint is accurate and to check if the evidence given justifies accepting the main diagnosis. It is also easy to see from such a structured 'Current past medical history' if all the necessary treatments have been given. The same can be done for all the other diagnoses. If there is doubt about the diagnoses because there is insufficient evidence then other diagnoses may also have to be considered and added to the list. One reason for such doubt would be if the patient still has symptoms that are slow to resolve. If there is doubt as to whether the answers are sensible, then the history and examination has to be repeated. If the same findings are discovered again, then they can be said to have been corroborated or replicated.

'Evidence' is of two types. The first type is the 'particular evidence' displayed in that particular situation for a particular patient. It has to be given with a time and place and in enough detail to allow a listener to question the witness or to repeat the observations so that they can be replicated along with the reasoning process and decision. (The same principles are used by the legal profession.) The second part of the evidence is experience from many similar past situations and their outcomes, which demonstrated that a high proportion were successful. This is 'general' evidence as opposed to the 'particular' evidence. For a treatment, it would consist of what happened to some patients on the treatment and to others on a placebo or something else. The problem is that such general or scientific evidence is not available for much of what we do in medicine especially when using different diagnostic criteria or 'gold standard' tests.

'General scientific evidence' is based on observations made on groups of individuals (who each have their own 'particular' observations). If a listener is going to accept such observations as 'general scientific evidence,' the results and methods have to be described in sufficient detail to be repeated by someone else and thus for the study result to be 'replicated' if necessary. If the study and its description is of high quality and published in a reputable journal (which reflects the quality) then the reader may not feel obliged to repeat it. One criterion is that there was a sensible hypothesis and thus a good reason for doing the study (i.e. that it was not just a chance observation). Another important criterion would be that the numbers of observations made were high, so that the statistical probability of replicating the study result was high (e.g. there was a 95% chance of getting a repeat result between two clinically acceptable 'confidence limits').

Modern medicine involves careful evidence-gathering and the use of imagination to decide on the best action. These actions are then explained to others using diagnoses and the evidence for those diagnoses. There is thus a private imaginative stage and then a public transparent stage to allow others to decide if they can agree. If it is not possible to provide a clear rationale in this way that can be understood by others who will be affected by an action, then the wisdom of the action should be reconsidered.

Differences of opinion about a diagnosis

Differences of opinion can sometimes cause consternation; a common reaction is that someone has to be wrong. Different opinions can all be valid if they are based on documented experience and framed as probability statements with a sensible element of doubt. For example, if a doctor makes a number of different predictions with 50% certainty and 50% turn out to be correct overall, then this shows good overall judgment. Different members of the team can thus hold different valid opinions about a diagnosis for a particular patient based on their different personal experiences. A doctor may be wrong about a prediction for a particular patient and yet be correct 75% of the time for such predictions with a 75% probability when they are all taken together in the long run. However, if a single opinion has to be adopted by a team in order to decide what should be done for a particular patient then traditionally, the opinion of the most senior member present is adopted (usually after this person has listened carefully to others).

If an opinion is totally certain, then it implies that all other opinions must be wrong. An opinion held with certainty also raises questions about the holder's judgment because in the long run, it is unlikely that 100% of predictions will be correct. An opinion may become distorted consciously or subconsciously because the holder stands to gain personally from its implementation. It is therefore important to be able to reassure patients and team members if there are differences of opinion. It is also important not to confuse opinions about outcomes with rules that a team has agreed to abide with. A team member may point out that a rule should be followed; this is not an overconfident opinion but a fact if it was agreed at a particular time and place. Overconfidence is also different to decisiveness. One can be decisive by choosing an option with a low probability of success because it represents the best of a number of poor options.

Differences of opinion may occur because the particular facts on which they are based are different. The first thing to do therefore when there is a difference of opinion is to check the particular facts for the patient and if necessary to review the methods and conventions used by the team to get agreement. This may allow facts to be replicated (see p682). The second thing is to clarify the personal and published experience on which the opinion and probability are based. This would include the facts that identified the group of patients who were followed and the details of outcomes such as the diagnostic criteria used or the treatment results.

Clarifying the facts often leads to agreement by revealing oversights and misunderstandings or pooling of experience. Meta-analysis is a technique for combining data from different publications. Bayesian statisticians also combine documented data with personal, undocumented subjective experience. Decision analysis can be used to ask patients' opinions about how they would feel personally about different outcomes so that this can be taken into account when interpreting the meta-analyses and the personal experiences of doctors.

Many opinions are straightforward and failure to hold some of them might be considered culpable (e.g. that bacterial meningitis should always be treated with antibiotics). There are also schools of thought and these are often represented by local guidelines (e.g. which antibiotic should be used as first line treatment). If teams agree to abide by such guidelines then differences of opinion are minimised and teamwork is made easier. Clinical audit is designed to detect poor performance that might be due to poor choice of guidelines for diagnosis or for treatment. However, there is less formal scientific evidence in the literature to guide us in choosing between diagnostic criteria than between treatments.

The blank pages in this book are there for you to express your own opinions, as in the other Oxford Handbooks.

Index

Reference values

Please note that the values and ranges vary among laboratories. Conventional units are used in some medical/scientific journals, and laboratories in some countries. Therefore both SI and conventional units are given.

Measurement	SI unit	Conventional unit	Conversion factor CF x C = SI
5- Hydroxyindole Acetic Acid (5-HIAA), urine	9.4–31.4µmol/day	1.8–6.0 mg/day	5.230
Alanine amino-transferase (ALT)	0–41 U/L	0–41 U/L	–
Albumin	35–50 g/l	3.5–5.0 g/dL	10
Alpha-fetoprotein	0–15 µg/L	0–15 ng/mL	1.0
Aspartate amino-transferase (AST)	10–40 U/L	10–40 U/L	–
Adrenocorticotrophin			
8 a.m.	2–11.5 pmol/L	9–52 pg/mL	0.2202
4 p.m.	1.1–8.2 pmol/L	5–37 pg/mL	
Aldosterone, serum			
Supine	50–250 pmol/L	2–9 ng/dL	27.74
Upright	80–970 pmol/L	3–35 ng/dL	
Alkaline phosphatase	40–129 U/L	40–129 U/L	–
Amylase	0.33–1.83 nkat/L	20–110 U/L	0.0167
Bicarbonate	22–30 mmol/L	22–30 mEq/L	1.0
Bilirubin, total	<17.1 µmol/l	<1.0 mg/dL	17.1
Calcitonin	<2.9 pmol/L	<10 pg/mL	0.29
Calcium, serum	2.23–2.63 mmol/L	8.9–10.5 mg/dL	0.2495
Ceruloplasmin	250–650 mg/L	25–65 mg/dL	10
Chloride	98–108 mmol/l	98–108 mEq/L	1.0
Cholesterol, total desirable	< 5.2 mmol/L	< 200 mg/dL	0.02586
Chorionic Gonado-trophin, human			
Non-pregnant	<5 IU/L	<5 mIU/mL	1.0
Pregnant	<100,000 IU/L	<100,000 mIU/mL	
Copper			
Serum	11–24 µmol/L	70–155 µg/dL	0.157
Urine	<0.94 µmol/day	<60 µg/day	0.0157
Cortisol, serum			
a.m.	140–700 nmol/L	5–25 µg/dL	27.59
4 p.m	96–280 nmol/L	4–10 µg/dL	
Cortisol, urine free	28–250 nmol/day	10–90 µg/day	2.8
C-peptide, serum	0.1–1.23 nmol/L	0.3–3.7 µg/L	0.331
Creatinine	62-106 µmol/l	0.70–1.20 mg/dL	88.40
Creatinine phosphokinase	25–145 U/L	25–145 mU/mL	1.0
Estradiol			
Male & postmeno-pausal F	37–220 pmol/L	10–60 ng/L	3.671
Menstruating F	<1.45 nmol/L	< 400 ng/L	0.0037
Ferritin	20–300 µg/L	20–300 ng/mL	1.0
Folate,			
Serum	6.4–49.5 nmol/L	2.8–21.8 ng/mL	2.27
Red blood cell	272–1530 nmol/L	120–674 ng/mL	
Follicle stimulating hormone			
Male	0.6–8.6 IU/L	0.6–8.6 mIU/mL	1.0
Female	4–13 IU/L	4–13 mIU/mL	
Postmenopausal F	20–138 IU/l	20–138 mIU/mL	